Lecture Notes in Computer Science   10551

Commenced Publication in 1973
Founding and Former Series Editors:
Gerhard Goos, Juris Hartmanis, and Jan van Leeuwen

More information about this series at http://www.springer.com/series/7412

M. Jorge Cardoso · Tal Arbel et al. (Eds.)

Graphs in Biomedical Image Analysis, Computational Anatomy and Imaging Genetics

First International Workshop, GRAIL 2017
6th International Workshop, MFCA 2017
and Third International Workshop, MICGen 2017
Held in Conjunction with MICCAI 2017
Québec City, QC, Canada, September 10–14, 2017
Proceedings

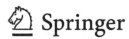
Springer

Editors
M. Jorge Cardoso
University College London
London
UK

Tal Arbel
McGill University
Montreal, QC
Canada

Workshop Editors *see next page*

ISSN 0302-9743   ISSN 1611-3349 (electronic)
Lecture Notes in Computer Science
ISBN 978-3-319-67674-6   ISBN 978-3-319-67675-3 (eBook)
DOI 10.1007/978-3-319-67675-3

Library of Congress Control Number: 2017953407

LNCS Sublibrary: SL6 – Image Processing, Computer Vision, Pattern Recognition, and Graphics

Printed on acid-free paper

This Springer imprint is published by Springer Nature
The registered company is Springer International Publishing AG
The registered company address is: Gewerbestrasse 11, 6330 Cham, Switzerland

Workshop Editors

First International Workshop on Graphs in Biomedical Image Analysis, GRAIL 2017

Enzo Ferrante
Imperial College London
London
UK

Aristeidis Sotiras 🔟
University of Pennsylvania
Philadelphia, PA
USA

Sarah Parisot
Imperial College London
London
UK

6th International Workshop on Mathematical Foundations of Computational Anatomy, MFCA 2017

Xavier Pennec
Inria Sophia
Sophia-Antipolis
France

Tom Fletcher
University of Utah
Salt Lake City, UT
USA

Sarang Joshi
University of Utah
Salt Lake City, UT
USA

Stanley Durrleman
Inria
Paris
France

Mads Nielsen
University of Copenhagen
Copenhagen
Denmark

Stefan Sommer
University of Copenhagen
Copenhagen
Denmark

Third International Workshop on Imaging Genetics, MICGen 2017

Adrian V. Dalca (iD)
Harvard Medical School
Massachusetts Institute of Technology
Boston, MA
USA

Nematollah K. Batmanghelich (iD)
University of Pennsylvania
Philadelphia, PA
USA

Mert R. Sabuncu (iD)
Cornell University
Ithaca, NY
USA

Li Shen (iD)
University of Indiana
Indianapolis, IN
USA

Preface GRAIL 2017

GRAIL 2017 was the first international workshop on Graphs in Biomedical Image Analysis, organized as a satellite event of the 20th International Conference on Medical Image Computing and Computer Assisted Intervention (MICCAI 2017) in Quebec, Canada. With this workshop we aimed to highlight the potential of using graph-based models for biomedical image analysis. Our goal was to bring together scientists that use and develop graph-based models for the analysis of biomedical images and encourage the exploration of graph-based models for difficult clinical problems within a variety of biomedical imaging contexts.

Graph-based models have been developed for a wide variety of problems in computer vision and biomedical image analysis. Applications ranging from segmentation, registration, classification, and shape modeling, to population analysis have been successfully encoded through graph structures, demonstrating the versatile and principled nature of graph-based approaches. Graphs are powerful mathematical structures which provide a flexible and scalable framework to model objects and their interactions in a readily interpretable fashion. As a consequence, an important body of work has been developed around different methodological aspects of graphs including, but not limited to, graphical models, graph-theoretical algorithms, spectral graph analysis, graph dimensionality reduction, and graph-based network analysis. However, new topics are also emerging as the outcome of interdisciplinary studies, shedding light on areas like deep-structured models and signal processing on graphs.

The GRAIL proceedings contain 7 high-quality papers of 8 to 11 pages that were pre-selected through a rigorous peer review process. All submissions were peer-reviewed through a double-blind process by at least 3 members of the Program Committee, comprising 18 experts in the field of graphs in biomedical image analysis. The accepted manuscripts cover a wide set of graph-based medical image analysis methods and applications, including probabilistic graphical models, neuroimaging using graph representations, machine learning for diagnosis and disease prediction, and shape modeling.

The proceedings of the workshop are published as a joint LNCS volume alongside other satellite events organized in conjunction with MICCAI. In addition to the LNCS volume, to promote transparency, the papers' reviews are publicly available on the workshop website (https://biomedic.doc.ic.ac.uk/miccai17-grail/) alongside their corresponding optional response to reviewers.

We wish to thank all the GRAIL 2017 authors for their participation and the members of the Program Committee for their detailed feedback and commitment to the workshop. We are very grateful to our sponsors CentraleSupelec and Inria for their valuable support.

September 2017

Enzo Ferrante
Sarah Parisot
Aristeidis Sotiras

Organization

Organizing Committee

Enzo Ferrante	Imperial College London, London, UK
Sarah Parisot	Imperial College London, London, UK
Aristeidis Sotiras	University of Pennsylvania, USA

Program Committee

Kayhan Batmanghelich	University of Pittsburgh and Carnegie Mellon University, USA
Michael Bronstein	University of Lugano, Switzerland; Tel Aviv University and Intel Perceptual Computing, Israel
Eugene Belilovsky	Inria, France and KU Leuven, Belgium
Christos Davatzikos	University of Pennsylvania, USA
Puneet K. Dokania	Oxford University, UK
Ben Glocker	Imperial College London, UK
Ali Gooya	University of Sheffield, UK
Mattias Heinrich	University of Luebeck, Germany
Dongjin Kwon	Stanford University, USA
Lisa Koch	ETH Zurich, Switzerland
Sofia Ira Ktena	Imperial College London, UK
Georg Langs	University of Vienna, Austria and MIT, USA
Jose Ignacio Orlando	Conicet and Unicen, Argentina
Ipek Oguz	University of Pennsylvania, USA
Yangming Ou	Harvard University, USA
Nikos Paragios	CentraleSupelec and Inria, France
Mert Sabuncu	Cornell University, USA
Christian Wachinger	LMU München, Germany

Preface MFCA 2017

This volume contains the proceedings of the Sixth International Workshop on Mathematical Foundations of Computational Anatomy (MFCA), which was held on September 14, 2017 in conjunction with the 20th International Conference on Medical Image Computing and Computer Assisted Intervention (MICCAI). The first workshop in the MFCA series was held in 2006 in Copenhagen, Denmark. This was followed by workshops in New York, USA, in 2008; Toronto, Canada, in 2011; Nagoya, Japan, in 2013; and Munich, Germany, in 2015[1].

The goal of computational anatomy is to analyze and to statistically model the anatomy of organs in different subjects. Computational anatomic methods are generally based on the extraction of anatomical features or manifolds which are then statistically analyzed, often through a non-linear registration. There are nowadays a growing number of methods that can faithfully deal with the underlying biomechanical behavior of intra-subject deformations. However, it is more difficult to relate the anatomies of different subjects. In the absence of any justified physical model, diffeomorphisms provide the most general mathematical framework for enforcing topological consistency. However, working with this infinite dimensional space raises some deep computational and mathematical problems, in particular for doing statistics. Likewise, modeling the variability of surfaces leads to relying on shape spaces that are much more complex than for curves. To cope with these, different methodological and computational frameworks have been proposed (e.g., using smooth left-invariant metrics, focusing on well-behaved subspaces of diffeomorphisms, or modeling surfaces using currents, etc.). The goal of the MFCA workshop is to foster interaction between researchers investigating the combination of geometry and statistics in non-linear image and surface registration in the context of computational anatomy from different points of view. A special emphasis is put on theoretical developments, with applications and results being welcomed as illustrations.

The 10 papers presented in this volume were carefully selected from a number of very high quality submissions following a thorough peer review process. All of the papers were presented as oral presentations, with ample time for in-depth discussions. We would like to thank the authors of the papers and the members of the Program Committee for their efforts in making a strong program for MFCA 2017.

September 2017

Xavier Pennec
Sarang Joshi
Mads Nielsen
Tom Fletcher
Stanley Durrleman
Stefan Sommer

---

[1] http://www.inria.fr/sophia/asclepios/events/MFCA06/.
http://www.inria.fr/sophia/asclepios/events/MFCA08/.
http://www.inria.fr/sophia/asclepios/events/MFCA11/.
http://www.inria.fr/sophia/asclepios/events/MFCA13/.
http://www.inria.fr/sophia/asclepios/events/MFCA15/.

Organization

Organizing Committee

Xavier Pennec	Inria Sophia-Antipolis, France
Sarang Joshi	University of Utah, USA
Mads Nielsen	University of Copenhagen, Denmark
Tom Fletcher	University of Utah, USA
Stanley Durrleman	Inria and Brain and Spine Institute ICM, Paris, France
Stefan Sommer	University of Copenhagen, Denmark

Program Committee

Stephanie Allassoniere	Ecole Polytechnique, France
Rachid Deriche	Inria, France
Ian Dryden	University of Nottingham, UK
Luc Florac	Eindhoven University of Technology, The Netherlands
Guido Gerig	New York University, USA
Polina Golland	Massachusetts Institute of Technology, USA
Susan Holmes	Stanford University, USA
Marco Lorenzi	Inria, France
Steve Marron	University of North Carolina, Chapel Hill, USA
Stephen Marsland	Massey University, New Zealand
Marc Niethammer	University of North Carolina, Chapel Hill, USA
Salvador Olmos	University of Saragossa, Spain
Kaleem Siddiqi	McGill University, Canada
Martin Styner	University of North Carolina, Chapel Hill, USA
Carole Twining	University of Manchester, UK
William M. Wells III	Massachusetts Institute of Technology and Harvard University, USA

Preface MICGen 2017

MICGen, MICCAI Workshop on Imaging Genetics (http://micgen.mit.edu), was held for the third time on September 10th, 2017, in conjunction with the Medical Image Computing and Computer Assisted Intervention (MICCAI) conference, in Quebec City, Canada. The first workshop was held at MICCAI 2014, at the Massachusetts Institute of Technology, Cambridge, MA, USA. MICGen brings together researchers and clinicians from various fields including medical genetics, computational biology, and medical imaging, presenting a forum for both fundamental concepts as well as state-of-the-art methods and applications. MICGen traditionally includes tutorial talks discussing fundamental concepts and challenges of imaging genetics, as well as oral presentations of accepted papers presenting novel methods or new applications. All researchers interested in imaging genetics, regardless of experience, are invited to attend.

Imaging genetics studies the relationships between genetic variation and measurements from anatomical or functional imaging data, often in the context of a disorder. While traditional genetic analyses are successful for deciphering simple genetic traits, imaging genetics can aid in understanding the underlying complex genetic mechanisms of multifaceted phenotypes. Specifically, imaging-based biomarkers are used as an intermediate or alternative phenotype that provides a rich quantitative characterization of disease. As large imaging genetics datasets are becoming available, their analysis poses unprecedented methodological challenges. MICCAI offers an ideal and timely opportunity to bring together people with different expertise and shared interests in this rapidly evolving field.

September 2017
Adrian V. Dalca
Nematollah K. Batmanghelich
Mert R. Sabuncu
Li Shen

Organization

Organizing Committee

Adrian V. Dalca	MGH, Harvard Medical School, and MIT, USA
Nematollah K. Batmanghelich	University of Pittsburgh, USA
Mert R. Sabuncu	Cornell University, USA
Li Shen	Indiana University School of Medicine, USA

Contents

Third International Workshop on Imaging Genetics, MICGen 2017

First International Workshop on Graphs in Biomedical Image Analysis, GRAIL 2017

Classifying Phenotypes Based on the Community Structure of Human Brain Networks

Anvar Kurmukov[1(✉)], Marina Ananyeva[2], Yulia Dodonova[1], Boris Gutman[3],
Joshua Faskowitz[3], Neda Jahanshad[3], Paul Thompson[3], and Leonid Zhukov[2]

[1] Kharkevich Institute for Information Transmission Problems, Moscow, Russia
kurmukovai@gmail.com
[2] National Research University Higher School of Economics, Moscow, Russia
[3] Imaging Genetics Center, Stevens Neuroimaging and Informatics Institute,
University of Southern California, Marina del Rey, USA

Abstract. Human anatomical brain networks derived from the analysis of neuroimaging data are known to demonstrate modular organization. Modules, or communities, of cortical brain regions capture information about the structure of connections in the entire network. Hence, anatomical changes in network connectivity (e.g., caused by a certain disease) should translate into changes in the community structure of brain regions. This means that essential structural differences between phenotypes (e.g., healthy and diseased) should be reflected in how brain networks cluster into communities. To test this hypothesis, we propose a pipeline to classify brain networks based on their underlying community structure. We consider network partitionings into both non-overlapping and overlapping communities and introduce a distance between connectomes based on whether or not they cluster into modules similarly. We next construct a classifier that uses partitioning-based kernels to predict a phenotype from brain networks. We demonstrate the performance of the proposed approach in a task of classifying structural connectomes of healthy subjects and those with mild cognitive impairment and Alzheimer's disease.

1 Introduction

Understanding disease-related changes in human brains has always been a challenge for neuroscience. A growing field of network science provides a powerful framework to study these changes [5]. This is because any shifts in brain anatomy or functioning are rarely confined to a single locus but rather affect the entire network system.

Human brain networks have been extensively studied in a recent decade. These networks, called connectomes, are constructed from neuroimaging data and represent either anatomical or functional connectivity between cortical brain regions. Several aspects of typical brain network organization have been described, including their modular structure. Modular structure of a network

© Springer International Publishing AG 2017
M.J. Cardoso et al. (Eds.): GRAIL/MFCA/MICGen 2017, LNCS 10551, pp. 3–11, 2017.
DOI: 10.1007/978-3-319-67675-3_1

means that its nodes tend to group into modules, or communities, with close within-group connections and sparse between-group connectivity. Meunier et al. [10] discuss why it is reasonable for human brains to be modular, and also review studies on the community structure of human connectomes. Alexander-Bloch et al. [1] demonstrate that brain network community structure differs between phenotypes (healthy subjects and those with childhood-onset schizophrenia).

This suggests that brain network community structure captures enough information about network topology to classify phenotypes associated with certain diseases. To test this hypothesis, one needs a framework to classify networks based on similarity in their partitions into communities. Recently, Kurmukov et al. [8] proposed such an algorithm. Its basic idea was to detect non-overlapping brain network communities, measure pairwise distances between the obtained network partitions and use these distances in a kernel classification framework. However, [8] only considered non-overlapping brain network communities and demonstrated the performance of the proposed method on a small dataset.

Although non-overlapping communities are more commonly studied in network neuroscience, a model of community structure that allows for overlapping offers a more realistic model of brain-network organization [13]. Some cortical areas are known to be heteromodal and to have a role in multiple networks; consistently with this, current theories on brain organization suggest that cognitive functions are organized into widespread, segregated, and overlapping networks. Thus, clarifying the overlapping structure of brain network communities remains a challenging and relatively unexplored research area.

In this study, we generalize the classification approach [8] by considering both non-overlapping and overlapping communities of cortical brain regions. We show how both types of partitions may be used to estimate distances between brain networks and run a kernel classifier on these distances. Based on a large Alzheimer's Disease Neuroimaging Initiative dataset, we question whether similarity in brain modular structure can help to differentiate subjects with different diagnoses and tackle this question with the proposed approach.

2   Similarity of Brain Network Community Structures

Clustering networks into communities has attracted much attention in graph theory. Here, we only briefly describe the algorithms that we used for partitioning brain networks into communities (both non-overlapping and overlapping), and discuss how community structures of different brain networks may be quantitatively compared.

2.1   Detecting Communities in Structural Brain Networks

We use two approaches to detect brain network community structure. Both approaches aim to identify communities, or groups of tightly anatomically connected cortical regions. The major difference is that the first approach separates brain network regions into unique, non-overlapping modules, while the second algorithm allows for nodes belonging to more than one community. Algorithms of the former type are much more common in graph theory, and hence much more widely used in applications including brain network analysis [10]. However, as discussed above, overlapping community structures offer more powerful description of human brain organization, although they are much rarer evaluated [13].

In this study, we use the Louvain method [2] to produce non-overlapping partitions of structural connectomes. Given a graph $G(E, V)$ with a set of edges E, a set of nodes V, and the adjacency matrix A, the algorithm divides nodes V into groups $\{V_1, V_2, ...V_k\}$ so that $V_1 \cup V_2 \cup ... \cup V_k = V$. Similarly to many other graph partitioning methods, it optimizes the so-called modularity by maximizing the number of intra-community connections and minimizing the number of inter-community links. The Louvain algorithm is a two-step iterative procedure. It starts with each node assigned to a separate cluster. In the first step, it moves each node i to a cluster of one of its neighbors j so that the gain in modularity is maximal. Once there is no such move that improves modularity, the algorithm proceeds to the second step, builds a new graph wherein nodes are clusters from the previous step, and reapplies the first step. Importantly, the Louvain method does not require any a-priori defined number of communities to be detected.

Second, we aim to estimate overlapping communities of structural brain networks. Two types of algorithms can accommodate this, differing in whether they use crisp or fuzzy assignment of nodes into communities. The former means that each node either belongs to each of the possible clusters or not, while the latter allows for a strength of belonging to a community. We detect fuzzy communities based on non-negative matrix factorization (NMF) [7]. Given a non-negative graph adjacency matrix A of size $n \times n$ (n being the number of nodes in brain network), we find its low-rank approximation

$$A \simeq WH, \qquad (1)$$

where W is of size $n \times k$ and H is $k \times n$. A parameter k is usually selected to be much smaller than n and stands for a number of communities to be detected. Elements h_{ij} of a normalized matrix H denote probability of a node i being in a community j. Unlike the first method, the NMF algorithm requires specifying the number of communities. In our computational experiments, we show results obtained for different values of k.

2.2 Measuring Distance Between Community Structures

We aim to evaluate similarity in community structure of brain networks stemming from different subjects, possibly with different diagnoses. Hence, we need to introduce a measure of distance between two partitions obtained from different brain networks. This becomes possible because nodes in connectomes (i.e., cortical regions) are uniquely labeled, and the set of labels is the same across connectomes obtained with the same parcellation atlas.

To estimate pairwise similarity of partitions of different brain networks we use two modifications of mutual information (MI) score. Let $U = \{U_1, U_2, \cdots U_l\}$

and $V = \{V_1, V_2, \cdots V_k\}$ be partitions of two networks G_U and G_V with the same sets of node labels, l and k be the number of clusters in the partitions U and V, respectively. MI between the partitions U and V is defined by:

$$MI(U,V) = \sum_{i=1}^{l} \sum_{j=1}^{m} P(i,j) \log \frac{P(i,j)}{P(i)P'(j)}, \tag{2}$$

For brain network partitions into non-overlapping communities, we use adjusted mutual information, AMI [12]. We measure similarity between partitions into overlapping communities based on normalized mutual information (NMI, [9]). A property of the latter measure is that it only accepts partitions into overlapping modules with crisp node assignment. To accommodate this, we binarize the community membership matrix H (1) using a threshold parameter; we demonstrate how the results of our computational experiments change depending on this parameter.

Both measures take values in $[0, 1]$, with the value of 1 indicating exactly the same partitions. We thus define a distance $\omega(G_U, G_V)$ between the community structures of networks G_U and G_V by:

$$\omega(G_U, G_V) = 1 - I(U, V), \tag{3}$$

where $I(U, V)$ is the index of similarity (AMI or NMI). Networks with the same community structure now have zero distance, and the maximum distance is close to 1.

3   Classifying Connectomes Based on their Community Structure

Since we obtained an optimal partition of each brain network into communities and introduced a measure of difference between community structures, we can proceed to the question of whether community structure of cortical brain regions provides enough information for differentiating between phenotypic classes. This question can be addressed in a machine learning framework.

Given a set of brain networks G_i (each with known community structure), class labels y_i, a training set of pairs (G_i, y_i) and the test set of input objects G_j, the task is to make a best possible prediction of the unknown class label y_j. Provided that we already defined a matrix of pairwise distances $\omega(G_U, G_V)$ (3), the most straightforward approach to classification is to convert the obtained distance matrix into a kernel and feed it to a kernel classifier. We accommodate this by exponentiating the obtained distances:

$$K(G_U, G_V) = e^{-\alpha\omega(G_U,G_V)}, \tag{4}$$

and run the support vector machines (SVM) classifier with the obtained kernel.

4 Experiments: Network-Based Alzheimer's Disease Classification

We argue that if the community structure of anatomical brain networks is affected by a disease in a certain manner, it should be possible to differentiate between healthy and diseased brain networks solely based on similarity in their community structures. In other words, brain networks stemming from the same class (e.g., obtained for healthy participants) should be more similar in their community structure than brain networks from different phenotypic classes (e.g., normal and diseased brains). Using the approach described in the previous sections, we test this hypothesis in a task of classifying Alzheimer's disease (AD), late- and early-stage mild cognitive impairment (LMCI and EMCI), and healthy participants (normal controls, NC).

4.1 Data and Network Construction

We use the Alzheimer's Disease Neuroimaging Initiative (ADNI2) database which comprises a total of 228 individuals (756 scans), with a mean age at baseline visit 72.9 ± 7.4 years, 96 females. Each individual has at least 1 brain scan and at most 6 scans. The data include 47 people with AD (136 AD scans), 40 individuals with LMCI (147 LMCI scans), 80 individuals with EMCI (283 EMCI scans), and 61 healthy participants (190 scans).

Corrected T1-weighted images were processed with Freesurfer's [4] recon-all pipeline to obtain a triangle mesh of the grey-white matter boundary registered to a shared spherical space, as well as corresponding vertex labels per subject. We used cortical parcellation based on the Desikan-Killiany (DK) atlas [3] which includes 68 cortical brain regions. T1w images were aligned (6-dof) to the 2 mm isotropic MNI 152 template. These were used as the template to register the average b_0 of the DWI images, in order to account for EPI related susceptibility artifacts. DWI images were also corrected for eddy current and motion related distortions. Rotation of b-vectors was performed accordingly. Tractography for ADNI data was then conducted using the distortion corrected DWI in 2-mm isotropic MNI 152 space. Probabilistic streamline tractography was performed using the Dipy [6] LocalTracking module and implementation of constrained spherical deconvolution (CSD) [11] with a spherical harmonics order of 6. Streamlines longer than 5 mm with both ends intersecting the cortical surface were retained.

Edge weights in the original cortical connectivity matrices were proportional to the number of streamlines detected by the algorithm. We binarize these weights by:

$$a_{ij}^{\text{binarized}} = \begin{cases} 1 & \text{if} \quad a_{ij} > 0 \\ 0 & \text{otherwise} \end{cases} \tag{5}$$

Thus, we only work with non-weighted graphs throughout the paper.

4.2 Experimental Setup

We obtain the best partition of each network into non-overlapping communities using the Louvain algorithm and compute a matrix of pairwise distances between partitions with the AMI metric. In parallel, we cluster each network into overlapping communities based on NMF and produce a matrix of pairwise NMI distances between these clusterings. This second algorithm requires two parameters (the number of communities and the cluster membership threshold), we report how the results of the overall pipeline change depending on their particular values. For purposes of comparison, we also compute pairwise distances between connectomes using the L_2 (Frobenius) norm.

For each of the three distance matrices, we compute a kernel by (4) and run an SVM classifier with this kernel. We vary the values of α in (4) from 0.01 to 10 and the penalty parameter of the classifier from 0.1 to 50; we only report the results obtained for the optimal values of these technical parameters.

We consider four binary classification tasks: AD versus NC, AD versus LMCI, LMCI versus EMCI, EMCI versus NC. We find optimal values for all parameters in the simplest task of classifying AD versus NC and keep them fixed in the remaining tasks. We use 10-fold cross-validation to train SVM on a subsample and make predictions for an unseen part of a sample. As the data include several networks for each subject, we use subjects rather than networks to split data into train and test and put all networks of the same subject into a respective category (thus avoiding data leakage).

We train the models on networks and next make a subject-based prediction as an average of predictions obtained for individual networks; this method of evaluation (subject-based rather than network-based) does not affect the reported results in any systematic way. We repeat the procedure 50 times with different data splits and report ROC AUC as a quality metric. All scripts are available at https://github.com/kurmukovai/GRAIL2017-communities.

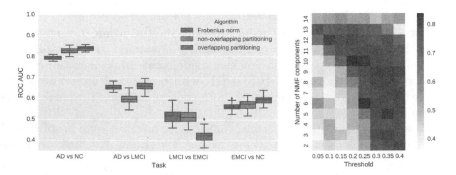

Fig. 1. Left: Classification results. Right: Results of classifying AD versus NC based on the overlapping community detection algorithm, depending on the number of components and the membership threshold; colorbar shows average ROC AUC values.

4.3 Results and Discussion

Figure 1 (left) shows the results of classifying AD, LMCI, EMCI and healthy controls based on $L2$-distance between the structural connectivity matrices of brain networks and on the distances representing similarity in brain community structures.

As expected, classifying AD versus NC was the simplest task, while for EMCI versus LMCI all algorithms only performed at chance level. For the tasks with reasonable overall classification quality, an algorithm based on overlapping community structures slightly outperformed the other algorithms. For AD versus NC, the model with overlapping communities provides an ROC AUC of 0.840 ± 0.010; the one based on non-overlapping communities gives an ROC AUC 0.828 ± 0.013. For this task, Fig. 1 (right) shows how the outcomes of the

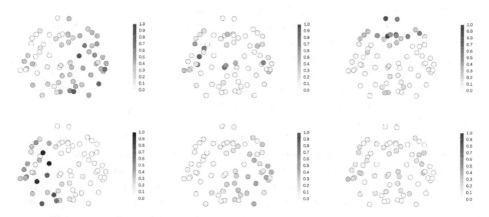

Fig. 2. Six overlapping communities: an example of a single network (healthy subject) with the nodes shown in their original 3D coordinates (axial view); color intensity is proportional to the strength of belonging to the respective community

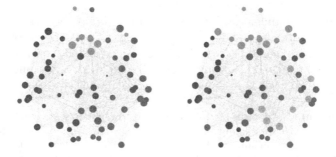

Fig. 3. Comparison of the non-overlapping (left) and overlapping (right) community structures obtained for the same example graph as in Fig. 3; node size is proportional to its degree (the number of edges coming from the respective node). Right plot is produced by selecting a single community for each node based on the maximal membership probability.

best-performing algorithm depend on the predefined number of clusters and the threshold of cluster membership used in computing the NMI distance. The best classification results are obtained with the community structure of six overlapping components, with membership probability thresholded at 0.25.

Figure 2 illustrates the obtained community structure based on a single example graph. Figure 3 compares the non-overlapping and the simplified overlapping community structures obtained for the same graph. The two algorithms seem to identify similar communities, but the outcome of the overlapping community detection algorithm retains more information on the underlying brain network structure.

5   Conclusions

Human brain networks show modular structure which arises based on the entire system of connections between cortical brain regions. Systematic shifts in connectivity patterns, for example those caused by a brain disease, may be expected to induce changes in the community structure of the macroscale brain networks. If true, that would produce similar modular structure in brain networks of individuals with the same phenotype (e.g., Alzheimer's disease) and different community structures in brain networks from different phenotypes (e.g., patients versus healthy controls).

In this study, we explored whether the community structure of anatomical human brain networks provides enough information to differentiate phenotypes of the respective individuals. We proposed a framework to compare both overlapping and non-overlapping community structures of brain networks within the machine learning settings. We demonstrated the performance of the proposed pipeline in a task of classifying Alzheimer's disease, mild cognitive impairment, and healthy participants. Algorithms based on the distances between partitions of brain networks slightly outperformed the baseline. Models that made full use of overlapping community structures performed slightly better than those based on non-overlapping community structures.

To sum up, the modular structure of anatomical brain networks seems to capture important information about the underlying network structure and can be useful in classifying phenotypes. Further studies are needed to study this idea on other phenotypic categories, and to specifically explore overlapping community structure of cortical regions in human anatomical brain networks.

Acknowledgments. The data used in preparing this paper were obtained from the Alzheimer's Disease Neuroimaging Initiative (ADNI) database. A complete listing of ADNI investigators and imaging protocols may be found at www.adni.loni.usc.edu.

The results of Sects. 2–5 are based on the scientific research conducted at IITP RAS and supported by the Russian Science Foundation under grant 17-11-01390.

References

1. Alexander-Bloch, A.F., Gogtay, N., Meunier, D., Birn, R., et al.: Disrupted modularity and local connectivity of brain functional networks in childhood-onset schizophrenia. Front. Syst. Neurosci. **4** (2010)
2. Blondel, V.D., Guillaume, J.L., Lambiotte, R., Lefebvre, E.: Fast unfolding of communities in large networks. J. Stat. Mech. Theory Exp. (2008)
3. Desikan, R.S., Ségonne, F., Fischl, B., Quinn, B.T., et al.: An automated labeling system for subdividing the human cerebral cortex on mri scans into gyral based regions of interest. Neuroimage **31**(3), 968–980 (2006)
4. Fischl, B.: Freesurfer. Neuroimage **62**(2), 774–781 (2012)
5. Fornito, A., Zalesky, A., Breakspear, M.: The connectomics of brain disorders. Nature Reviews. Neurosci. **16**, 159–172 (2015)
6. Garyfallidis, E., Brett, M., Amirbekian, B., Rokem, A., et al.: Dipy, a library for the analysis of diffusion mri data. Front. Neuroinformatics **8**, 8 (2014)
7. Kuang, D., Ding, C., Park, H.: Symmetric nonnegative matrix factorization for graph clustering. In: The 12th SIAM International Conference on Data Mining, pp. 106–117 (2012)
8. Kurmukov, A., Dodonova, Y., Zhukov, L.E.: Classification of normal and pathological brain networks based on similarity in graph partitions. In: 2016 IEEE 16th International Conference Data Mining Workshops (ICDMW), pp. 107–112 (2016)
9. McDaid, A.F., Greene, D., Hurley, N.: Normalized mutual information to evaluate overlapping community finding algorithms (2011)
10. Meunier, D., Lambiotte, R., Bullmore, E.T.: Modular and hierarchically modular organization of brain networks. Frontiers of Neuroinformatics **4** (2010)
11. Tax, C.M., Jeurissen, B., Vos, S.B., Viergever, M.A., Leemans, A.: Recursive calibration of the fiber response function for spherical deconvolution of diffusion mri data. Neuroimage **86**, 67–80 (2014)
12. Vinh, N.X., Epps, J., Bailey, J.: Information theoretic measures for clusterings comparison: variants, properties, normalization and correction for chance. J. Mach. Learn. Res., 2837–2854 (2010)
13. Wu, K., Taki, Y., Sato, K., et al.: The overlapping community structure of structural brain network in young healthy individuals. PLoS One **6** (2011)

Autism Spectrum Disorder Diagnosis Using Sparse Graph Embedding of Morphological Brain Networks

Carrie Morris and Islem Rekik$^{(\boxtimes)}$

BASIRA Lab, CVIP Group, School of Science and Engineering,
Computing, University of Dundee, Dundee, UK
irekik@dundee.ac.uk
http://www.basira-lab.com

Abstract. Autism Spectrum Disorder (ASD) is a neurodevelopmental disorder involving a complex cognitive impairment that can be difficult to diagnose early enough. Much work has therefore been done investigating the use of machine-learning techniques on functional and structural connectivity networks for ASD diagnosis. However, networks based on the morphology of the brain have yet to be similarly investigated, despite research findings that morphological features, such as cortical thickness, are affected by ASD. In this paper, we first propose modelling morphological brain connectivity (or graph) using a set of cortical attributes, each encoding a unique aspect of cortical morphology. However, it can be difficult to capture for each subject the complex pattern of relationships between morphological brain graphs, where each may be affected simultaneously or independently by ASD. In order to solve this problem, we therefore also propose the use of high-order networks which can better capture these relationships. Further, since ASD and normal control (NC) high-dimensional connectomic data might lie in different manifolds, we aim to find a low-dimensional representation of the data which captures the intrinsic dimensions of the underlying connectomic manifolds, thereby allowing better learning by linear classifiers. Hence, we propose the use of sparse graph embedding (SGE) method, which allows us to distinguish between data points drawn from different manifolds, even when they are too close to one another. SGE learns a similarity matrix of the connectomic data graph, which then is used to embed the high-dimensional connectomic features into a low-dimensional space that preserves the locality of the original data. Our ASD/NC classification results outperformed several state-of-the-art methods including statistical feature selection, and local linear embedding methods.

1 Introduction

Autism Spectrum Disorder (ASD) is a neurodevelopmental disorder characterized by varied impairments in cognitive function, including difficulties with social communication and interaction, language, and restricted, repetitive behaviours. This has made diagnosing the disorder a challenging task [1]. However, aided by recent

© Springer International Publishing AG 2017
M.J. Cardoso et al. (Eds.): GRAIL/MFCA/MICGen 2017, LNCS 10551, pp. 12–20, 2017.
DOI: 10.1007/978-3-319-67675-3_2

technological and methodological advances in neuroimaging tools, there has been growing interest in understanding how ASD can alter the connectivity between different regions within the brain, and how this information may be leveraged to help diagnose the disorder with greater accuracy [2]. The two most widely used measures of brain connectivity used for investigating ASD in the literature are functional connectivity and structural connectivity, derived from functional magnetic resonance imaging (fMRI) and diffusion tensor imaging (DTI) respectively, with literature reviews available for both types of data [3, 4]. For example, all 77 studies discussed in [5]'s review of using machine learning on connectomes (networks of the brain) to predict clinical outcomes used functional and/or structural connectivity networks to do so. Despite this growing body of research on such networks, however, there is still a gap in the literature where morphological networks have not been explored to the same degree. This gap needs to be filled, considering there are studies that indicate morphological features of the brain, such as cortical thickness, can be affected in neurological disorders, including ASD [6, 7]. As such, the use of networks based on morphological data in neurological disorder diagnosis, using machine learning, could prove fruitful. Further, such networks have not been used to investigate ASD in the literature so far. In this study, we will therefore aim to define several networks based on the morphology or geometry of the cortical surface of ASD and NC subjects, and investigate their use in diagnosing ASD using machine learning techniques.

Different morphological views of the cortical surface (e.g. cortical thickness and mean curvature) may also have different relationships between them, where they could be affected simultaneously or independently in different regions of the brain by ASD. As a result, there could be a very complex pattern of how ASD affects the different morphological views of the brain. The easiest and most commonly employed method for exploring such relationships is simply to concatenate the multiple networks together so that the data from each view is included in the overall set of data for each subject, unaltered [5]. However, recent research on Alzheimer's Disease has found better results when using High Order Networks (HONs) [8]. These are constructed from low-order (e.g. functional connectivity) networks by, for each view or network, extracting the correlations between different pairs of brain regions, then calculating the correlation between these values across all views, for each pair of brain regions. This method therefore better allows us to capture the higher-order relationships between different views of the brain. However, it has yet to be applied to ASD data in machine learning research, and so, with this study, we also aim to contribute to the literature on the use of such HONs when investigating ASD. One potential problem with the use of HONs, however, is that the networks produced are very large and, as a result, computationally expensive. To mitigate this, feature selection or dimensionality reduction is necessary. Noting that ASD morphological changes between brain regions might be very subtle, the manifolds where both ASD and healthy connectomic data lie might be very close and challenging to embed into a low-dimensional space. To address this problem, we further propose a classification framework based on a *sparse graph embedding of connectomic data* using the method developed in [9]. Specifically, we use graph embedding of the HONs, which would allow us to (1) explore the high-order relationships without having to deal with overly large networks, (2) learn the features that are most discriminative in classifying and diagnosing ASD, and (3) investigate the effectiveness of SGE as a dimensionality reduction technique on our data, as compared to other state-of-the-art methods.

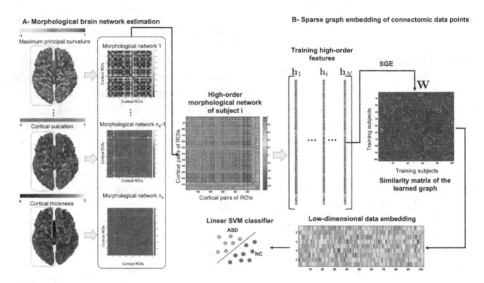

Fig. 1. *High-order sparse graph embedding (SGE) of high-order brain networks for classifying autism spectrum disorder (ASD) and healthy brains.* (A) For each subject i, we construct n_a low-order morphological networks for each cortical attribute. Then, we merge these into a high-order network represented by a feature vector $\mathbf{h}_i$. (B) Given the high-order feature matrix of all subjects, we use sparse graph embedding [9] to learn a sparse similarity matrix $\mathbf{W}$ of a graph $\mathcal{G}$ which models the relationship between data points lying in different connectomic manifolds. Next, we embed the graph into a low-dimensional space where a linear SVM classifier is trained.

2 Proposed Sparse Graph Embedding of High-Order Morphological Brain Networks for Autism Classification

In this section, we present our sparse graph embedding (SGE) of high-order morphological brain networks for ASD classification using the SMCE method proposed in [9]. We denote matrices by boldface capital letters, e.g., $\mathbf{X}$, and scalars are denoted by lowercase letters, e.g., x. For easy reference, we have summarized the major mathematical notations in Table 1. Figure 1 illustrates

Table 1. Major mathematical notations used in this paper.

Mathematical notation	Definition
$\mathbf{C}_i^a = (V_C, E_C)$	Low-order brain network graph $\mathbb{R}^{n_r \times n_r}$ of a single subject i for cortical attribute a
V_C	Nodes or brain ROIs of size n_r
E_C	Edges connecting pairs of brain ROIs in a single subject
n_a	Number of cortical attributes
$\mathbf{H}_i = (V_H, E_H)$	High-order brain network graph of a single subject i
V_H	A node represents a pair of brain ROIs
E_H	Edges connecting two pairs of brain ROIs in a single subject
$\mathbf{h}_i$	High-order connectomic feature vector $\in \mathbb{R}^D$ of subject i derived from brain graph $\mathbf{H}_i$
N	Number of training subjects
K	Number of manifolds
$\mathcal{M}_l$	Manifold where similar connectomic data points lie
d_l	Intrinsic dimension of manifold $\mathcal{M}_l$
$\mathcal{G} = (V_\mathcal{M}, E_\mathcal{M})$	Similarity graph of connectomic data points nested in different manifolds $\{\mathcal{M}_l\}_{l=1}^K$
$\check{\mathbf{D}}_i$	Normalized distance matrix in $\mathbb{R}^{D \times N-1}$ between current data point $\mathbf{h}_i$ and other data points
$\mathbf{Q}_i$	Positive-definite diagonal proximity inducing matrix
α_i	A sparse vector whose $d_l + 1$ nonzero elements correspond to $d_l + 1$ neighbours of $\mathbf{h}_i \in \mathcal{M}_l$
$\mathbf{w}_i$	Weight vector in $\mathbb{R}^N$ associated with the i-th point
$\mathbf{W}$	Similarity matrix in $\mathbb{R}^{N \times N}$ of graph $\mathcal{G}$

the proposed pipeline for ASD/NC classification in four major steps: (1) construction of low-order morphological networks, (2) construction of high-order morphological network, (3) connectomic feature extraction, and (4) sparse graph learning and embedding to reduce the dimension of the extracted features for our target classification task.

Low-order morphological network construction. For each subject i and each cortical attribute a (e.g., cortical thickness), we build a brain graph $\mathbf{C}_i^a = (V_C, E_C)$, where each node in V_C represents a cortical region of interest (ROI), and each edge in E_C connecting two ROIs R_p and R_q is defined as $\mathbf{C}_i(p,q) = |\hat{x}_p - \hat{x}_q|$, where $\hat{x}_p$ denotes the average of the cortical attribute across all vertices in region R_p. Given n_a cortical attributes, we generate for each cortical hemisphere n_a morphological brain graphs $\{\mathbf{C}_a\}_{a=1}^{n_a}$.

High-order morphological network construction (HON). We note that ASD might affect not only region-to-region morphological brain connections on a low-order level, but also high-order relationships between pairs of ROIs, where complex interactions between sets of ROIs might be affected. Hence, we propose constructing a high-order morphological network to integrate into a single, larger brain graph $\mathbf{H}_i = (V_H, E_H)$ all low-order brain graphs $\{\mathbf{C}_a\}_{a=1}^{n_a}$ of *both* hemispheres. Each node in V_H denotes a *pair* of ROIs and each edge in E_H connecting two pairs or ROIs (p, q) and (p', q') denotes the Pearson Correlation coefficient between vectors $\mathbf{y_{pq}}$ and $\mathbf{y_{p'q'}}$, where $\mathbf{y_{pq}}$ corresponds to the connectivity strength between the p-th and q-th ROIs across all $2n_a$ brain networks in both hemispheres.

Feature Extraction. We propose two types of features: high-order features (HON), and concatenated low-order features (CON). Noting that all brain graphs are symmetric, for each subject i, we represent its high-order brain graph as a matrix $\mathbf{H}_i$, then concatenate its upper triangle elements into a long feature vector $\mathbf{h}_i$. The weights on the diagonal are set to zero to avoid self-connectedness. For low-order brain graphs $\{\mathbf{C}_a\}_{a=1}^{n_a}$, we simply concatenate the upper triangle elements across all cortical attributes into a feature vector (termed as CON). To address the issue of 'high-dimensional features vs.a low sample size' in classification, we propose embedding our high-dimensional connectomic features into a low-dimensional space where we can efficiently train a linear classifier through learning a sparse graph.

Sparse graph embedding (SGE) using connectomic brain features for ASD classification. Since ASD and NC high-dimensional connectomic data might lie in different manifolds, we aim to find a low-dimensional representation of the data which captures the intrinsic dimensions of the underlying connectomic manifolds, thereby allowing better learning by classifiers. However, since morphological brain changes can be very subtle in autistic subjects compared with healthy brains, their data manifolds can be very close to each other. Hence, estimating a low-dimensional embedding that allows us to distinguish between data points drawn from different manifolds is challenging. To solve this problem, Elhamifar *et al.* proposed a robust algorithm for sparse manifold clustering and embedding (SMCE) that efficiently handles multiple manifolds that are very close to each other [9]. This is achieved through encouraging a sparse selection of nearby connectomic points that lie in the same manifold and spanning a low-dimensional affine subspace. Unlike typical dimensionality reduction methods such as local linear embedding (LLE), which builds a neighbourhood graph by connecting each data point to a *fixed* number of nearest points, SMCE learns a graph neighbourhood automatically, thereby allowing the neighbourhood size on the manifold to vary. This better handles variation in the density of data points on the manifold.

Leveraging the strengths of the SMCE method, we then propose our sparse graph embedding (SGE) framework for the low-dimensional representation of the high-order connectomic brain manifolds of ASD and NC subjects (Fig. 1). Given N training high-order feature vectors $\{\mathbf{h}_i \in \mathbb{R}^D\}_{i=1}^N$ lying in K different manifolds $\{\mathcal{M}_{l=1}^K\}$ of intrinsic dimensions $\{d_l\}_{l=1}^K$, we build a similarity graph $\mathcal{G} = (V_\mathcal{M}, E_\mathcal{M})$, where each node in $V_\mathcal{M}$ represents a feature vector $\mathbf{h}$ derived from a brain graph $\mathbf{H}$. Our goal is to learn sparse connections in graph $\mathcal{G}$ through connecting each point to a few neighbouring points with appropriate weights such that the selected neighbouring points are from the same manifold. This is achieved through solving a sparse optimization function that selects for each connectomic point $\mathbf{h}_i \in \mathcal{M}_l$ *a few* neighbouring points that span a low-dimensional affine subspace passing near $\mathbf{h}_i$:

$$\min_{\alpha_i} \lambda ||\mathbf{Q}_i \alpha_i||_1 + \frac{1}{2} ||\check{\mathbf{D}}_i \alpha_i||_2^2 \ s.t. \ \mathbf{1}^T \alpha_i = 1, \tag{1}$$

where $\alpha_i^T \triangleq [\alpha_{i1} \ldots \alpha_{iN}]$ denotes a solution whose $d_l + 1$ nonzero elements correspond to $d_l + 1$ neighbours of $\mathbf{h}_i \in \mathcal{M}_l$. $\check{\mathbf{D}}_i$ represents the normalized distance matrix between current data point $\mathbf{h}_i$ and other points: $\check{\mathbf{D}}_i \triangleq [\frac{\mathbf{h}_1 - \mathbf{h}_i}{||\mathbf{h}_1 - \mathbf{h}_i||_2} \cdots \frac{\mathbf{h}_N - \mathbf{h}_i}{||\mathbf{h}_N - \mathbf{h}_i||_2}] \in \mathbb{R}^{D \times N - 1}$. L_1 sparsity penalty constrains points closer to $\mathbf{h}_i$ to be less penalised than points that are further away. $\mathbf{Q}_i$ is a proximity inducing positive-definite diagonal matrix, which favours the selection of close points to the current point $\mathbf{h}_i$ through assigning smaller weights to them. We define its diagonal elements as $\frac{||\mathbf{h}_j - \mathbf{h}_i||_2}{\sum_{t \neq i} ||\mathbf{h}_t - \mathbf{h}_i||_2} \in (0, 1]$). The trade-off parameter λ balances the sparsity solution (first term) and the affine reconstruction error (second term).

After solving Eq. 1, we define a weight vector $\mathbf{w}_i^T = [w_{i1} \ldots w_{iN}] \in \mathbb{R}^N$ associated with the i-th point as: $w_{ii} = 0$ and $w_{ij} \triangleq \frac{\alpha_{ij} / ||\mathbf{h}_j - \mathbf{h}_i||_2}{\sum_{t \neq i} \alpha_{it} / ||\mathbf{h}_t - \mathbf{h}_i||_2}$, $j \neq i$. Ideally, non-zero elements of $\mathbf{w}_i$ will correspond to sparse neighbours of $\mathbf{h}_i$ which belong to the same manifold. Next, we use these weights to define edges in the similarity graph $\mathcal{G}$ where a node $\mathbf{h}_i$ connects to node $\mathbf{h}_j$ with weight $|w_{ij}|$. Ideally, points in the same manifold will belong to the same connected component in the learned graph $\mathcal{G}$. Ultimately, we define the similarity matrix $\mathbf{W} \triangleq [|\mathbf{w}_1| \ldots |\mathbf{w}_N|]$ in $\mathbb{R}^{N \times N}$ of the manifold graph $\mathcal{G}$, which groups points from the same manifold into a block-by-block matrix structure. We then generate the local embedding of the connectomic features by taking the last eigenvectors of the normalized Laplacian matrix associated with each cluster in $\mathbf{W}$. In the training stage, we learn $\mathbf{W}_{tr}$ for all training subjects. Then we use the produced low-dimensional features to train a linear support vector machine (SVM) classifier. In the testing stage, we map the testing subject to a low-dimensional space (with same dimension) through estimating a new $\mathbf{W}_{ts}$ that includes training and testing samples.

3 Results and Discussion

Evaluation dataset and method parameters. We used leave-one-out cross validation to evaluate the proposed classification framework on 102 subjects (59 ASD and 43 NC) from Autism Brain Imaging Data Exchange (ABIDE I)[1] public dataset, each with structural T1-w MR image [10]. We used FREESURFER

---

[1] http://fcon_1000.projects.nitrc.org/indi/abide/.

to reconstruct both right and left cortical hemispheres for each subject from T1-w MRI. Then we parcellated each cortical hemisphere into 35 cortical regions using Desikan-Killiany Atlas. For each subject, we generated $n_a = 4$ cortical morphological networks: $\mathbf{C}^1$ denotes the maximum principal curvature brain view, $\mathbf{C}^2$ denotes the mean cortical thickness brain view, $\mathbf{C}^3$ denotes the mean sulcal depth brain view, and $\mathbf{C}^4$ denotes the mean of average curvature. For SGE parameters, we set $\lambda = 10$. For both LLE and SGE, we used nested grid-search to estimate the low dimension of the feature embedding (9 for SGE and 50 for LLE).

Method evaluation and comparison methods. We compared our method with three state-of-the-art methods: (RAW) where we directly input the raw connectomic brain features, (t-test) where we perform dimensionality reduction using statistical feature selection, and (LLE) where we perform a local linear embedding of the connectomic features to produce a compact and low-dimensional representation of feature vectors. Since both CON and HON feature vectors are high-dimensional, we propose a preliminary dimensionality reduction step through representing each network by a clustering coefficients (CC) feature vector. This will allow us to benchmark our method against the recent connectomic classification framework proposed in [8] where they first concatenated the clustering coefficients of the functional HON (CC(HON)) and CON features (i.e., CC(HON) + CON), then performed t-test for feature selection to train an SVM classifier for Alzheimer's disease diagnosis. We further evaluated all methods using combinations of different feature types: (1) HON, (2) CON, (3) CC(HON), (4) HON + CON, and (5) CC(HON) + CON. All results are presented in Table 2 and Fig. 2. Our method produced the best ASD/NC classification accuracy (61.76%) when using (CC(HON) + CON) features, which largely outperformed t-test using (CC(HON) + CON) as in [8].

Table 2. ASD/NC classification results using our method and different comparison methods.

Features	Accuracy (%)	Sensitivity (%)	Specificity (%)
View 1 (Raw)	51.9608	48.8372	54.2373
View 2 (Raw)	53.9216	44.1860	61.0169
View 3 (Raw)	47.0588	37.2093	54.2373
View 4 (Raw)	47.0588	41.8605	50.8475
CON (Raw)	52.9412	37.2093	64.4068
HON (Raw)	52.9412	44.1860	59.3220
CC(HON) (Raw)	46.0784	32.5581	55.9322
HON + CON (Raw)	53.9216	46.5116	59.3220
CC(HON) + CON (Raw)	51.9608	39.5349	61.0169
CC(HON) (T-Test)	47.0588	32.5581	57.6271
HON + CON (T-test)	55.8824	37.2093	69.4915
CC(HON) + CON (T-test)	52.9412	37.2093	64.4068
CC(HON) (LLE)	58.8235	60.4651	57.6271
HON + CON (LLE)	50.9804	55.8140	47.4576
CC(HON) + CON (LLE)	43.1373	32.5581	50.8475
CC(HON) (SGE)	52.9412	62.7907	45.7627
HON + CON (SGE)	50	51.1628	49.1525
CC(HON) + CON (SGE)	61.7647	62.7907	61.0169

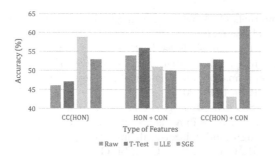

Fig. 2. *ASD/NC classification accuracies for our method (SGE) and other comparison methods using combinations of different connectomic feature types.* We compared our method with three state-of-the-art methods: (RAW) where we directly input the raw connectomic brain features, (t-test) where we perform dimensionality reduction using statistical feature selection, and (LLE) where we perform a local linear embedding of the connectomic features to produce a compact and low-dimensional representation of feature vectors. Our method produced the best ASD/NC classification accuracy when using (CC(HON) + CON) features, which significantly outperformed t-test using (CC(HON) + CON) as in [8].

4   Conclusion

We proposed a sparse graph learning framework for classifying disordered brain connectivities based on the morphology of cortical hemispheres. Specifically, we estimated a local embedding of high-order and low-order morphological brain networks for distinguishing between autistic and healthy brains. Given that morphological brain changes are subtle in ASD patients, our results are promising. Instead of performing the local embedding of data points for each feature type independently, we will further extend our method to jointly embed different feature types nested in multiple views of the same manifold (e.g., ASD data manifold).

References

1. Lord, C., Cook, E.H., Leventhal, B.L., Amaral, D.G.: Autism spectrum disorders. Neuron **28**, 355–363 (2000)
2. Anagnostou, E., Taylor, M.J.: Review of neuroimaging in autism spectrum disorders: what have we learned and where we go from here. Mol. Autism **2**, 4 (2011)
3. Philip, R.C., Dauvermann, M.R., Whalley, H.C., Baynham, K., Lawrie, S.M., Stanfield, A.C.: A systematic review and meta-analysis of the fmri investigation of autism spectrum disorders. Neurosci. Biobehav. Rev. **36**, 901–942 (2012)
4. Stanfield, A.C., McIntosh, A.M., Spencer, M.D., Philip, R., Gaur, S., Lawrie, S.M.: Towards a neuroanatomy of autism: a systematic review and meta-analysis of structural magnetic resonance imaging studies. Eur. Psychiatry **23**, 289–299 (2008). Neuroimaging

5. Brown, C., Hamarneh, G.: Machine learning on human connectome data from MRI (2016). arXiv:1611.08699v1
6. Cauda, F., Costa, T., Nani, A., Fava, L., Palermo, S., Bianco, F., Duca, S., Tatu, K., Keller, R.: Are schizophrenia, autistic, and obsessive spectrum disorders dissociable on the basis of neuroimaging morphological findings? A voxel-based meta-analysis. Autism Res. **10**, 1079–1095 (2017)
7. Khundrakpam, B.S., Lewis, J.D., Kostopoulos, P., Carbonell, F., Evans, A.C.: Cortical thickness abnormalities in autism spectrum disorders through late childhood, adolescence, and adulthood: a large-scale mri study. Cereb. Cortex **27**, 1721 (2017)
8. Chen, X., Zhang, H., Gao, Y., Wee, C.Y., Li, G., Shen, D., the Alzheimer's Disease Neuroimaging Initiative: High-order resting-state functional connectivity network for mci classification. Hum. Brain Mapp. **37**, 3282–3296 (2016)
9. Elhamifar, E., Vidal, R.: Sparse manifold clustering and embedding, pp. 55–63 (2011)
10. Mueller, S.G., Weiner, M.W., Thal, L.J., Petersen, R.C., Jack, C., Jagust, W., Trojanowski, J.Q., Toga, A.W., Beckett, L.: The Alzheimer's Disease Neuroimaging Initiative. Neuroimaging Clin. North Am. **10**, 869–877 (2005)

Topology of Surface Displacement Shape Feature in Subcortical Structures

Amanmeet Garg$^{(\boxtimes)}$, Donghuan Lu, Karteek Popuri, and Mirza Faisal Beg

Simon Fraser University, 8888 University Drive, Burnaby, Canada
aga46@sfu.ca

Abstract. The shape of anatomical structures in the brain has been adversely influenced by neurodegenerative disorders. However, the shape feature covariation between regions (e.g. subfields) of the structure and its change with disease remains unclear. In this paper, we present a first work to study the topology of the *surface displacement* shape feature via its persistence homology timeline features and model the polyadic interactions between the shape across the subfields of subcortical structures. Specifically, we study the caudate and pallidum structures for *Shape Topology* change with Parkinson's disease. The shape topology features show statistically significant group level difference and good prediction performance in a repeated hold out stratified training experiment. These features show promise in their potential application to other neurological conditions and in clinical settings with further testing on larger data cohorts.

Keywords: Topological data analysis · Shape topology · Parkinson's disease · Caudate · Pallidum

1   Introduction

Neurodegeneration in Parkinson's disease (PD) has shown morphology change in subcortical (deep gray matter, substantia nigral area) structures where shape [2,4] of the structures was found to be adversely affected in Parkinson's patients. Additionally, topology of functional and structural networks has shown strong differences in Parkinson's patients in comparison to healthy individuals. However, little is known for the covariation of shape across the subfields of anatomical structures in the brain. This highlights the need to study the topology of the shape networks in brain subcortical structures. In this work, we study the topology via a novel topology data analysis method and test the features for their ability to differentiate between groups, and utility as a disease marker. Additionally, we compare these novel features with classical network features commonly studied in the scientific literature. On the lines of our previous work [2] we study the caudate and pallidum structures in both hemispheres.

The shape of an object is the geometry information retained after removal of position, orientation, and scaling (size) of an object. The change in shape

© Springer International Publishing AG 2017
M.J. Cardoso et al. (Eds.): GRAIL/MFCA/MICGen 2017, LNCS 10551, pp. 21–30, 2017.
DOI: 10.1007/978-3-319-67675-3_3

of anatomical structures has been previously observed in our work with Parkinson's disease [2]. The structures inside the brain are closely located and often have touching boundaries. The shape change or deformation on one surface (e.g. medial boundary of caudate) is expected to influence the other surfaces (e.g. lateral boundary of the caudate) of the structure. This leads us to question, *Is there an interaction of shape change between the surface subfields of a structure?*. We model this question as a topological data analysis problem where we study the topology of the surface displacement (SurfDisp) shape feature indexed on the geometry (nodes, group of vertices) on the structure. It is important to note that we do not develop a new shape feature, rather, our focus is to study the co-variation of shape and derive topological features for this information.

In this work, we address this question by studying the inter-regional co-variation of shape in the subcortical (deep gray matter) structures in the brain due to neurodegeneration. To this end, we apply the previously developed shape analysis framework and further model the topology of the network of interaction between subfields on the structure. The surface deformation based SurfDisp shape feature is our signal of interest where the difference in SurfDisp is a measure of covariation (similarity) between two regions within the structure. We compute the multiscale homology feature (persistence homology) of the induced Vietoris-Rips simplicial complex on the underlying topology of the SurfDisp network. We present experiments to test the ability of these features to differentiate between the disease and healthy groups on a group level and correctly classify previously unseen subjects.

2   Methods

The central aim of this work is to quantify the inter-regional covariation of shape between the surface subfields within the subcortical structures via the shape topology features. These features utilize the SurfDisp data as their signal of interest and model the topology of shape in brain structures. Here we describe each module of our pipeline followed by the statistical analysis and classification experiments.

2.1   Shape Feature

The SurfDisp shape feature is obtained via a template injection approach where a population average template for each structure is injected into the surface of corresponding structure in each subject via non linear registration. This results in vertex wise correspondence between the surfaces of the template and target subjects. Further, the vector between the vertices of the reference (template) and the target surface is projected along the template surface normal to obtain the SurfDisp feature. The complete mathematical details of the SurfDisp method are available in our prior work in analysis of shape change in subcortical structures [2]. Specifically, for a structure with m vertices we obtain a surface displacement s_i at each vertex for a total of m values per subject.

2.2 Shape Topology

The shape topology models the polyadic (many-to-many) interaction between the subfields on the surface of subcortical structures for covariation of shape (SurfDisp). To obtain such information we first obtain a reduced dimensionality representation of the shape data via adaptive parcellation, followed by a network filtration computed for each structure to obtain the homology of the shape topology space. The workflow is visually represented in the Fig. 1.

Adaptive Parcellation: The SurfDisp data inherently resides in a high dimensional space with large number of vertices per structure in comparison to the number of subjects in the data cohort. In order to mitigate the effects of curse of dimensionality and retain the computational tractability of the persistent homology features we perform adaptive parcellation by computing a patchwise averaged representation of the surface. In this, we begin by computing n patches (represented by their centroids) on the surface of the structure of the template as clusters of neighbouring vertices where 3D coordinates of a vertex form the input. The averaging is based on the assumption that neighbouring vertices exhibit similar form of shape change which differs from far and distant vertices. For each patch we compute the average SurfDisp value s_i resulting in n values per subject. As a result, m SurfDisp values (one per vertex) are converted into $n << m$ value (one per patch). The resultant matrix (subject × features) acts as an input to the persistent homology computation pipeline as outlined below. For each subject with n patches, we compute the distance $d_{ij} = s_i - s_j, i, j = 1, 2, \cdots, n$ resulting in a $n \times n$ square symmetric distance matrix D yielding a weighted undirected graph G.

Network Filtration: In complex network analysis, the threshold to obtain a binary graph from a weighted graph is a parameter often selected based on the suitability to the application at hand, thus, limiting its generalizability. To circumvent this issue, we construct a network filtration with a monotonically increasing set of threshold values to obtain a set of binary undirected networks with different levels of network sparsity. This approach has the advantage of providing a complete set of network topology characteristics from a fully disconnected network to a fully connected network.

   A weighted undirected brain graph G is thresholded at a value ε_k to yield a binary undirected graph G_k. Upon changing the threshold $\varepsilon_1 < \varepsilon_2 < \cdots < \varepsilon_k < \cdots < \varepsilon_n$ we get a hierarchical sequence of n binary undirected graphs $G_1 \subseteq G_2 \subseteq \cdots \subseteq G_k \subseteq \cdots \subseteq G_n$ termed as a *Network Filtration*. A graph originates from a distance matrix D where, each entry d_{ij} is the connection strength between the nodes i and j. Each D is converted into an adjacency matrix A_k where, $\{a_{ij} = 1 | d_{ij} < \varepsilon_k, 0\, otherwise\}$ for a chosen threshold ε_k giving the graph G_k. We compute the features of nodal degree, clustering coefficient and local efficiency for each network in the filtration. For a detailed mathematical description of these features, the reader is guided to the seminal work by Rubinov and Sporns [7].

The inter-patch distance for each subject varies depending on the brain size rendering the graph filtration generated based on the raw distance values influenced by the scale of the overall brain size in addition to the relative inter-regional distances whose alterations with disease are of interest. Thus, in order to overcome such scale-related differences, we normalize the values of the inter-patch distance for each individual to the range of $[0, 1]$ prior to the generation of a graph filtration. This enables a comparison of the network and topology features across subjects and groups by potentially reducing the affect of scale variation of the brain size.

2.3   Persistent Homology

The central idea behind the theory of persistent homology (PH) is to build a sequence of nested subsets on a space of simplicial complexes, studied at different resolutions. For our work, the Vietoris-Rips (VR) complex completely defined by the underlying 1-skeleton is induced on a symmetric distance matrix of pairwise distances between points in a point cloud.

A VR complex is defined on a metric space M for a specific distance value γ by forming a k-simplex for every finite set of $k + 1$ points that has diameter at most γ. For a set of k nodes in the point cloud, the VR complex has at most $(k - 1)$ simplices, enabling the geometry networks to obtain higher dimensional interactions limited in binary networks to 1-dimensional simplices (edges). Monotonically increasing values of the scale parameter ε_k lead to a VR filtration where $VR_{\varepsilon_1} \subseteq VR_{\varepsilon_2} \cdots \subseteq VR_{\varepsilon_k} \cdots \subseteq VR_{\varepsilon_n}$. For each filtered persistence module of the VR complex we obtain the tuples (b_i, d_i), with $b_i < d_i$ commonly known as a *birth-death pairs* of a k-dimensional simplex in the filtration. The length $d_i - b_i$ provides information of persistence of a k-simplex where long persistence times are suggestive of signal and short persistence times indicate towards noise.

Persistence diagrams: A *persistence diagram (PDia)* is a two dimensional representation of the birth and death times of the k-simplices in a given point cloud, where the horizontal axis is the birth time b_i and the vertical axis is the death time $d_i > b_i$. Each tuple (b_i, d_i) for a simplicial complexes is represented as a point in the 2-dimensional space. An overlay of persistence diagrams from two different point clouds enables comparison of two point clouds where a strong topological difference will be visible as a segregation of points in the PD space, and a strong overlap of points would suggest a topological similarity between the point clouds. Informally, a PD is a scatter plot of the persistence timelines where the x-axis is the birth time and the y-axis is the death time.

Persistence Landscapes: A persistence landscape (PL) for each $\{(b_i, d_i)\}_{i=1}^{n}$ is a sequence of functions $\lambda_k : \mathbb{R} \to [0, \infty], k = 1, 2, 3, \ldots$ where $\lambda_k(x)$ is the k-th largest value of $\{f_{b_i, d_i}(x)\}_{i=1}^{n}$ [1]. For every birth-death pair (b, d) we define a piecewise linear function $f_{(b,d)} : \mathbb{R} \to [0, \infty]$ such as:

$$f_{(b,d)} = \begin{cases} 0, & if\ x \notin (b,d), \\ x - b & if\ x \in (b, \frac{b+d}{2}], \\ -x + d & if\ x \in (\frac{b+d}{2}, b). \end{cases}$$

For a set of persistence landscapes $\lambda^1, \ldots, \lambda^N$ we compute the average landscape as $\bar{\lambda} = \sum_{j=1}^{N} \frac{1}{N} \lambda^j$.

Persistence Landscape Kernel: The distance between two persistence landscapes $\mathbb{L} = \{\mathbb{L}_k\}$ and $\mathbb{L}' = \{\mathbb{L}'_k\}$ can be obtained as the L^p norms for $1 < p < \infty$ which is defined as,

$$\|\mathbb{L}_k - \mathbb{L}'_k\|_p = \left[\sum_{k=1}^{K} \int \|\mathbb{L}_k - \mathbb{L}'_k\|_p^p \right]^{\frac{1}{p}} \tag{1}$$

and for $p = 2$, the L_2 distance between two persistence landscapes acts as a kernel metric between them named as a PL kernel [1].

Persistence Scale Space Kernel: The persistence scale space kernel (PSSK) [6] represents the multiset of points in a persistence diagram as a sum of dirac delta functions centered at each point. This enables the representation of points in persistence diagrams in a Hilbert space thereby supporting computation of a kernel between two point. Briefly, for two persistence diagrams F and G we compute the PSSK kernel ($k_\sigma(F, G)$) as:

$$k_\sigma(F, G) = \frac{1}{8\pi\sigma} \sum_{p \in F, q \in G} \exp^{-\frac{\|p - q\|^2}{8\sigma}} - \exp^{-\frac{\|p - \bar{q}\|^2}{8\sigma}} \tag{2}$$

where each $p = (b_i, d_i)$, $q = (b_j, d_j)$ and $\bar{q} = (d_j, b_j)$. For two persistence timelines represented as persistence diagrams we can compute the kernel matrix between all data groups.

2.4 Experiments

We tested the classical network features and persistence homology (PL & PDia) features for group level difference and their ability to predict previously unseen subjects in experiments as outlined below.

Group difference analysis: For the two groups of persistence landscapes $\mathbb{L}^1, \ldots, \mathbb{L}^N$ and $\mathbb{L}^1, \ldots, \mathbb{L}^M$, let δ be the true L_p distance between their average PLs, $\overline{\mathbb{L}_N}$ and $\overline{\mathbb{L}_M}$. We permute the group labels and compute the group level average landscapes $\overline{\mathbb{L}_N}$ and $\overline{\mathbb{L}_M}$ and find the corresponding L_p distance between them. The p-value of the statistical test equals the proportion of random permutations in which the distance between $\overline{\mathbb{L}_N}$ and $\overline{\mathbb{L}_M}$ is greater than the true difference.

For the classical network features of nodal degree, local efficiency and clustering coefficient for the graphs in the filtration for each subject, we test the

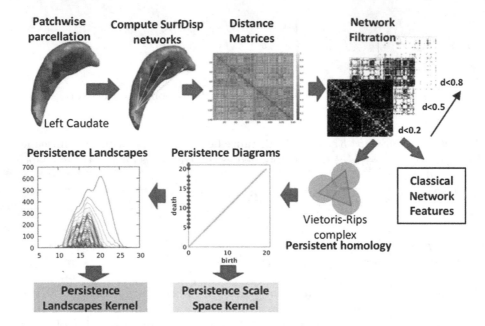

Fig. 1. Method workflow for the shape topology networks.

group level difference between the features in the two groups in a Hotelling's T2 test in a permutation testing experiment (2000 permutations) after PCA dimensionality reduction into a reduced dimensionality space. The experiment tests for the hypothesis that the feature values originate from two distributions with same mean value, rejecting the hypothesis at $\alpha = 0.05$ and p-value < 0.05.

Classification experiment: To test the ability of the network and PH features to correctly classify unseen subjects, we trained a kernel support vector machine classifier with a radial basis function (RBF) kernel for the complex network features, the PL kernel for the PL features and the PSSK kernel for the PDia features. The classifier was trained in a random and repeated holdout stratified training experiment with parameter tuning for the RBF and PSSK kernels. Results for the accuracy, sensitivity, specificity and F1-measure are reported for each classification experiment.

Computational tools: We input the distance matrices for the geometry networks in the package *Perseus* with the parameter (*distmat*) to compute the PH of the Vietoris-Rips complex for each brain point cloud from the inter-patch distance matrices [5]. We obtain birth-death pairs (b_i, d_i) for the k-dimensional simplices for $k = 0, 1, 2, 3$. A recent *persistence landscapes* toolbox was released for research use by [1] enabling computation and statistical inference of the persistence landscapes. The number of landscapes λ^i varies dependent upon the underlying persistence diagrams which inherently depend on the birth-death pairs (b_i, d_i). Further, we perform permutation testing on the persistence landscapes in the two groups for 2000 random group assignments.

2.5 Imaging and Demographics

Imaging data for this work was obtained from the publicly available database provided under the Parkinson's Progressive Markers Initiative (*PPMI*). Detailed protocol for image acquisition and quality control for the study is available at the website www.ppmi-info.org. The two groups with De Novo PD patients (n = 189, age = 68.02 ± 4.77, 115M/74F) and healthy controls (CN) (n = 137, age = 63.85 ± 7.46, 75M/62F) were selected and analysed through the method as described above. The original T1 MRI images were first preprocessed to obtain the segmentation labels for the subcortical structures via a multi-template registration based segmentation method (FS+LDDMM [3]). The segmentation outlines and surfaces were quality controlled prior to the computation of SurfDisp shape feature.

3 Results

The homology of the SurfDisp feature only had 0-dimensional PH features, higher dimensional homology features were not present in the SurfDisp networks for all structures. The persistence landscapes showed statistically significant difference between the two groups for all structures (Table 1). The local efficiency (L-caud,L-Pall), clustering coefficient (R-caud) and nodal degree (L-pall) were significantly different between the two groups. The PL kernel showed poor performance in classification experiments, on the contrary, the PSSK kernel showed good performance (ACC = 74.9, 75.1) for left and right pallidum (Table 2). The classical network features were unable to correctly classify subjects in the two groups (Table 3).

Table 1. Group level difference performance of the surface displacement network features in the permutation testing experiment to differentiate Parkinson's disease and healthy groups.

Feature	Caudate		Pallidum	
	L	R	L	R
Persistence landscape β_0	0*	0*	0*	0*
Local effficiency	0.030*	0.333	0.0064*	0.482
Clustering coefficient	0.80	0.028*	0.121	0.261
Nodal degree	0.231	0.003	0.049*	0.5829

Table 2. Classification performance of persistence homology features of surface displacement networks in Parkinson's disease.

PL

	Sens	Spec	F1	Accuracy
lcaud	0.495	0.510	0.615	49.753
rcaud	0.503	0.471	0.618	49.727
lpall	0.495	0.494	0.613	49.506
rpall	0.496	0.527	0.617	50.156

PSSK

	Sens	Spec	F1	Accuracy
lcaud	0.533	0.473	0.642	52.195
rcaud	0.465	0.480	0.585	46.766
lpall	0.883	0.145	0.847	**74.91**
rpall	0.886	0.141	0.852	**75.01**

caud: caudate, pall: pallidum
PL: persistence landscape kernel,
PSSK: persistence scale space kernel,
Sens: sensitivity, Spec: specificity,
F1: F1-measure, Acc: accuracy.

Table 3. Classification performance of classical network features of surface displacement networks in Parkinson's disease.

		Sens	Spec	F1	nPCs	Acc
lcaud	2	0.603	0.425	0.661	63.920	55.524
	3	0.568	0.466	0.611	8.420	54.095
	4	0.567	0.553	0.653	50.850	56.333
rcaud	1	0.471	0.678	0.590	82.560	52.610
	2	0.571	0.381	0.599	11.850	52.067
	3	0.528	0.547	0.619	61.190	53.333
lpall	1	0.595	0.466	0.662	49.030	56.029
	2	0.686	0.331	0.675	5.900	59.105
	3	0.544	0.519	0.630	47.010	53.724
rpall	1	0.499	0.508	0.592	36.740	50.143
	2	0.372	0.650	0.433	3	44.571
	3	0.530	0.514	0.619	34.640	52.552

(1) Clustering Coefficient, (2) Nodal Degree,
(3) Local Efficiency
Sens: sensitivity, Spec: specificity,
F1: F1-measure, Acc: accuracy.

4   Discussion and Conclusion

In this work, we aimed to quantify the inter-regional covariation of shape between subfields of subcortical structures. To this end, we computed the persistence homology and classical network analysis features for SurfDisp data indexed on the surface of the structures. It is interesting to note that the SurfDisp data on the subcortical structures only showed a 0-dimensional homology, whereas, higher dimensional homology was not present with the Vietoris-Rips complex. This can be attributed to the small distribution of values in the surface displacement data, where the 0-dimensional homology is present and the 1, 2 & 3 dimensional homology components are not present. Additionally, we can infer that the SurfDisp point cloud connectivity grows through the filtration in a single large connected component, possibly attributable to small spread of SurfDisp values in the data space.

The focus of this work was to test performance of the PH features in comparison to classical network features. In the statistical experiments, significant group level difference was found in the persistence landscapes and some network features for the structures. However, the classification performance was subpar and was unable to correctly predict previously unseen subjects. However, the PSSK kernel for the right and left pallidum showed good performance to correctly classify subjects. This suggests that the PL features contain information that is distinguishable on a group level, however, share a strong overlap for it to identify individual subjects. Thus, suggesting that the approximation of the persistence diagrams to persistence landscapes potentially leads to loss of information, which is otherwise captured by the PSSK kernel.

In this work our goal was to quantify and study the inter-regional co-variation of shape change in subcortical structures with brain abnormalities. The topology of the underlying data space was quantified in the persistence homology features and studied for their strengths to identify group level and subject level differences due to brain abnormalities. The results suggest a robust ability of the method and its derived features to differentiate on a group level. The features did not show a consistent and strong performance to predict individual subjects suggestive of wide variability between subjects overpowering the differences between subjects. Future work on bigger data cohorts is expected to enhance the subject level prediction of disease conditions. The feature is sensitive to disease and brain abnormalities as it is able to successfully differentiate between groups, where, on average, large changes can be observed. However, the prediction of disease via correct classification of individuals depends upon the sensitivity of the feature to changes within a subject.

The PH features computed in the current work showed moderate performance to predict individual subjects in a machine learning model. This can be associated with the averaging of features into small number of patches to obtain connectivity between SubCortical surface ROIs. Further, the surface displacement feature has both outward (positive) and inward (negative) deformation of the surface. Thus, smaller patches are needed to avoid the averaging affect on large patches potentially reducing the sensitivity of the SurfDisp data.

In the current work, we limited to large patch size due to the limits of tractability of the persistence homology computation. Further development of computationally efficient algorithms would greatly solve this limitation is expected to yield state-of-the-art performance in prediction of disease.

This is a first work to study the persistence homology of a shape feature for subcortical structures and can potentially benefit from newer methodological extensions. We studied the SurfDisp shape feature, however, the general nature of the Shape topology method enables its applicability to other shape features such as spherical harmonics, initial momentum an the like. Further extensions to include more complex distance functions or better homology features can potentially improve it application in clinical settings.

Acknowledgment. Data used in the preparation of this article were obtained from the Parkinson's Progression Markers Initiative (PPMI) database (http://www.ppmi-info.org/data). For up-to-date information on the study, visit www.ppmi-info.org. The authors acknowledge and thank the Natural Sciences and Engineering Research Council (NSERC), Michael Smith Foundation for Health Research (MSFHR), Canadian Institute of Health Research (CIHR), Brain Canada and MITACS Canada for their generous funding support.

References

1. Bubenik, P.: Statistical topological data analysis using persistence landscapes. J. Mach. Learn. Res. **16**, 25 (2015)
2. Garg, A., Appel-Cresswell, S., Popuri, K., McKeown, M.J., Beg, M.F.: Morphological alterations in the caudate, putamen, pallidum, and thalamus in Parkinson's disease. Front. Neurosci. **9**(March), 1–14 (2015)
3. Khan, A., Wang, L., Beg, M.: Freesurfer-initiated fully-automated subcortical brain segmentation in MRI using large deformation diffeomorphic metric mapping. NeuroImage **41**(3), 735–746 (2008)
4. McKeown, M.J., Uthama, A., Abugharbieh, R., Palmer, S., Lewis, M., Huang, X.: Shape (but not volume) changes in the thalami in Parkinson disease. BMC Neurol. 8, 8, January 2008
5. Mischaikow, K., Nanda, V.: Morse theory for filtrations and efficient computation of persistent homology. Discrete Comput. Geom. **50**(2), 330–353 (2013)
6. Reininghaus, J., Huber, S., Bauer, U., Kwitt, R.: A stable multi-scale kernel for topological machine learning. In: Proceedings of the IEEE Computer Society Conference on Computer Vision and Pattern Recognition, vol. 07, pp. 4741–4748, 12 June 2015
7. Rubinov, M., Sporns, O.: Complex network measures of brain connectivity: uses and interpretations. NeuroImage **52**(3), 1059–1069 (2010)

Graph Geodesics to Find Progressively Similar Skin Lesion Images

Jeremy Kawahara, Kathleen P. Moriarty, and Ghassan Hamarneh$^{(\boxtimes)}$

Medical Image Analysis Lab, Simon Fraser University, Burnaby, Canada
{jkawahar,kmoriart,hamarneh}@sfu.ca

Abstract. Skin conditions represent an enormous health care burden worldwide, and as datasets of skin images grow, there is continued interest in computerized approaches to analyze skin images. In order to explore and gain insights into datasets of skin images, we propose a graph based approach to visualize a progression of similar skin images between pairs of images. In our graph, a node represents both a clinical and dermoscopic image of the same lesion, and an edge between nodes captures the visual dissimilarity between lesions, where dissimilarity is computed by comparing the image responses of a pretrained convolutional neural network. We compute the geodesic/shortest path between nodes to determine a path of progressively visually similar skin lesions. To quantitatively evaluate the quality of the returned path, we propose metrics to measure the number of transitions with respect to the lesion diagnosis, and the progression with respect to the clinical 7-point checklist. Compared to baseline experiments, our approach shows improvements to the quality of the returned paths.

Keywords: Graph geodesics · Skin lesions · Visualizing similar images

1 Introduction

Globally, skin conditions are the fourth most common cause of healthy years lost due to disability [6], and represent the most common reason for a patient to visit their general practitioner in studied populations [16]. Skin conditions such as malignant melanoma, a common cancer, can be fatal [14]. Many groups recognize the potential for computerized systems to analyze skin lesions and help reduce the burden on health care, and much work has gone into developing computerized systems to diagnose skin disorders [13]. Typically, such systems take as input a skin lesion image, and output either a discrete label or the probability that this lesion has a particular diagnosis. For example, Estevan et al. [5] used a human designed taxonomy to partition clinically similar images into classes that have a similar number of samples. They fine-tuned a Convolutional Neural Network pretrained over ImageNet [15] to classify skin lesions, and achieved results comparable to human dermatologists. While knowing the probability that the image contains a particular type of skin lesion is a worthwhile goal, a disadvantage to this approach is that it is a "black box", where the user gains no insights into the automated diagnosis or of the underlying dataset of skin images.

© Springer International Publishing AG 2017
M.J. Cardoso et al. (Eds.): GRAIL/MFCA/MICGen 2017, LNCS 10551, pp. 31–41, 2017.
DOI: 10.1007/978-3-319-67675-3_4

A different approach from classification that offers some insights into the dataset or diagnosis is to adopt an image retrieval based approach. For example, Bunte et al. [3] extracted colour features from clinical skin images, learned a supervised transformation of these features, and retrieved images in a dataset based on the k nearest neighbours to these features. These returned images can be displayed to the user, giving insights into the appearance of similarly diseased images and allow the diagnosis to be inferred. Kawahara et al. [10] displayed a network graph visualization based on the nearest neighbours to a single query image, which allow users to efficiently search the space of similar lesion images.

Another approach to visualize *general images* was proposed by Hegde et al. [7], where rather than retrieving the k nearest images to a single query image, their approach uses two query images (a source and target) to retrieve a list of images that progress in visual similarity between the two images. They accomplish this by representing images as nodes in a graph, where the edges between nodes indicate their pair-wise distance, and the geodesic (shortest path) between source and target nodes represents a visually smooth progression of images. A similar approach for *general images* was recently implemented online [12], which is based on an experimental visualization tool as part of Google Arts and Culture [11]. In other works, representing images as nodes to find an optimal path between nodes has been used to guide subject-template brain registration in MR images [8].

In this work, we apply a similar method to find images of skin lesions that visually progress between a source and target lesion. This visualization approach may be useful for clinicians who wish to find reference images of hard to classify, visually challenging "borderline" cases across types of skin diseases (e.g., note the visually challenging aspects in distinguishing clark nevus from melanoma in Fig. 1 *bottom row*). Another use may be to show or predict the visual progression over time between a low-risk benign lesion to a malignant lesion (e.g., progression in Fig. 3 *bottom row*). This may give insights into the progression of the disease (e.g., Clark/Dysplastic nevi is potentially a precursor to melanoma and studies estimate that 20–30% of melanomas come from nevi [4]), or serve as a useful reference for patients to monitor and compare the progression of their own lesion. In these potential applications, the target images could be from either a set of predefined reference images, or the geodesics to each of the nearest unique diseases could be automatically shown.

To the best of our knowledge, this is the first work that has applied geodesic paths to visualize skin lesion images. In contrast to previous work [7,8,11,12], we propose to let each node in our graph represent images from two modalities (a dermoscopic and a clinical image), where the edge weights are influenced by both types of images. We apply an exponential function to the pair-wise dissimilarity measures, and show how this results in longer paths of higher quality without risking disconnected graphs. Finally, we propose measures to quantitatively evaluate the quality of our paths, which is lacking in prior work. These proposed quality measures are particularly important as without them, we would need to qualitatively inspect each path.

2   Methods

A skin lesion can be captured by both a dermatoscope (producing a *dermoscopic* image x_d), and a photo camera (producing a *clinical* image x_c), where the dermoscopic images show a more standardized view of the lesion, and the clinical images are non-standardized and often show additional contextual information (e.g., the body part the lesion is on) not available in the dermoscopic images. Given a dataset of skin lesions, the i-th skin lesion is represented by a dermoscopic and clinical pair of images $(x_d^{(i)}, x_c^{(i)})$. We create a graph where each pair of images $(x_d^{(i)}, x_c^{(i)})$ are represented by a single node $v^{(i)}$, and an edge $e^{(ij)}$ encodes the dissimilarity between nodes i and j. Our goal is to find a set of nodes $(v_0^{(s)}, v_1^{(i)}, \ldots, v_{R-1}^{(j)}, v_R^{(l)})$ of an unknown length R such that the initial node $v_0^{(s)}$ is a given source node (the superscript identifies the lesion, and the subscript indicates the position in the returned path), the R-th node is a given target node $v_R^{(t)}$, and the intermediate nodes $(v_1^{(i)}, \ldots, v_{R-1}^{(j)})$ represent lesions that visually progress between the source and target nodes. We find these intermediate nodes using Dijkstra's algorithm, which computes the geodesic between the source and target and returns a path of nodes representing a progression of visually similar lesions.

The key components that we now examine in detail are how to: extract image features that capture the salient properties of skin images, compute local dissimilarity between pairs of skin lesion images, weigh and connect the node edges using multi-modal images, and quantitatively evaluate the quality of the returned paths.

Skin Images as Deep Pretrained Neural Nets Responses. The responses of skin images with deep convolutional neural networks pretrained over ImageNet [15] have shown to be effective feature vectors for skin lesion classification despite the differences in appearance between skin lesions and natural images [9]. We use a similar approach to compute feature vectors as in [9], and for a particular image, extract the responses from the first fully connected layer of VGG16 [17], and average the responses over a set of predefined image augmentations,

$$\Phi(x)_m = \frac{1}{|\Pi|} \sum_{\pi \in \Pi} \phi(\pi(x - \mu))_m \tag{1}$$

where π is a function to augment an image (e.g., left-right flip); Π is the set of $|\Pi|$ number of image augmentations; $\phi(\cdot)_m$ extracts the m-th response of the first fully connected layer of VGG16; and, μ represent the mean pixel over the training data from ImageNet, which is subtracted from the skin lesion image x. The resulting feature vector $\Phi(x)$ represents a single lesion image by averaging the augmented responses over a single image, without increasing the dimensions of the feature vector.

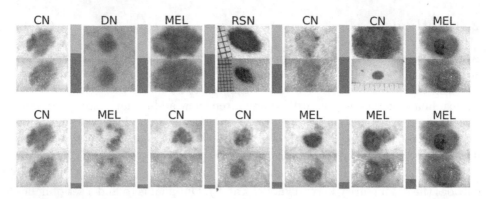

Fig. 1. An example random path (*top*) and geodesic returned from the proposed method (*bottom*), where the *leftmost* and *rightmost* image represent the source and target nodes, respectively. The dermoscopic image is shown above the clinical image in each row. The *magenta bar* indicates the dissimilarity between adjacent images, where a higher bar indicates that they are more dissimilar. (Color figure online)

Local Image Dissimilarity. Given two feature vectors $u, v \in \mathbb{R}^M$ (which represent the responses of two skin images), we compute the dissimilarity between them as the cosine distance raised to the p-th power,

$$\mathcal{D}(u, v) = \left(1 - \frac{\sum_i^M u_i v_i}{\sqrt{\sum_i^M u_i^2}\sqrt{\sum_i^M v_i^2}} \right)^p \tag{2}$$

where setting $p \neq 1$ non-linearly changes the dissimilarity between vectors. By using a high p (e.g., $p = 4$), we assign very low values to edges connecting similar images, thus encouraging geodesics to pass through nearby nodes of similar images, avoiding very short paths even in the case of complete graphs, i.e., fully connected graphs (further discussed in the Results section). Other distance measures are possible (e.g., L_1, L_2), and we found them to give empirically similar results. Figure 1 shows the dissimilarity between pairs of images (dissimilarity is displayed in magenta using $p = 1$ for clarity).

Multi-modal Edge Weights. We define the edge weight $e^{(ij)}$ between nodes i and j as a weighted sum based on both the dermoscopic and clinical images,

$$e^{(ij)} = \alpha \mathcal{D}(\Phi(x_d^{(i)}), \Phi(x_d^{(j)})) + (1 - \alpha)\mathcal{D}(\Phi(x_c^{(i)}), \Phi(x_c^{(j)})) \tag{3}$$

where $\mathcal{D}(\cdot)$ is a function that computes the dissimilarity (Eq. 2) between the feature vectors $\Phi(\cdot)$ computed in Eq. 1; and α weighs the influence of the dermoscopic and clinical images ($0 \leq \alpha \leq 1$). Increasing α causes an edge to be more influenced by the dermoscopic image than the clinical image, which may be desired as dermoscopic images contain more salient lesion properties.

Node Connectivity. To form the graph, we must decide on the connectivity of nodes. This can be done by connecting the k nearest neighbours (where nearest is defined via Eq. 2) to each node with an edge. However, choosing k is challenging as a large k (e.g., a complete graph) increases computational complexity and can lead to very short paths being returned when a direct edge exists between any pair of source and target nodes. Too small a k can lead to disconnected graphs, where no path exists between the source and target nodes. In the Results, we experiment with different values of k and show that by setting a high value of p in Eq. 3, the returned paths remain longer even in the case of complete graphs.

Surrogate Measures of Path Quality. While we provide qualitative results through visualizing the returned paths (Fig. 3), we also propose the following measures to quantitatively evaluate the quality of the returned paths. We define a *quality path* as a smooth visual progression of images. However, this definition is hard to precisely define and directly measure. Thus we propose a surrogate measure that uses the diagnoses of the lesions, as skin lesion datasets are often accompanied with a corresponding clinical diagnosis $y^{(i)}$ (e.g., melanoma, nevus), indicating the disease type of the i-th lesion $x^{(i)}$, where $y^{(i)}$ is an attribute of node $v^{(i)}$. Our assumption is that lesions with the same diagnosis will likely be visually similar, and that a high quality path will have a smooth progression with respect to the lesion diagnosis. In order to give a high cost to paths that frequently change neighbouring labels, we define the *transition cost* as,

$$\text{trans}(v_0^{(s)}, v_1^{(i)}, \ldots, v_{R-1}^{(j)}, v_R^{(t)}) = \frac{1}{R-1} \sum_{r=1}^{R} \left(1 - \delta(y_r^{(a)} - y_{r-1}^{(b)})\right) \qquad (4)$$

where R is the number of nodes in the returned path; and $y_r^{(i)}$ indicates the skin lesion diagnosis for the r-th returned path node corresponding to node $v_r^{(i)}$ (e.g., $y_0^{(s)}$ and $y_R^{(t)}$ correspond to the labels of the source and target nodes $v_0^{(s)}, v_R^{(t)}$ respectively). The Dirac delta function $\delta(\cdot)$ returns 1 if the two labels have the same class, and 0 otherwise.

Our second surrogate quality measure quantifies the progression of the 7-point score between the source and target nodes. The 7-point score is a clinical measure of melanoma based on the visual presence of seven criteria (e.g., irregular streaks) within a lesion. The weighted sum of these seven criteria form the 7-point score $\hat{y} \in \mathbb{Z}$ [1], where $\hat{y}^{(i)}$ is an attribute of node $v^{(i)}$. We assume that a quality path will have 7-point scores that smoothly progress from a low to high score, as higher scores indicate the presence of lesion more indicative of melanoma (and vice versa). We define the *progression cost* as,

$$\text{progress}(v_0^{(s)}, \ldots, v_R^{(t)}) = \frac{1}{R} \sum_{r=1}^{R} \left(\max\left[\left(\text{sgn}(\hat{y}_0^{(s)} - \hat{y}_R^{(t)})(\hat{y}_r^{(i)} - \hat{y}_{r-1}^{(j)})\right), 0\right]\right) \quad (5)$$

where sgn(z) returns the sign of the difference between the source and target node scores,

$$\text{sgn}(z) = \begin{cases} 1, & \text{if } z = 0 \\ \frac{z}{|z|}, & \text{otherwise.} \end{cases} \tag{6}$$

This measure returns a cost of 0 if the 7-point score consistently decreases, increases, or remains constant along the path between the source and target nodes, and penalizes by the magnitude of the change otherwise. This approach, however, will always compute a 0 cost if the path only consists of the source and target nodes. As this is a degenerate case, we ignore the progression costs for paths of length two when computing results, and note that this measure is biased to return lower costs for shorter paths, and is thus most informative when comparing paths with the same number of nodes.

3   Results

Data. We test our proposed approach and surrogate measures using the Interactive Atlas of Dermoscopy [2] skin dataset. This dataset contains 1011 cases of skin lesions, where all but four cases are captured by both a clinical x_c and dermoscopic x_d image (in the four cases missing x_c, we set $x_c = x_d$). Each case has a class label y that represents a known lesion diagnosis, and a 7-point score $\hat{y}$. The diagnosis y can take on one of the 15 class labels: basal cell carcinoma (BCC), blue nevus (BN), clark nevus (CN), combined nevus (CBN), congenital nevus (CGN), dermal nevus (DN), dermatofibroma (DF), lentigo (LT), melanoma (MEL), melanosis (MLS), miscellaneous (MISC), recurrent nevus (RN), reed or spitz nevus (RSN), seborrheic keratosis (SK), and vascular lesion (VL). The 7-point score $\hat{y} \in \mathbb{Z}$ ranges between 0 and 7 (in this dataset), where a higher score indicates the lesion has visual properties more indicative of melanoma. The lesion diagnosis and the 7-point score are only used to quantify the quality of the returned paths, and are not used to form the graph. We randomly select a set of 1000 pairs of source and target nodes which are used across all experiments.

Recovering Synthetic Paths. We start by testing if our proposed approach can recover the path of images created by a progressive synthetic transformation. To do this, we crop the image by removing 15% of the pixels at the borders of the images, and repeat this five times. This progressively enlarges the lesion over a series of five images. We added these five synthetic images to our dataset, select the original image as the source and the final synthetic image as the target ($p = 4$ and $k = 30$). We find our approach not only recovers all synthetic images, but it recovers the correct sequence of synthetic images, i.e. in the order they were synthesized (Fig. 2), indicating that this approach and the feature vectors are sensitive to scale despite the CNN being trained on images at multiple scales.

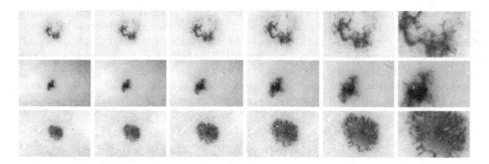

Fig. 2. Synthetic examples: Here the *leftmost* images represent the source nodes, which belong to the original (non-enlarged) dermoscopic images in the dataset. The *rightmost* images represent target nodes, which were the last of the progressively enlarged images. The returned geodesic path is represented by the images in between. Note that the returned geodesic included all five synthetic images, in proper order of increasing enlargement.

Retrieving Paths from a Complete and Non-complete Graphs. For our first experiment, in Table 1 **row 1.1** (*complete graph with p = 1*) we report results using a complete graph (i.e., $k = 1011$) using only the dermoscopic images (i.e., $\alpha = 1$ in Eq. 1) and setting $p = 1$ in Eq. 3. We observe that when using a complete graph, the returned paths often consist of only the source and target nodes as their shared edge yields the shortest path. This experiment highlights the need to either prune the edges in the graph or modify the edge weights. Following the approach of [12], we form a new graph where each node is connected to its $k = 30$ neighbours. **Row 1.2** (*non-complete graph with p = 1*) shows that restricting the node connectivity increases the number of nodes in the returned path and improves the transition cost (note that the progression cost performs worse as it is biased towards paths with fewer nodes, and is thus most informative when comparing paths with a similar number of nodes).

Paths with Exponential Edge Weights. While decreasing node connectivity (i.e., lowering k) results in longer paths, care must be taken when choosing k, as reducing k increases the risk of forming disconnected graphs where no path exists between a source and target node. Thus instead of pruning edges, our next experiment (**row 1.3** *complete graph with p = 4*) shows how applying an exponential function (i.e., $p = 4$ in Eq. 3) to the dissimilarity function results in longer paths of higher quality even in a complete graph. By removing the need to prune graphs (i.e., choose k), we guarantee a path to exist, while still preventing short paths. If we are not concerned with disconnected graphs, we can combine edge pruning using k neighbours with the increased p, to match the computational efficiency of a pruned graph without penalty to quality (**row 1.4** *non-complete graph with p = 4*). For the remaining experiments, we use $p = 4$ and non-complete graphs with $k = 30$, as our graphs remained connected.

Table 1. Quantitative results of the returned paths using the proposed surrogate quality measures. The *Img.* column indicates if the input was a dermoscopic image x_d, clinical image x_c, or included both. k represents the number of nearest neighbours used to form edges that connect nodes. *Aug.* indicates if the image was augmented or not when forming the image feature vector. *Trans., Progress.,* indicates the average and standard deviation transition and progression cost as defined in the text. *Num. Path* shows the average and standard deviation number of nodes in the computed path.

Exp.	Img.	Aug.	p	k	Ordered	Trans.	Progress.	Num. Path
1.1	x_d	✗	1	1011	min-path	0.76 ± 0.42	0.10 ± 0.19	2.02 ± 0.13
1.2 [12]	x_d	✗	1	30	min-path	0.64 ± 0.34	0.23 ± 0.26	3.59 ± 0.85
1.3	x_d	✗	4	1011	min-path	0.56 ± 0.26	0.37 ± 0.20	8.11 ± 2.87
1.4	x_d	✗	4	30	min-path	0.56 ± 0.26	0.37 ± 0.20	8.12 ± 2.87
1.5	x_d	✓	4	30	min-path	0.55 ± 0.25	0.35 ± 0.17	9.16 ± 3.62
1.6	–	–	–	–	random	0.76 ± 0.19	0.54 ± 0.24	9.16 ± 3.62
1.7	x_d	✓	–	–	linear	0.58 ± 0.25	0.44 ± 0.21	9.16 ± 3.62
1.8	x_c	✗	4	30	min-path	0.65 ± 0.18	0.46 ± 0.20	10.64 ± 5.08
1.9	x_d, x_c	✗	4	30	min-path	0.45 ± 0.24	0.34 ± 0.19	7.90 ± 3.27
1.10	x_d, x_c	✓	4	30	min-path	0.45 ± 0.23	0.34 ± 0.17	8.86 ± 3.73

Comparing Random and Linearly Interpolated Path. In **row 1.5** (*augmented images*) we augment the feature vector with left-right image flips (Eq. 1), which results in longer geodesics paths and minor improvements to the path quality. We form a path with an equal number of nodes as those returned in the geodesic path in the previous experiment (from row 1.5) by randomly sampling nodes (without replacement). As the labels in our dataset are highly imbalanced, these random paths give us a baseline quality score (**row 1.6** *random paths*). We also compare our method by ignoring the graph, and instead using linearly interpolated feature vectors between the source and target feature vectors. These interpolated feature vectors are uniformly separated to match the number of returned nodes in row 1.5. The nearest unique neighbour to this interpolated feature vector is used to form the path. **Row 1.7** (*linear paths*) shows that this approach yields paths of worse quality when compared to using graph geodesics. We highlight that the graph geodesic approach has the additional advantage of automatically determining the number of nodes in the path, whereas the linearly interpolated approach requires this to be specified (we set it equal to the length of the geodesic path).

Using Clinical Image Features. In **row 1.8** (*clinical images*) we use only the clinical image (i.e., $\alpha = 0$ in Eq. 3) and notice a marked decrease in the quality of the paths when compared to dermoscopic images. This is expected since dermoscopic images are more standardized and focused on the lesion, while

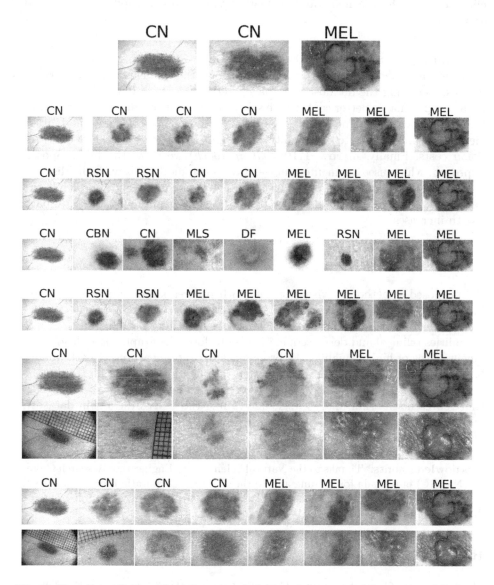

Fig. 3. Visualizing Paths. The *leftmost* and *rightmost* dermoscopic images are the given source (clark nevus) and target (melanoma) node, where the images in each row in between them correspond to the computed geodesic/minimal path. Each row, starting from the *top* to *bottom* row, correspond to the following experiments in Table 1: 1.2 (*non-complete graph with* $p = 1$), 1.4 (*non-complete graph with* $p = 4$), 1.5 (*augmented images*), 1.6 (*random paths*), 1.7 (*linear paths*), 1.9 (*dermoscopic and clinical images*), and 1.10 (*full approach*). The geodesic of Experiments 1.9 and 1.10 incorporates clinical images, shown directly below the dermoscopic images.

clinical images have a non-standard field of view and can capture background artifacts.

Combining Dermoscopic and Clinical Image Features. In **row 1.9** (*dermoscopic and clinical images*) we include both the clinical and dermoscopic images, weighting the dermoscopic images higher (i.e., $\alpha = 0.8$ in Eq. 3) as the dermoscopic images better capture the salient lesion features and avoid irrelevant background artifacts. The returned paths now respect both imaging modalities, yielding improvements to the quality of the paths, most noticeable with transition costs. Finally, in **row 1.10** (*full approach*) we show the full proposed approach, which uses augmented images from both modalities with the dissimilarity measure raised to the power of $p = 4$ on a non-complete graph. While the path quality measures remain similar to the previous experiment, the total path length increases.

4 Conclusions

We proposed a method to visualize a smooth progression of similar skin lesion images between two skin lesions. Our graph geodesic based approach applies an exponential dissimilarity function and considers information from multiple modalities (clinical and dermoscopic images) to form the graph edges, leading to longer paths of higher quality. We proposed surrogate measures of path quality based on the diagnostic labels of the skin lesions to quantitatively assess the resulting paths. Future work would explore how to improve the feature vectors that represent the skin images (e.g., fine-tuning the CNN over a skin dataset), and examine how to make the progression quality measure less sensitive to the length of the path.

Acknowledgments. Thanks to the Natural Sciences and Engineering Research Council (NSERC) of Canada for funding and to the NVIDIA Corporation for the donation of a Titan X GPU used in this research. Thanks to Sara Daneshvar for preparing the data used in this work.

References

1. Argenziano, G., Fabbrocini, G., Carli, P., Vincenzo, D.G., Sammarco, E., Delfino, M.: Epiluminescence microscopy for the diagnosis of doubtful melanocytic skin lesions. Comparison of the ABCD rule of dermatoscopy and a new 7-point checklist based on pattern analysis. Arch. Dermatol. **134**(12), 1563–1570 (1998)
2. Argenziano, G., Soyer, H.P., Giorgio, V.D., Piccolo, D., Carli, P., Delfino, M., Ferrari, A., Hofmann-Wellenhof, R., Massi, D., Mazzocchetti, G., Scal-venzi, M., Wolf, I.H.: Interactive atlas of dermoscopy: a tutorial (Book and CD-ROM) (2000)
3. Bunte, K., Biehl, M., Jonkman, M.F., Petkov, N.: Learning effective color features for content based image retrieval in dermatology. Pattern Recogn. **44**(9), 1892–1902 (2011)

4. Duffy, K., Grossman, D.: The dysplastic nevus: from historical perspective to management in the modern era: Part I. Historical, histologic, and clinical aspects. J. Am. Acad. Dermatol. **67**(1), 1–27 (2012)
5. Esteva, A., Kuprel, B., Novoa, R.A., Ko, J., Swetter, S.M., Blau, H.M., Thrun, S.: Dermatologist-level classification of skin cancer with deep neural networks. Nature **542**(7639), 115–118 (2017)
6. Hay, R.J., Johns, N.E., Williams, H.C., Bolliger, I.W., Dellavalle, R.P., Margolis, D.J., Marks, R., Naldi, L., Weinstock, M.A., Wulf, S.K., Michaud, C., Murray, J.L.C., Naghavi, M.: The global burden of skin disease in 2010: an analysis of the prevalence and impact of skin conditions. J. Invest. Dermatol. **134**, 1527–1534 (2014)
7. Hegde, C., Sankaranarayanan, A.C., Baraniuk, R.G.: Learning manifolds in the wild. J. Mach. Learn. Res. 5037 (2012)
8. Jia, H., Wu, G., Wang, Q., Wang, Y., Kim, M., Shen, D.: Directed graph based image registration. In: Suzuki, K., Wang, F., Shen, D., Yan, P. (eds.) MLMI 2011. LNCS, vol. 7009, pp. 175–183. Springer, Heidelberg (2011). doi:10.1007/978-3-642-24319-6_22
9. Kawahara, J., BenTaieb, A., Hamarneh, G.: Deep features to classify skin lesions. In: IEEE ISBI, pp. 1397–1400 (2016)
10. Kawahara, J., Hamarneh, G.: Image content-based navigation of skin conditions. In: World Congress of Dermatology (2015)
11. Klingemann, M., Doury, S.: X Degrees of Separation (2016). https://artsexperiments.withgoogle.com/xdegrees/
12. Kogan, G.: Shortest path between images (2017). https://github.com/ml4a/ml4a-guides/blob/master/notebooks/image-path.ipynb
13. Korotkov, K., Garcia, R.: Computerized analysis of pigmented skin lesions: a review. Artif. Intell. Med. **56**(2), 69–90 (2012)
14. Markovic, S., Erickson, L.A., Rao, R., Creagan, E.T., et al.: Malignant melanoma in the 21st century, Part 1: epidemiology, risk factors, screening, prevention, and diagnosis. Mayo Clin. Proc. **82**(3), 364–380 (2007)
15. Russakovsky, O., Deng, J., Su, H., Krause, J., Satheesh, S., Ma, S., Huang, Z., Karpathy, A., Khosla, A., Bernstein, M., Berg, A.C., Fei-Fei, L.: ImageNet large scale visual recognition challenge. Int. J. Comput. Vision (IJCV) **115**(3), 211–252 (2015)
16. Schofield, J.K., Fleming, D., Grindlay, D., Williams, H.: Skin conditions are the commonest new reason people present to general practitioners in England and Wales. Br. J. Dermatol. **165**, 1044–1050 (2011)
17. Simonyan, K., Zisserman, A.: Very deep convolutional networks for large-scale image recognition. In: International Conference on Learning Representations Learning Representations (ICLR) (2015)

Uncertainty Estimation in Vascular Networks

Markus Rempfler[1,2]([✉]), Bjoern Andres[3], and Bjoern H. Menze[1,2]

[1] Institute for Advanced Study, Technical University of Munich, Munich, Germany
markus.rempfler@tum.de
[2] Department of Informatics, Technical University of Munich, Munich, Germany
[3] Bosch Center for Artificial Intelligence (BCAI), Renningen, Germany

Abstract. Reconstructing vascular networks is a challenging task in medical image processing as automated methods have to deal with large variations in vessel shape and image quality. Recent methods have addressed this problem as constrained maximum a posteriori (MAP) inference in a graphical model, formulated over an overcomplete network graph. Manual control and adjustments are often desired in practice and strongly benefit from indicating the uncertainties in the reconstruction or presenting alternative solutions. In this paper, we examine two different methods to sample vessel network graphs, a perturbation and a Gibbs sampler, and thereby estimate marginals. We quantitatively validate the accuracy of the approximated marginals using true marginals, computed by enumeration.

1 Introduction

Vessel segmentation and centerline extraction is a longstanding problem in computer vision [1]. From a medical perspective, segmenting and tracking vessels is crucial for planning and guiding several types of interventions. Several recent methods, however, have focussed on reconstructing vessel network graphs [2–6]. Analysing vascular graphs is expected to give insights into various biological properties, e.g. the relation between vascular remodeling processes and neurological diseases or pharmaceutical treatments [7]. These methods formulate the task as MAP inference in a constrained probabilistic model over a (super-)graph of candidate vasculature, where the solution encodes the subgraph that is most likely to represent the underlying vasculature. Variations of this approach include joint-tasks such as anatomical labeling of vasculature [6] or artery-vein separation [5].

As in many applications, exploring multiple solutions or even marginal distributions would be preferable over mere point estimates – either to present local uncertainty to the end user or to pass it over to the next stage of the processing pipeline. An automated reconstruction can be inspected and, if needed, edited by

Electronic supplementary material The online version of this chapter (doi:10. 1007/978-3-319-67675-3_5) contains supplementary material, which is available to authorized users.

M.J. Cardoso et al. (Eds.): GRAIL/MFCA/MICGen 2017, LNCS 10551, pp. 42–52, 2017.
DOI: 10.1007/978-3-319-67675-3_5

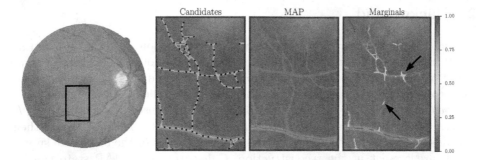

Fig. 1. Illustration of the uncertainty quantification in vasculature graphs from a 2D retinal image (**left**). Recent methods reconstruct the network from an overcomplete graph of candidate vessels (**second**, graph in green) by calculating the MAP state (**third**, graph in red) in a probabilistic model. Approximating marginal distributions (**right**) enables us to quantify the uncertainty in the network graph, which is valuable information for manual inspection and correction. Two examples are indicated with black arrows: In the first, the model is uncertain whether it is a furcation or a crossing, while in the second, a connection is not contained in the MAP but still has a high marginal probability. (Color figure online)

an expert. In such a workflow, the controlling expert benefits from an indication of the uncertainty in the presented reconstruction (cf. Fig. 1). To this end, recent work investigated how to find the m-best diverse solutions to the MAP problem in conditional random fields (CRFs) to explore a variety of highly probable assignments [8,9]. This approach, however, increases the computational complexity of the discrete optimization further. Alternatively, Markov chain Monte Carlo (MCMC) methods can be used to sample from probabilistic models [10,11]. While being well established for many statistical inference tasks, they are often considered expensive and difficult to parametrize for typical problems in computer vision. Papandreou and Youille [12] presented the idea to introduce local perturbations and solve for the MAP estimate of the perturbed model repeatedly to generate samples. They identify a perturbation distribution which allows to estimate marginal densities of the original Gibbs distribution while leveraging the computational efficiency of available discrete solvers. This idea was extended to a broader problem class in [13], while the theoretical framework was further developed in [14–17]. A few empirical studies investigated the effectiveness of such perturbation models in typical segmentation problems [15,18,19].

In this paper, we extend recent graph-based methods for reconstructing vascular networks that rely on integer progamming. We adapt two sampling approaches for the underlying probabilistic model, a perturbation sampler based on [12–15] and a Gibbs sampler based on [10,20]. They enable estimates of marginal distributions and a straight-forward way to quantify uncertainty in properties calculated from the resulting network graphs. To deal with the difficulty of validating the quality of the approximated marginals, we compare the approximated marginals to the true marginals, calculated by enumeration.

2   Background

Several recent methods for vessel network reconstruction pose the problem as MAP inference in a (constrained) probabilistic model over a supergraph composed of candidate vessels [2–6]. In short, such a candidate supergraph is typically constructed by detecting points that are likely to lie on a vessel centerline, composing the nodes $v \in V$ of the graph, and then inserting an edge $e \in E$ for each path that connects two nodes in close proximity. The MAP state then encodes a subgraph and thereby represents which parts of the candidate supergraph are present in the reconstruction. Calculating this MAP state can be formulated as an integer linear program (ILP) and solved by a branch-and-cut procedure. In the remainder of this section, we first describe such probabilistic model for vessel graphs and its MAP estimator. Details on the particular choice of candidate graph construction used in this study can be found in Sect. 4.

Probabilistic Model. Given a (directed) candidate graph $G = (V, E)$, we define a measure of probability $P(\mathbf{X} = \mathbf{x}|\Omega, I, \Theta)$ over possible vessel networks within G, encoded by $\mathbf{x} \in \{0, 1\}^E$. These indicator variables then encode whether an edge e is present in the solution ($x_e = 1$) or not ($x_e = 0$). We denote the set of *feasible* solutions as Ω, the image evidence as I and the model parameters as Θ. The measure of probability can be defined as:

$$P(\mathbf{x}|\Omega, I, \Theta) \propto P(\Omega|\mathbf{x}) \prod_{ij \in E} P(x_{ij}|I, \Theta) \prod_{C \in \mathcal{C}(G)} P(x_C|\Theta), \qquad (1)$$

$$\text{where } P(\Omega|\mathbf{x}) \propto \begin{cases} 1 & \text{if } \mathbf{x} \in \Omega, \\ 0 & \text{otherwise} \end{cases}. \qquad (2)$$

We identify three parts: First, $P(\Omega|\mathbf{x})$ is the uniform prior over all feasible solutions. Second, $P(x_e|I, \Theta)$ is the local evidence for an edge, i.e. the *unaries*. Third, $P(x_C|\Theta)$ corresponds to joint-events C that form higher-level potentials, and $\mathcal{C}(G)$ denotes the set of all events at any possible location within G. $x_C = 1$ indicates that the particular event C occurred.

In [2–6], these different parts have been chosen depending on the particular image datasets and target application of the reconstructed vasculature. For this study, we will impose the following constraints: each node can have at most one incoming edge and at most two outgoing edges. Furthermore, we do not allow the solution to contain circles. These three types of constraints define our Ω. As higher-level events x_C, we consider *appearance*, *termination* and *bifurcation* in each node, leaving us with at most $3|V|$ possible events in $\mathcal{C}(G)$. These events can be represented with binary indicator variables x_C and a set of $3|V|$ auxiliary constraints that tie their state to the original edge variables $\mathbf{x}$ upon which they depend. Note that the number of involved edge variables of a particular type of event varies with its location within G: For example, a bifurcation event at node v involves all x_e of potential outgoing edges $e \in \delta^-(v)$. We denote the set of auxiliary constraints necessary for higher-level events as Ω_A in the remainder of this section. The description of both Ω and Ω_A in terms of linear inequalities can be found in the supplement.

MAP Estimator. Using the bilinear representation of the pseudo-boolean probability functions $P(x_{ij}|I,\Theta)$ and $P(x_C|\Theta)$, we can formulate the MAP estimator to (1) as ILP:

$$\text{minimize} \quad \sum_{(i,j)\in E} w_{ij}x_{ij} + \sum_{C\in\mathcal{C}(G)} w_C x_C \tag{3}$$

$$\text{s.t.} \quad \mathbf{x} \in \Omega, \ [\mathbf{x},\mathbf{x}_C] \in \Omega_A, \ x \in \{0,1\} , \tag{4}$$

where $w_{ij} = -\log\frac{P(x_{ij}=1|I,\Theta)}{1-P(x_{ij}=1|I,\Theta)}$ and $w_C = -\log\frac{P(x_C=1|\Theta)}{1-P(x_C=1|\Theta)}$. The constraint $\mathbf{x} \in \Omega$ is due to $P(\Omega|\mathbf{x})$ and $[\mathbf{x},\mathbf{x}_C] \in \Omega_A$ ties auxiliary variables for the events to the edge variables $\mathbf{x}$. Finally, all variables are binary. This ILP can be optimized with the branch-and-cut algorithm. Certain types of constraints contained in Ω may consist of an extensive number of inequalities (e.g. the cycle free constraint). In this case, we employ a lazy constraint generation strategy: Whenever the solver arrives at an integral solution $\mathbf{x}'$, we check for violated constraints in the corresponding solution, add them if required and reject $\mathbf{x}'$. If no violation is found, i.e. $\mathbf{x}'$ is already a feasible solution, then it is accepted as new current solution $\mathbf{x}^*$. For our set of constraints Ω, we use this scheme for the cycle constraints, where we identify strongly connected components efficiently with [21] and add the violated constraints for the cycles within them. All other constraints for incoming and outgoing edges, as well as auxiliaries can be added to the optimization model from the start.

3 Uncertainty Estimation by Means of Sampling

3.1 Perturbation Sampler

Following the work of [12,14,15], a perturbation model is induced by perturbing the energy function of a random field and solving for its (perturbed) MAP state:

$$P(\hat{\mathbf{x}}|I,\Theta) = P_\gamma(\hat{\mathbf{x}} \in \underset{\mathbf{x}\in\Omega}{\arg\min} E(\mathbf{x};I,\Theta) + \gamma(\mathbf{x})), \tag{5}$$

where $E(\mathbf{x},I,\Theta)$ is the energy function of the random field and $\gamma(\mathbf{x})$ is the perturbation. It was shown that if the full potential table is perturbed with IID Gumbel-distributed samples of zero mean, then the perturbation model and the Gibbs model coincide [12]. In practice, this is not feasible. The full potential table may be too large and it destroys local Markov structure, rendering optimization difficult. However, it was shown in several studies that even first order Gumbel perturbations yield sufficiently good approximations [12,15]. In this case, only the unary potentials are perturbed and hence, the perturbation $\gamma(\mathbf{x})$ becomes:

$$\gamma(\mathbf{x}) = \sum_{i=1}^{N}\sum_{l\in\mathcal{L}} \gamma_i^l \mathbb{1}(x_i = l), \tag{6}$$

with γ_i^k being IID samples from the Gumbel distribution [22] with zero mean and variance $\frac{\pi^2}{6}$, and $\mathbb{1}(.)$ is the indicator function. Sampling from the perturbation model then boils down to drawing a new perturbation $\gamma(\mathbf{x})$ and determining the new MAP state. Having a procedure to sample efficiently from the model enables us to estimate marginal distributions of variables (and variable subsets) as well as derived measures of uncertainty. We refer the interested reader to [12–16] for further information on perturbation models.

We next derive the first-order perturbed objective for the MAP estimator in (3). First, we note that two states will need two independent gumbel samples $\gamma_{ij}^1, \gamma_{ij}^0$ according to (6). Our MAP estimator, however, uses only one binary variable to encode both states. We use again the bilinear representation of the pseudo-boolean functions to find that perturbing the unaries adds a difference of the two independent gumbel samples, i.e. $\Delta\gamma_{ij} = (\gamma_{ij}^1 - \gamma_{ij}^0)$, to the original weight w_{ij}. The first-order perturbed objective of (3) is thus:

$$\sum_{(i,j)\in E} (w_{ij} + \Delta\gamma_{ij})x_{ij} + \sum_{C\in\mathcal{C}(G)} w_C x_C. \tag{7}$$

Drawing a sample from our probabilistic model therefore boils down to constructing a new perturbed objective (with a new set of $\Delta\gamma_{ij}$) and optimizing the according ILP with the original constraints (4) and (7) instead of (3). This can be implemented by changing the coefficients of the optimization problem for each new perturbation. We note that we can warm-start the optimization with the previous solution and that we can keep previously generated constraints since they are not depending on the weights but only on the structure of G and thus, remain valid.

3.2 Gibbs Sampler

As alternative to the perturbation sampling, we employ a Gibbs sampler [10], a method of the MCMC family. We apply the following two modifications described in [20] to obtain a *metropolized* variant of the Gibbs sampler, which is expected to be more efficient for discrete problems. (1) variables are sampled in random-scan fashion within each sweep, and (2) the acceptance probability is replaced with the Metropolis-Hastings acceptance probability

$$\alpha = \min\left(1, \frac{1 - \pi(x_e|\mathbf{x}_{\backslash e})}{1 - \pi(x'_e|\mathbf{x}_{\backslash e})}\right), \tag{8}$$

where $\pi(x_e|\mathbf{x}_{\backslash e})$ and $\pi(x'_e|\mathbf{x}_{\backslash e})$ are the conditional probabilities of current and proposed state. To cope with the extra constraints of Ω, we can employ the same procedures to identify violated constraints as within the branch-and-cut algorithm. In this case, however, it suffices to check only those constraints which involve the changed variable(s). Changes that render the state infeasible with respect to Ω have a zero probability and will thus always be rejected. Auxiliary variables x_C for higher-level events need not to be sampled but can be determined directly from the current state $\mathbf{x}$ using the relationship encoded by the auxiliary constraints Ω_A. After a burn-in period of 1000 sweeps, we run one sweep for each sample.

4 Experiments and Results

We conduct our experiments on retinal images [23]. In the first part of this section, we detail on the preprocessing, i.e. the candidate vessel graph construction. In the second part, we then present both quantitative and qualitative results of the two sampling approaches. We address the difficulty of validating marginal distribution estimates by computing exact marginals on smaller problem instances, where brute-force enumeration of all states is computationally possible.

Candidate Graph Construction. As a first step, we need to propose vasculature in terms of an overcomplete candidate graph $G = (V, E)$. We rely on the following scheme to achieve this, which is mainly based on [2,3,24]:

1. *Centerline detection.* We compute a centerline score $f_{cl}(I)$ for the entire image using a regression approach based on [24]. High centerline scores indicate the presence of the centerline of the vessel.
2. *Candidate node selection.* We construct a collection of candidate nodes V by iteratively selecting the locations with the highest value in the centerline measure map and suppressing its neighbourhood within a radius r_{sup} until no more locations with a value larger than θ_T are left.
3. *Connection of candidates.* Next, we reconnect previously selected candidate nodes to its N closest neighbours using Dijkstra's algorithm on the centerline score map. A connection between two nodes $i, j \in V$ then forms an edge $(i, j) \in E$ in the vessel candidate graph. Connections that pass through a third candidate node are discarded as they would introduce unnecessary redundance. To save computation time, we limit the maximum search radius to r_s.

In these experiments, we set $r_{sup} = 5\,\mathrm{px}$ and $\theta_T = 0.3 \max f_{cl}(I)$ for the candidate selection, and $N = 4$ and $r_s = 30\,\mathrm{px}$ for the edge construction. We use a discriminative path classifier to estimate $P(x_{ij} = 1|I)$, i.e. how likely edge $ij \in E$ belongs to the graph or not, which is then used to calculate the weights w_{ij}. To this end, we use gradient boosted decision trees with 5 features calculated along the path: length, tortuosity, cumulative f_{cl}, min f_{cl} and standard deviation of f_{cl}. Additional details on both centerline regressor and path classifier can be found in the supplement. For each class of events, appearance, termination and bifurcation, we introduce one parameter θ^a, θ^t and θ^b as constant weight for the respective event happening at a given node, and set them to $\theta^a = 0.5$, $\theta^t = 0.1$ and $\theta^b = 0.1$.

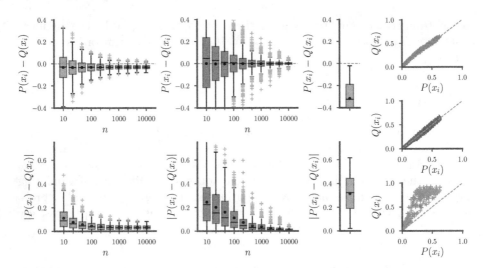

Fig. 2. Comparison of the approximated marginals $Q(x_i)$ with the exact marginals $P(x_i)$ calculated by brute force enumeration of all states. Approximates are obtained from the perturbation sampler (**blue**), from the Gibbs sampler (**red**), and from the raw classifier probability (**orange**). The figure shows deviation $P(x_i) - Q(x_i)$ (**top row**) and absolute deviation $|P(x_i) - Q(x_i)|$ (**bottom row**) of the marginal estimate with increasing number of samples n. Boxplots denote the median with a black bar, the mean value with a black dot and outliers with a grey cross. **Right column:** Scatter plot of exact marginal probabilities $P(x_i)$ versus approximated marginal probabilities $Q(x_i)$. We observe that the perturbation sampler converges to an absolute bias of about 0.032 on average and has the tendency to overestimate the marginal probabilites slightly. The Gibbs sampler does not exhibit such a systematic bias, but needs more samples to reduce its variance. Using the probabilistic output of the local classifier as an approximate to the marginals is considerably less accurate than both sampling approaches. (Color figure online)

Comparison. In order to quantitatively validate the marginals that we approximate by using the perturbation sampler, we set up a series of 15 small test graphs with $|E| \leq 20$ from the test images of [23], such that we are able to enumerate all feasible states and thereby obtain exact marginals by brute force. We then compare these exact marginals to the approximate marginals obtained by both perturbation and Gibbs sampler. We solve the ILP of our MAP estimator by the branch-and-cut algorithm of [25] and implement the lazy constraint generation as callback. We use the default relative optimality gap of 10^{-4}.

In Fig. 2, we compare the approximated marginals from our perturbation sampler with exact marginals. We sample 10000 samples per case in total and repeat the experiment 5 times. We observe that the absolute deviation of the approximated from the exact marginals converges already at about 1000 samples to an absolute error of $|P(x_i) - Q(x_i)| \approx 0.032$ on average and the perturbation sampler shows a tendency to overestimate the marginal probabilities. Such a systematic bias is to be expected, as we apply a low-order perturbation instead

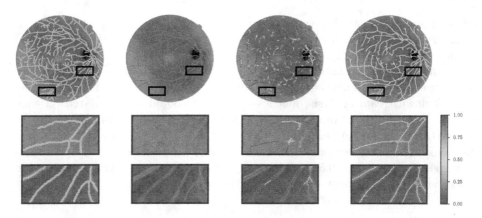

Fig. 3. Visualisation of the vascular network graphs overlaid on the (grey-scale) input image. **From left to right:** Pixel-based centerline obtained by skeletonizing the ground truth segmentation, MAP reconstruction, approximated marginals using the perturbation sampler, and the Gibbs sampler. The colorbar applies only to the marginals of two right columns, where we show the marginal $P(x_{ij} = 1 \vee x_{ji} = 1)$, i.e. the probability of either edge being active, for better visibility. We find that the marginals of the perturbation sampler indicate uncertainty in small bifurcations and point out the (possible) presence of weak terminal branches, which would be discarded if we only consider the MAP solution. The Gibbs sampler displays overall a higher uncertainty on such large graphs.

of the (intractable) full perturbation. The Gibbs sampler does not exhibit such systematic bias, yet shows a larger variance when fewer samples are aquired. With 10000 samples, its mean absolute approximation error is 0.012 and therefore better than the perturbation sampler. Wilcoxon signed-rank tests for each fixed number of samples n indicate that the approximation errors of perturbation and Gibbs sampler are significantly different ($p < 0.001$), with the exception of $n = 1000$ where both show similar errors. Using the probabilities of the path classifier directly as an approximate marginal is considerably worse than both sampling approaches. Note that the exact marginals for our test cases do not exhibit very high values (cf. Fig. 2, right column) due to the fact that for these small graphs, often no direction is strongly dominating and thus, several solutions that contain similar physical paths but in different orientations are competing.

A qualitative visualisation of the approximated marginals on complete graphs is given in Fig. 3. We draw 100 perturbation samples, which we found a reasonable trade-off between computation time and informativeness of the marginals, and slightly increase the relative optimality gap to $5 \cdot 10^{-3}$ to prevent the branch-and-cut solver from spending too much time proofing optimality. From the Gibbs sampler, we draw 10000 samples after a burn-in period of 1000. We find that the marginals from the Gibbs sampler display overall a higher uncertainty in the graph than the perturbation samples, which could be due to more difficult transitions between different modi of the distribution and would likely require adapted sampling parametrization or even an extension of the set of allowed transformations. In both cases, thresholding the marginal distributions $P(x_e)$ has no guarantee to satisfy all constraints and is therefore not recommended for obtaining a single reconstruction. To improve a reconstruction, an interactive procedure using the uncertainties (and individual samples) would be advisable, and for downstream analysis, metrics of interest should be calculated on each sample. Regarding computation time, the average runtime per sample is 7.85 s for the perturbation and approximately 0.01 s for the Gibbs sampler (not including any additional overhead caused by the burn in period). The perturbation sampler spends on average 0.5 % of its runtime in the lazy constraint generation where violated cycle inequalities are identified.

5   Conclusion

We adapted two sampling approaches for vascular network graph reconstruction models, a perturbation sampler and a Gibbs sampler. Our experiments confirm the expected systematic bias of the perturbation sampler due to the computationally cheaper low-order perturbations. The Gibbs sampler, on the other hand, exhibits an unbiased behaviour but instances with varying properties might require an appropriately adapted parametrization. The perturbation approach benefits from not having a burn in period, which renders it considerably easier to use on large instances. Both approaches were shown to be more informative than the predictive probabilities of local classifier and can be used to approximate marginals or determine the uncertainty in network graph properties. Beyond this, the two sampling procedures could be employed within a Bayesian model selection framework or for maximum-likelihood hyperparameter estimation.

Acknowledgements. With the support of the Technische Universität München – Institute for Advanced Study, funded by the German Excellence Initiative (and the European Union Seventh Framework Programme under grant agreement n° 291763).

References

1. Lesage, D., Angelini, E., Bloch, I., Funka-Lea, G.: A review of 3D vessel lumen segmentation techniques: Models, features and extraction schemes. Med. Image Anal. **13**(6), 819–845 (2009)
2. Türetken, E., Benmansour, F., Andres, B., Glowacki, P., Pfister, H., Fua, P.: Reconstructing curvilinear networks using path classifiers and integer programming. IEEE Trans. Pattern Anal. Mach. Intell. **38**(12), 2515–2530 (2016)
3. Rempfler, M., Schneider, M., Ielacqua, G.D., Xiao, X., Stock, S.R., Klohs, J., Székely, G., Andres, B., Menze, B.H.: Reconstructing cerebrovascular networks under local physiological constraints by integer programming. Med. Image Anal. **25**(1), 86–94 (2015)

4. Rempfler, M., Andres, B., Menze, B.H.: The minimum cost connected subgraph problem in medical image analysis. In: Ourselin, S., Joskowicz, L., Sabuncu, M.R., Unal, G., Wells, W. (eds.) MICCAI 2016. LNCS, vol. 9902, pp. 397–405. Springer, Cham (2016). doi:10.1007/978-3-319-46726-9_46

5. Payer, C., Pienn, M., Bálint, Z., Shekhovtsov, A., Talakic, E., Nagy, E., Olschewski, A., Olschewski, H., Urschler, M.: Automated integer programming based separation of arteries and veins from thoracic CT images. Med. Image Anal. **34**, 109–122 (2016)

6. Robben, D., Türetken, E., Sunaert, S., Thijs, V., Wilms, G., Fua, P., Maes, F., Suetens, P.: Simultaneous segmentation and anatomical labeling of the cerebral vasculature. Med. Image Anal. **32**, 201–215 (2016)

7. Klohs, J., Baltes, C., Princz-Kranz, F., Ratering, D., Nitsch, R.M., Knuesel, I., Rudin, M.: Contrast-enhanced magnetic resonance microangiography reveals remodeling of the cerebral microvasculature in transgenic arcaβ mice. J. Neurosci. **32**(5), 1705–1713 (2012)

8. Batra, D., Yadollahpour, P., Guzman-Rivera, A., Shakhnarovich, G.: Diverse M-best solutions in markov random fields. In: Fitzgibbon, A., Lazebnik, S., Perona, P., Sato, Y., Schmid, C. (eds.) ECCV 2012. LNCS, vol. 7576, pp. 1–16. Springer, Heidelberg (2012). doi:10.1007/978-3-642-33715-4_1

9. Kirillov, A., Savchynskyy, B., Schlesinger, D., Vetrov, D., Rother, C.: Inferring M-best diverse labelings in a single one. In: IEEE International Conference on Computer Vision (ICCV), pp. 1814–1822 (2015)

10. Geman, S., Geman, D.: Stochastic relaxation, Gibbs distributions, and the bayesian restoration of images. IEEE Trans. Pattern Anal. Mach. Intell. PAMI **6**(6), 721–741 (1984)

11. Koller, D., Friedman, N.: Probabilistic Graphical Models: Principles and Techniques. MIT press (2009)

12. Papandreou, G., Yuille, A.L.: Perturb-and-MAP random fields: using discrete optimization to learn and sample from energy models. In: International Conference on Computer Vision 2011, pp. 193–200 (2011)

13. Tarlow, D., Adams, R.P., Zemel, R.S.: Randomized optimum models for structured prediction. In: Proceedings of the Fifteenth International Conference on Artificial Intelligence and Statistics, vol. 22, pp. 1221–1229 (2012)

14. Hazan, T., Jaakkola, T.: On the partition function and random maximum a-posteriori perturbations. In: Proceedings of the 29th International Conference on Machine Learning (ICML-12), pp. 991–998 (2012)

15. Hazan, T., Maji, S., Jaakkola, T.: On sampling from the gibbs distribution with random maximum a-posteriori perturbations. In: Advances in Neural Information Processing Systems, pp. 1268–1276 (2013)

16. Orabona, F., Hazan, T., Sarwate, A., Jaakkola, T.: On measure concentration of random maximum a-posteriori perturbations. In: International Conference on Machine Learning, pp. 432–440 (2014)

17. Gane, A., Hazan, T., Jaakkola, T.: Learning with maximum a-posteriori perturbation models. In: Artificial Intelligence and Statistics, pp. 247–256 (2014)

18. Alberts, E., Rempfler, M., Alber, G., Huber, T., Kirschke, J., Zimmer, C., Menze, B.H.: Uncertainty quantification in brain tumor segmentation using CRFs and random perturbation models. In: 2016 IEEE 13th International Symposium on Biomedical Imaging (ISBI), pp. 428–431 (2016)

19. Meier, R., Knecht, U., Jungo, A., Wiest, R., Reyes, M.: Perturb-and-MPM: quantifying segmentation uncertainty in dense multi-label CRFs. CoRR abs/1703.00312 (2017). http://arxiv.org/abs/1703.00312

20. Liu, J.S.: Monte Carlo Strategies in Scientific Computing. Springer, New York (2001)
21. Mehlhorn, K., Näher, S., Sanders, P.: Engineering DFS-based graph algorithms. CoRR abs/1703.10023 (2017). http://arxiv.org/abs/1703.10023
22. Gumbel, E.J.: Statistical theory of extreme values and some practical applications: a series of lectures. No. 33, US Govt. Print. Office (1954)
23. Staal, J.J., Abramoff, M.D., Niemeijer, M., Viergever, M.A., Van Ginneken, B.: Ridge based vessel segmentation in color images of the retina. IEEE Trans. Med. Imaging **23**(4), 501–509 (2004)
24. Sironi, A., Türetken, E., Lepetit, V., Fua, P.: Multiscale centerline detection. IEEE Trans. Pattern Anal. Mach. Intell. **1**, 1–14 (2015)
25. Gurobi Optimization, Inc.: Gurobi Optimizer Reference Manual (2017). http://www.gurobi.com

Extraction of Airways with Probabilistic State-Space Models and Bayesian Smoothing

Raghavendra Selvan[1]([✉]), Jens Petersen[1], Jesper H. Pedersen[2], and Marleen de Bruijne[1,3]

[1] Department of Computer Science,
University of Copenhagen, Copenhagen, Denmark
`raghav@di.ku.dk`
[2] Department of Cardio-Thoracic Surgery RT, Rigshospitalet,
University Hospital of Copenhagen, Copenhagen, Denmark
[3] Departments of Medical Informatics and Radiology, Erasmus MC,
Rotterdam, The Netherlands

Abstract. Segmenting tree structures is common in several image processing applications. In medical image analysis, reliable segmentations of airways, vessels, neurons and other tree structures can enable important clinical applications. We present a framework for tracking tree structures comprising of elongated branches using probabilistic state-space models and Bayesian smoothing. Unlike most existing methods that proceed with sequential tracking of branches, we present an exploratory method, that is less sensitive to local anomalies in the data due to acquisition noise and/or interfering structures. The evolution of individual branches is modelled using a process model and the observed data is incorporated into the update step of the Bayesian smoother using a measurement model that is based on a multi-scale blob detector. Bayesian smoothing is performed using the RTS (Rauch-Tung-Striebel) smoother, which provides Gaussian density estimates of branch states at each tracking step. We select likely branch seed points automatically based on the response of the blob detection and track from all such seed points using the RTS smoother. We use covariance of the marginal posterior density estimated for each branch to discriminate false positive and true positive branches. The method is evaluated on 3D chest CT scans to track airways. We show that the presented method results in additional branches compared to a baseline method based on region growing on probability images

Keywords: Probabilistic state-space · Bayesian smoothing · Tree segmentation · Airways · CT

1 Introduction

Segmentation of tree structures comprising of vessels, neurons, airways etc. are useful in extraction of clinically relevant biomarkers [1,2]. The task of extracting

© Springer International Publishing AG 2017
M.J. Cardoso et al. (Eds.): GRAIL/MFCA/MICGen 2017, LNCS 10551, pp. 53–63, 2017.
DOI: 10.1007/978-3-319-67675-3_6

trees, mainly in relation to vessel segmentation, has been studied widely using different methods. A successful class of these methods are based on techniques from target tracking. Perhaps the most used tracking strategy is to proceed from an initial seed point, make local-model fits to track individual branches in a sequential manner and perform regular branching checks [3,4]. Such methods are prone to local anomalies and can prematurely terminate if occlusions are encountered. The method in [3] can overcome such problems to a certain extent using a deterministic multiple hypothesis testing approach; however, it is a semi-automatic method requiring extensive manual intervention and can be computationally expensive. In [4], vessel tracking on 2D retinal scans is performed using a Kalman filter. They propose an automatic seed point detection strategy using a matched filter. From each of these seed points vessel branches are progressively tracked using measurements that are derived from the image data. A gradient based measurement function is employed which fails in low-contrast regions of the image, which are predominantly regions with thin vessels. Another major class of tracking algorithms are based on a stochastic formulation of tracking [5,6] using some variation of particle filtering. Particle filter-based methods are known to scale poorly with dimensions of the state space [1].

In spirit, we propose an exploratory method like particle filter-based methods, with a salient distinction that the proposed method can track branches from several seed points across the volume. We use linear Bayesian smoothing to estimate branch states, described using Gaussian densities. Thus, the method inherently provides an uncertainty measure, which we use to discriminate true and false positive branches. Further, unlike particle filter-based methods, the proposed method is fast, as Bayesian smoothing is implemented using the RTS (Rauch-Tung-Striebel) smoother [7] involving only a set of linear equations.

2   Method

We formulate tracking of branches in tree structures using probabilistic state-space models, commonly used in target tracking and control theory [7]. The proposed method takes image data as input and outputs a collection of disconnected branches that taken together forms the tree structure of interest. We first process the image data to obtain a sequence of measurements and track all possible branches individually using Bayesian smoothing. We then use covariance estimates of individual branches to output a subset of the most likely branches yielding the tree structure of interest. Details of this process are described below.

2.1   Tracking Individual Branches

We assume the tree structure of interest, $\mathbf{X}$, to be a collection of T independent random variables $\mathbf{X} = \{\mathbf{X}_1, \mathbf{X}_2, \ldots, \mathbf{X}_T\}$, where individual branches are denoted $\mathbf{X}_i$. Each branch $\mathbf{X}_i$ of length L_i is treated as a sequence of states, $\mathbf{X}_i = [\mathbf{x}_0, \mathbf{x}_1, \ldots, \mathbf{x}_{L_i}]$. These states are assumed to obey a first-order Markov assumption, i.e.,

$$p(\mathbf{x}_k|\mathbf{x}_{k-1}, \mathbf{x}_{k-2}, \ldots, \mathbf{x}_0) = p(\mathbf{x}_k|\mathbf{x}_{k-1}). \tag{1}$$

The state vector has seven random variables,

$$\mathbf{x}_k = [x, y, z, r, v_x, v_y, v_z]^T, \tag{2}$$

describing a tubular segment centered at Euclidean coordinates $[x, y, z]$, along an axis given by the direction vector $[v_x, v_y, v_z]$ with radius r.

The observed data, image $\mathbf{I}$, is processed to be available as a sequence of vectors. We model the measurements as four dimensional state vectors consisting only of position and radius. This is accomplished using a multi-scale blob detector [8]. The input image $\mathbf{I}$ with N_v voxels is transformed into a sequence of N measurements, with position and radius information, denoted $\mathbf{Y} = [\mathbf{y}_0, \ldots, \mathbf{y}_N]$, where each $\mathbf{y}_i = [x, y, z, r]^T$. This procedure applied to the application of tracking airway trees is described in Sect. 2.5.

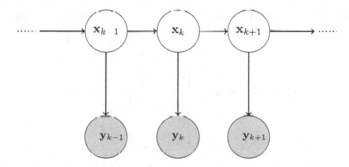

Fig. 1. Bayesian network view of the relation between the underlying true states, $\mathbf{x}_i$, and the measurements, $\mathbf{y}_i$, for a single branch.

2.2 Process and Measurement Models

Transition from one tracking step to another within a branch is modelled using the process model. We use a process model that captures our understanding of how individual branches evolve between tracking steps and has similarities with the model used in [4]. We assume first-order Markov independence in state transitions from (1), captured in the process model below:

$$\mathbf{x}_k = \mathbf{F}\mathbf{x}_{k-1} + \mathbf{q} = \begin{bmatrix} 1 & 0 & 0 & 0 & \Delta & 0 & 0 \\ 0 & 1 & 0 & 0 & 0 & \Delta & 0 \\ 0 & 0 & 1 & 0 & 0 & 0 & \Delta \\ 0 & 0 & 0 & 1 & 0 & 0 & 0 \\ 0 & 0 & 0 & 0 & 1 & 0 & 0 \\ 0 & 0 & 0 & 0 & 0 & 1 & 0 \\ 0 & 0 & 0 & 0 & 0 & 0 & 1 \end{bmatrix} \begin{bmatrix} x_{k-1} \\ y_{k-1} \\ z_{k-1} \\ r_{k-1} \\ v_{x\,k-1} \\ v_{y\,k-1} \\ v_{z\,k-1} \end{bmatrix} + \mathbf{q} \tag{3}$$

where $\mathbf{F}$ is the process model function and $\mathbf{q}$ is the process noise. $\mathbf{q}$ is assumed to be a zero mean Gaussian density, i.e., $\mathbf{q} \sim N(\mathbf{0}, \mathbf{Q})$, with process covariance, $\mathbf{Q}_{7\times7}$, acting only on direction and radius components of the state vector,

$$\mathbf{Q}_{[4:7,4:7]} = \sigma_q^2 \Delta \times \mathbf{I}_{4\times4}, \tag{4}$$

where only the non-zero part of the matrix is shown and σ_q^2 is the process variance. The parameter Δ can be seen as step size between tracking steps. As (3) is a recursion, the initial point (seed point), $\mathbf{x}_0$, comprising of position, scale and orientation information is provided to the model. Seed points are assumed to be described by Gaussian densities, $\mathbf{x}_0 \sim N(\hat{\mathbf{x}}_0, \mathbf{P}_0)$, with mean $\hat{\mathbf{x}}_0$ and covariance $\mathbf{P}_0$. We present an automatic strategy to detect such initial seed points in Sect. 2.5.

The measurement model describes the relation between each of the 4-D measurements, $\mathbf{y}_k$ in the sequence, $\mathbf{Y} = [\mathbf{y}_1, \ldots, \mathbf{y}_N]$, and the state vector, $\mathbf{x}_k$, as shown in Fig. 1. A simple linear measurement model captures this relation,

$$\mathbf{y}_k = \mathbf{H}\mathbf{x}_k + \mathbf{m} = \begin{bmatrix} 1 & 0 & 0 & 0 \\ 0 & 1 & 0 & 0 \\ 0 & 0 & 1 & 0 \\ 0 & 0 & 0 & 1 \\ 0 & 0 & 0 & 0 \\ 0 & 0 & 0 & 0 \\ 0 & 0 & 0 & 0 \end{bmatrix} \begin{bmatrix} x_k \\ y_k \\ z_k \\ r_k \\ v_{x_k} \\ v_{y_k} \\ v_{z_k} \end{bmatrix} + \mathbf{m} \tag{5}$$

where $\mathbf{y}_k$ are observations generated by true states of the underlying branch at step k, $\mathbf{H}$ is the measurement function. $\mathbf{m} \sim N(\mathbf{0}, \mathbf{R})$ is the measurement noise with covariance $\mathbf{R}$ that is a diagonal matrix with entries, $[\sigma_{m_x}^2, \sigma_{m_y}^2, \sigma_{m_z}^2, \sigma_{m_r}^2]$, which correspond to variance in the observed position and radius, respectively. All possible measurement vectors obtained from the image are aggregated into the measurement variable $\mathbf{Y}$.

2.3 Bayesian Smoothing

The state-space models presented above enable us to estimate branches using the posterior distributions, $p(\mathbf{X}_i|\mathbf{Y})\forall i = [0, \ldots, T]$, using standard Bayesian methods. We employ Bayesian smoothing as all the measurements are available at once, when compared to sequential observations that are more common in object tracking applications. Due to a linear, Gaussian process and measurement models, Bayesian smoothing can be optimally performed using the RTS smoother [7]. RTS smoother uses two Bayesian filters to perform forward filtering and backward smoothing. Forward filtering is identical to performing Kalman filtering and consists of sequential prediction and update with observed information of the state variable. Once a branch is estimated using forward filtering, the saved states are used to perform backward smoothing using a Kalman-like filter which improves state estimates by incorporating additional information from future steps. Standard equations for an RTS smoother are presented below [7].

Table 1. Standard RTS smoother equations

Forward Filtering		Backward Smoothing	
$\hat{\mathbf{x}}_{k\|k-1} = \mathbf{F}\hat{\mathbf{x}}_{k-1\|k-1}$	(6)		
$\mathbf{P}_{k\|k-1} = \mathbf{F}\mathbf{P}_{k-1\|k-1}\mathbf{F}^T + \mathbf{Q}$	(7)	$\mathbf{G}_k = \mathbf{P}_{k\|k}\mathbf{F}^T\mathbf{P}_{k+1\|k}^{-1}$	(13)
$\mathbf{v}_k = \mathbf{y}_k - \mathbf{H}\hat{\mathbf{x}}_{k\|k-1}$	(8)	$\hat{\mathbf{x}}_{k\|L} = \hat{\mathbf{x}}_{k\|k} + \mathbf{G}_k(\hat{\mathbf{x}}_{k+1\|L} - \hat{\mathbf{x}}_{k+1\|k})$	
$\mathbf{S}_k = \mathbf{H}\mathbf{P}_{k\|k-1}\mathbf{H}^T + \mathbf{R}$	(9)		(14)
$\mathbf{K}_k = \mathbf{P}_{k\|k-1}\mathbf{H}^T\mathbf{S}_k^{-1}$	(10)	$\mathbf{P}_{k\|L} = \mathbf{P}_{k\|k} - \mathbf{G}_k(\mathbf{P}_{k+1\|k} - \mathbf{P}_{k+1\|L})\mathbf{G}^T$	
$\hat{\mathbf{x}}_{k\|k} = \hat{\mathbf{x}}_{k\|k-1} + \mathbf{K}_k\mathbf{v}_k$	(11)		(15)
$\mathbf{P}_{k\|k} = \mathbf{P}_{k\|k-1} - \mathbf{K}_k\mathbf{S}_k\mathbf{K}_k^T$	(12)		

Forward Filtering. Equations in the first column of Table 1 are used to perform prediction and update steps of the forward filtering. In the prediction step, process model is used to predict states at the next step. Mean $\hat{\mathbf{x}}_{k|k-1}$ and covariance $\mathbf{P}_{k|k-1}$ estimates of the predicted Gaussian density, i.e., of state k conditioned on the previous state, denoted with subscript $k|k-1$, are computed in (6) and (7). In the update step, described in (8)–(12), predicted density is associated with a measurement vector to obtain posterior density. First, the new information from measurement $\mathbf{y}_k$ is computed using (8) and is aptly called the "innovation", denoted as $\mathbf{v}_k$. Uncertainty in the new information, innovation covariance $\mathbf{S}_k$, is computed in (9). Then, predicted mean is adjusted with weighted innovation and predicted covariance is adjusted with weighted innovation covariance to obtain the posterior mean and covariances, in (11) and (12), respectively. The weighting computed in (10), denoted as $\mathbf{K}_k$, is the Kalman gain which controls the extent of information fusion from process and measurement models.

We continue estimation of the posterior density (described by posterior mean and covariance) in a sequential manner for the branch until no new measurements exist for updating. After the final update step, a sequence of posterior mean estimates $[\hat{\mathbf{x}}_{0|0}, \ldots, \hat{\mathbf{x}}_{L_i|L_i}]$ and posterior covariance estimates $[\mathbf{P}_{0|0}, \ldots, \mathbf{P}_{L_i|L_i}]$, obtained from the forward filter are saved, for further use by the backward smoother.

Backward Smoothing. The smoothed estimates are obtained by running a backward filter starting from the final tracked state of the forward filter. The intuition behind backward smoothing is that the uncertainty in making predictions in the forward filtering can be alleviated using information from future steps. It is implemented using the equations in the second column of Table 1.

Gating. When performing the RTS smoother recursions, the forward filter expects a single measurement vector for the update step. We employ rectangular and ellipsoidal gating to reduce the number of measurements handled during the update step [9].

First, we perform simple rectangular gating which is based on excluding measurements that are outside a rectangular region around the predicted measurement $\mathbf{H}\hat{\mathbf{x}}_{k|k-1}$ in Eq. (8) using the following condition:

$$|\mathbf{y}_i - \mathbf{H}\mathbf{x}_{k|k-1}| \leq \kappa \times \mathrm{diag}(\mathbf{S}_k), \forall \mathbf{y}_i \in \mathbf{Y} \tag{6}$$

where $\mathbf{S}_k$ is the covariance of the predicted measurement in Eq. (9). The rectangular gating coefficient, κ, is usually set to a value ≥ 3 [9]. Rectangular gating localises the number of candidate measurements relevant to the current tracking step. To further narrow down on the best candidate measurement for update, we follow rectangular gating with ellipsoidal gating [9]. With ellipsoidal gating we accept the measurements within the ellipsoidal region of the predicated covariance, using the following rule:

$$(\mathbf{H}\mathbf{x}_{k|k-1} - \mathbf{y}_i)^T \mathbf{S}_k^{-1}(\mathbf{H}\mathbf{x}_{k|k-1} - \mathbf{y}_i) \leq G \tag{7}$$

where G is the rectangular gating threshold, obtained from the gating probability P_g, which is the probability of observing the measurement within the ellipsoidal gate,

$$P_g = 1 - \exp\left(-\frac{G}{2}\right). \tag{8}$$

2.4   Tree as a Collection of Branches

Once a branch is smoothed and saved using Bayesian smoothing described previously, we process new seed points and start tracking branches until no further seed points remain to track from. This procedure yields a collection of disconnected branches. The next task is to obtain a subset of likely branches that represent the tree structure of interest by discarding false positive branches.

Validation of Tracked Branches. An advantage of using Bayesian smoothing to track individual branches is that apart from estimating the branch states from the image data (using the smoothed posterior mean estimates), we can also quantify the uncertainty of the estimation at each tracking step (using the smoothed posterior covariance estimates). Thus, we have the possibility of aggregating this uncertainty over the entire branch to validate them. We explore this notion to create a criterion for accepting or rejecting branches.

By aggregating variance for all tracking steps in each branch, we obtain a measure of the quality of branches. A straightforward approach is to use total variance, obtained using the trace of each of the smoothed posterior covariance matrices. We average the sum total variance over the length of each branch, l_i, to obtain a score, μ_i, which is then thresholded by a cut-off μ_c to qualify the branches,

$$\mu_i = \frac{\sum_{k=1}^{l_i} \mathrm{Tr}(\mathbf{P}_{k|k})}{l_i}. \tag{9}$$

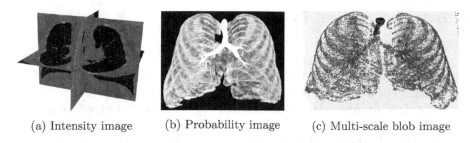

(a) Intensity image   (b) Probability image   (c) Multi-scale blob image

Fig. 2. The pipeline of image representations, ultimately showing the multi-scale representation.

2.5 Application to Airways

The proposed method for tracking tree structures can be applied to track airways, vessels or other tree structures encountered in image processing applications. We focus on tracking airways from lung CT data and present the specific strategies used to implement the proposed method.

Multi-scale Representation. The measurement model discussed in Sect. 2.2 assumes a 4-D state vector as measurements to the RTS smoother. This is achieved by first computing an airway probability image using a k-Nearest Neighbour voxel classifier trained to discriminate between airway and background, described in [11]. Blob detection with automatic scale selection [8] for different scales, $\sigma_s = (1, 2, 4, 8, 12)$ mm, is performed on the probability image to obtain the 4D state measurements as blob position and radius. Indistinct blobs are removed if the absolute value of the normalized response at the selected scale, σ_s^*, is less than a threshold [8]. This makes the representation sparse, $N << N_v$, and the tracking more efficient than if performed at voxel-level. An example of the sparse representation can be found in Fig. 2.

Initialisation of Branches. The multi-scale representation of the image data discussed above also provides a response corresponding to the best scale. As this response is normalised for scales, we incorporate this information in selecting the initial seed point for every branch. We start tracking from the seed point with the largest scale and the largest response. The initial direction information is obtained from eigen value analysis of the Hessian matrix computed at the corresponding scale provided in the measurement vector. Once a branch is tracked along the initial direction, we track from the same seed point but in the opposite direction. Thus, if a seed point is obtained from the middle of a branch we can track it bidirectionally. After tracking in both directions, all the involved measurements including the seed point are removed from the measurement vector, and the next best candidate seed point is chosen and tracking commences from there. The tracking procedure on the entire image is complete when no more seed points are available.

3   Experiments and Results

3.1   Data

The evaluation was carried out on 32 low-dose CT chest scans from a lung cancer screening trial [10]. Training and test sets comprising of 16 images each were randomly obtained from the data set. All scans have a resolution of approximately $1\,\text{mm} \times 0.78\,\text{mm} \times 0.78\,\text{mm}$. The reference segmentations consist of expert verified union over the results of two previous methods [11,12]. The proposed method is compared with region growing on the probability images.

3.2   Error Measure, Initial Parameters and Tuning

We use an error measure defined as the average of two distances, $d_{err} = (d_{FP} + d_{FN})/2$. The first distance, d_{FP}, captures the false positive error and is the average minimum Euclidean distance from segmentation centerline points to reference centerline points. d_{FN} similarly defines the false negative error, as the average minimum Euclidean distance from reference centerlines points to segmentation centerline points.

There are several parameters related to the RTS smoother that need to be initialised. These parameters were tuned using the training set and fixed for the evaluation on the test set to: standard deviations of the process noise, $\sigma_q = 0.3$, measurement noise on radius $\sigma_{m_r} = 1\,\text{mm}$ and measurement noise on position $(\sigma_{m_x}, \sigma_{m_y}, \sigma_{m_z}) = 2\,\text{mm}$. The initial covariance, $\mathbf{P}_0$ across branches was set to $\mathbf{I}_{7\times7}$. The most crucial parameter in the proposed method is the threshold parameter μ_c presented in Sect. 2.4. The threshold to validate branches is tuned to be $\mu_c = 2.0$. The gating probability was set to a high value, $P_g = 0.99$ [9].

3.3   Results

Figure 3 illustrates features of the proposed method by visualising centerlines overlaid on the reference segmentation. Influence of the threshold parameter μ_c is illustrated with the segmentation results for a single volume without any threshold (seen in Fig. 3a) and after applying the tuned threshold (seen in Fig. 3b). Evidently, thresholding the average total variance of a branch eliminates false positive branches.

The final output obtained from the method is a collection of disconnected branches. While such collection of branches are still useful in extracting biomarkers, for evaluation purposes we merge the results obtained with the segmentations from region growing on probability images and extract centerlines from the merged segmentation using 3D thinning, as seen in Fig. 3a and b. This also allows us to demonstrate the improvement our method provides by extracting peripheral airway branches, which are typically the challenging ones. One such combined result is shown in Fig. 3c, where the yellow centerlines correspond to region growing and blue one is the combined result.

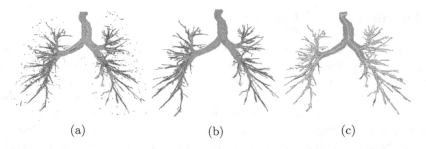

(a)   (b)   (c)

Fig. 3. Visualisation of the centerlines extracted using the proposed method before and after thresholding to discard false positive branches overlaid on the reference segmentation, shown in (a) and (b) respectively. The combined results from the proposed method and region growing on probability is shown as the blue centerline in (c).

Table 2. Performance comparison on the test set

Method	d_{FP} (mm)	d_{FN} (mm)	d_{err} (mm)	Std.Dev. (mm)
RG	0.423	3.579	2.001	0.208
(RTS+RG)$_1$	0.449	2.102	1.276	0.187
(RTS+RG)$_2$	0.401	2.658	1.529	0.165

Performance on the test set for two different scenarios of the proposed method is reported in Table 2 along with the numbers for region growing on probability images. The result for the best performing region growing on probability images is denoted with RG and those obtained by combining the proposed method with region growing are denoted as RTS+RG. We first combine the proposed method with the best performing region growing case (with minimum d_{err}) results and it is denoted as (RG+RTS)$_1$. We observe an improvement of about 36% on d_{err}. It is to be noted, there is substantial reduction in d_{FN}, indicating that many branches missed by region growing are now segmented. There is a very small increase in false positives which could also be due to the missing branches in the reference segmentation; however, the net result is a large improvement. To test whether the proposed method can simultaneously reduce the number of false positives and false negatives compared to region growing, we merge the proposed method with the region growing result that yields non-optimal d_{err}, and do observe a reduction in both d_{FP} and d_{FN} when compared to the best performing RG as seen in the entries for (RG+RTS)$_2$.

The computational expense for running the proposed method is small. The largest chunk of it is used in generating the multi-scale representation of the images, which is in the range of 10–15 s per volume. Tracking using the RTS smoother and obtaining the segmentation takes about 4 s on a laptop with 8 cores and 32 GB memory running Debian operating system.

4   Discussion and Conclusions

We presented an automatic method for tracking tree structures, in particular airways, using probabilistic state-space models and Bayesian smoothing. We demonstrated that branches can be tracked individually from across the volume, starting from several seed points. This approach of tracking branches from across the volume has the advantage that even in the presence of occlusions, such as mucous plugging or image acquisition noise, the chances of detecting branches beyond the occlusions are higher. An inherent measure of uncertainty in the branch estimates has been presented due to the Bayesian nature of the method. We demonstrated the use of thresholding this uncertainty measure to discriminate detected branches. The use of sparse representation of voxels in the image using blob detection makes the method computationally efficient.

A possible limitation with the proposed method is that it yields a disconnected tree structure. For applications where this is an issue, one can enforce a global connectivity constraint on the disconnected set of branches to obtain fully connected tree as done in [13] or similar. It is also possible to derive biomarkers directly from the disconnected branches, as shown in [14].

We performed an evaluation of the results obtained from the proposed method by combining it with the results from region growing on probability images. We showed that there is substantial improvement in the segmentation results, indicating that the exploratory approach taken up in our method has potential in improving tree segmentations.

Acknowledgements. This work was funded by the Independent Research Fund Denmark (DFF) and Netherlands Organisation for Scientific Research (NWO).

References

1. Lesage, D., et al.: A review of 3D vessel lumen segmentation techniques: Models, features and extraction schemes. Med. Image Anal. **13**(6), 819–45 (2009)
2. Lo, P., et al.: Extraction of airways from CT (EXACT'09). IEEE Trans. Med. Imaging **31**(11), 2093–107 (2012)
3. Friman, O., et al.: Multiple hypothesis template tracking of small 3D vessel structures. Med. Image Anal. **14**(2), 160–71 (2010)
4. Yedidya, T., et al.: Tracking of blood vessels in retinal images using Kalman filter. In: Computing: Techniques and Applications, Digital Image, pp. 52–58 (2008)
5. Florin, C., Paragios, N., Williams, J.: Particle filters, a quasi-monte carlo solution for segmentation of coronaries. In: Duncan, J.S., Gerig, G. (eds.) MICCAI 2005. LNCS, vol. 3749, pp. 246–253. Springer, Heidelberg (2005). doi:10.1007/11566465_31
6. Lesage, D., et al.: Adaptive particle filtering for coronary artery segmentation from 3D CT angiograms. Comput. Vis. Image Underst. **151**, 29–46 (2016)
7. Särkkä, S.: Bayesian Filtering and Smoothing. Cambridge University Press, New York (2013)
8. Lindeberg, T.: Feature detection with automatic scale selection. Int. J. Comput. Vis. **30**(2), 79–116 (1998)

9. Bar-Shalom, Y., Willett, P.K., Tian, X.: Tracking and Data Fusion. YBS publishing, Dedham (2011)
10. Pedersen, J.H., et al.: The Danish randomized lung cancer CT screening trial-overall design and results of the prevalence round. J. Thorac. Oncol. **4**, 608–614 (2009)
11. Lo, P., et al.: Vessel-guided airway segmentation based on voxel classification. In: First International Workshop on Pulmonary Image Analysis, MICCAI (2008)
12. Lo, P., Sporring, J., Pedersen, J.J.H., Bruijne, M.: Airway tree extraction with locally optimal paths. In: Yang, G.-Z., Hawkes, D., Rueckert, D., Noble, A., Taylor, C. (eds.) MICCAI 2009. LNCS, vol. 5762, pp. 51–58. Springer, Heidelberg (2009). doi:10.1007/978-3-642-04271-3_7
13. Graham, M.W., et al.: Robust 3-D airway tree segmentation for image-guided peripheral bronchoscopy. IEEE Trans. Med. Imaging **29**, 982–997 (2010)
14. Sørensen, L., Lo, P., Dirksen, A., Petersen, J., de Bruijne, M.: Dissimilarity-based classification of anatomical tree structures. In: Székely, G., Hahn, H.K. (eds.) IPMI 2011. LNCS, vol. 6801, pp. 475–485. Springer, Heidelberg (2011). doi:10.1007/978-3-642-22092-0_39

Detection and Localization of Landmarks in the Lower Extremities Using an Automatically Learned Conditional Random Field

Alexander Oliver Mader[1,2,3](✉), Cristian Lorenz[3], Martin Bergtholdt[3],
Jens von Berg[3], Hauke Schramm[1,2], Jan Modersitzki[4], and Carsten Meyer[1,2,3]

[1] Institute of Computer Science, Kiel University of Applied Sciences, Kiel, Germany
`alexander.o.mader@fh-kiel.de`
[2] Department of Computer Science, Faculty of Engineering,
Kiel University, Kiel, Germany
[3] Department of Digital Imaging, Philips Research, Hamburg, Germany
[4] Institute of Mathematics and Image Computing, Lübeck University,
Lübeck, Germany

Abstract. The detection and localization of single or multiple landmarks is a crucial task in medical imaging. It is often required as initialization for other tasks like segmentation or registration. A common approach to localize multiple landmarks is to exploit their spatial correlations, e.g., by using a conditional random field (CRF) to incorporate geometric information between landmark pairs. This CRF is usually applied to resolve ambiguities of a localizer, e.g., a random forest or a deep neural network. In this paper, we apply a random forest/CRF combination to the task of jointly detecting and localizing 6 landmarks in the lower extremities, taken from a dataset of 660 X-ray images. The dataset is challenging since a significant number of images does not show all the landmarks. Furthermore, 11.3% of the target landmarks are altered by prostheses or pathologies.

To account for this, we introduce a "missing" label for each landmark (represented by a node in the CRF). Moreover, instead of manually specifying the CRF model by selecting suitable potential functions and the graph topology, we suggest to automatically optimize both in a learning framework. Specifically, we define a pool of potential functions and learn their CRF weights (relative contributions), in addition to the potential values in case of missing landmarks. Potentials with a low weight are removed, thus optimizing the graph topology. Detailed evaluations on our database show the feasibility of our approach. Our algorithm removed on average 23 of the initial 51 CRF potentials, and correctly detected and localized (within 10 mm tolerance) on average 92.8% of the landmarks, with individual rates ranging from 90.0% to 97.4%.

1 Introduction

The automatic localization of landmarks in medical images is a crucial task. It is clinically required, inter alia, for the purposes of diagnosis, surgical planning,

© Springer International Publishing AG 2017
M.J. Cardoso et al. (Eds.): GRAIL/MFCA/MICGen 2017, LNCS 10551, pp. 64–75, 2017.
DOI: 10.1007/978-3-319-67675-3_7

and post-operative assessment. Because of the large amount of variability and outliers in medical data, the automatic and accurate localization of landmarks is comparably hard. It becomes harder, when a landmark's presence is not guaranteed (e.g., due to a restricted field of view). In this case, each landmark has to be detected before it can be localized.

Many approaches have been proposed to solve the task of localizing spatially correlated landmarks. Often, first a "landmark localizer" is used to generate a (pseudo) probability map for each landmark over the image domain. To this end, e.g., random forests [6,7,14,18], decision trees [2], deep convolutional neural networks [15], and the discriminative generalized Hough transform [16] have been used. Then, a conditional random field (CRF) is often applied to select the globally optimal configuration for all landmarks, characterized by the largest joint posterior probability [2,6,14,18]. The posterior probability of the CRF is generally expressed by an energy, which is parameterized by potential functions (often unary or binary). The unary potentials of the CRF are related to the locations of individual landmarks and are defined based on the localizer output. Binary potentials model the spatial relations between two landmarks, assuming a specific topology (i.e., graph connectivity). Both the potentials (e.g., distance [2], vector [6], vector field profiles [5], etc.) and the topology are often selected in a heuristic manner. Potentials of higher arity are possible, but seldomly used due to computational complexity [12,19]. Only few papers explicitly learn the weights of the CRF potentials, i.e., their relative contribution to the joint posterior probability, let alone address the possibility of missing landmarks due to, e.g., a restricted field of view. Among them [2], which includes a heuristic penalty for a false miss. To compute the globally optimal landmark configuration based on the CRF model, various inference algorithms [19] can be applied.

In this paper, we automatically learn essential components of a CRF – including the possibility of missing landmarks – to automatically detect (i.e., determine whether a landmark is present in the current image) and localize (i.e., specify the position of a landmark present in the current image) six landmarks of the lower extremities in a database of 660 X-ray images with significant fractions of missing landmarks due to restricted field of view. Specifically, we define a pool of potential functions, the weights of which are – together with the values of potentials in case of missing landmarks – automatically learned. Starting from a fully connected graph, potentials with low weights are removed. In this way, the graph topology can be automatically optimized. Applying our method, on average 23 of the initially 51 CRF potentials were removed, and (on average) 92.8% of the landmarks were correctly detected and (if present) localized within 10 mm tolerance.

2   Related Work

Various approaches have been proposed to detect and localize a set of landmarks. Here, we briefly summarize the contributions that are closest to our work. Random forests have been used to generate landmark localization hypotheses, e.g., in [6,14,18]. Donner et al. [6] use a random forest/Hough forest combination to first classify the image into candidate regions for each landmark, which are then aggregated by the Hough forest to generate precise location hypotheses. In contrast, [14,18] use the random forest to directly regress (pseudo) probability maps for the location of each landmark, based on local and global [18] or only local [14] image features, followed by a non-maximum suppression (NMS). Other approaches include decision trees based on a set of image features [2], deep convolutional networks [15] and the discriminative generalized Hough transform [16]. The CRF is generally based on unary potentials (based on the localizer output) and heuristically motivated binary potentials, e.g., distance [2], vector [6], vector field profiles [5], etc. Bergtholdt et al. [2] associate the CRF potentials with weights which are automatically learned using maximum likelihood (ML) based on the posterior probabilities of the training data. They also account for missing landmarks by assigning heuristically motivated values for the corresponding potentials, the weights of which are also learned (involving a heuristic parameter for false misses). However, the ML criterion may stress the influence of outliers, requiring corresponding weightings in case of a large amount of incorrect localization hypotheses. Moreover, a ML approach quickly becomes infeasible with increasing number of combinations in terms of computational complexity. Bergtholdt et al. [2] uses a fully connected graph, and thus does not exploit the potential of simplifying the graph topology for a reduced computational complexity. In contrast, [6] defined the CRF graph topology heuristically based on the differential entropy of the distribution of relative landmark distances calculated on the training data. This may not be optimal if other features than the relative distance are used to characterize landmark pairs.

In this work, we define a pool of CRF potential functions (currently unary and binary, but generally of any arity) and associate a weight with each potential function and each landmark pair (generally each landmark subset). Starting from a fully connected graph, we automatically learn the potential weights together with the values of the potentials in case of missing landmarks. Potentials with low weights are removed, thus optimizing the CRF graph topology. In contrast to [2], we use a max-margin approach (considering only the best incorrect configuration of all landmarks in addition to the correct configuration) in an energy-based formulation [13]. For efficiency reasons (short training and test times, moderate number of annotated training images required), our landmark localizer is based on regression trees [14]. However, any other localizer generating (pseudo) probability maps for each landmark can be used instead (including a deep neural network).

The task of localizing six landmarks of the lower extremities has been addressed before in [8,16,17] using the discriminative generalized Hough transform. However, they only addressed the localization task, i.e., only considering landmarks known to be contained in the image. Thus, they are not able to cope with missing landmarks.

3   Methods

The task is to detect and localize – if present – up to N different landmarks in an image. We solve this problem in two steps: First, landmark-specific regression tree ensembles rating local image features are used to generate n localization hypotheses $\hat{\mathcal{X}}_i = \{\hat{\mathbf{x}}_{i,1}, \ldots, \hat{\mathbf{x}}_{i,n}\}$ for each landmark $i \in \{1, \ldots, N\}$. Second, the unary information of the localizer is combined with binary information rating spatial features between landmarks and jointly modeled in a CRF. An additional "missing" state is introduced to solve the detection problem and all required parameters are automatically learned in a gradient descent optimization. Finally, a common CRF inference technique is applied to find the best selection $\hat{\mathbf{S}} \in \{0, 1, \ldots, n\}^N$ out of all possible selections $\mathcal{S}$. For each landmark, one or no localization hypothesis is selected, effectively solving the detection and localization in one inference step.

Section 3.1 introduces the regression-tree-ensemble-based localizer, followed by the joint formulation of weighted knowledge sources in a CRF in Sect. 3.2. Finally, the optimization step used to learn all CRF parameters and to reduce the number of necessary potential functions is illustrated in Sect. 3.3.

3.1   Landmark Localization Using Regression Tree Ensembles

The goal of the first step is to predict (as accurately as possible) candidate positions for each landmark based on local context only. At this stage we tolerate confusions as long as any (not necessarily the first) of the $n = 15$ best localization hypotheses is correct, since they will be resolved in the second step. The basic idea is to transform an image $\mathbf{I} : \mathbb{R}^2 \to \mathbb{R}$ into a pseudo (not normalized) probability map $\widetilde{\mathbf{P}}_i : \mathbb{R}^2 \to \mathbb{R}^+$ in which the location of the highest value $\hat{\mathbf{x}}_{i,1} = \arg\max_{\mathbf{x}} \widetilde{\mathbf{P}}_i(\mathbf{x})$ corresponds to the most likely predicted position of the target landmark i. For efficiency reasons, we use random forests, which only need a small or moderate number of annotated training images. As in [14], for each landmark i, an ensemble of $K = 96$ decision tree regressors [4] is used to transform feature vectors $\mathbf{f}_i^k(\mathbf{x})$, computed for a certain position $\mathbf{x}$ in image $\mathbf{I}$ for the k-th regression tree, into pseudo probabilities $\widetilde{p}_i^k(\mathbf{x})$. This is done for all pixels in the image and averaged over all trees k to form the pseudo probability map $\widetilde{\mathbf{P}}_i$. Finally, NMS with a minimal distance between peaks of 3 pixels is applied to find local maxima. The n best local maxima are used as localization hypotheses $\hat{\mathcal{X}}_i = \{\hat{\mathbf{x}}_{i,1}, \ldots, \hat{\mathbf{x}}_{i,n}\}$ for each landmark i.

To extract the feature vector $\mathbf{f}_i^k(\mathbf{x})$ for a certain pixel $\mathbf{x}$ we use a BRIEF-like [3] approach. Each tree in the ensemble is associated with an individual sampling mask to extract $F = 128$ pixel intensity values from a local patch. The mask is obtained by sampling locations from $\mathbf{X} \sim$ i.i.d. $\mathcal{N}\left(\mathbf{0}, \frac{1}{25}\begin{pmatrix} A_1^2 & 0 \\ 0 & A_2^2 \end{pmatrix}\right)$ with $\mathbf{A} = (a_1\ a_2)$ being the patch size; in our experiments $\mathbf{A} = (351\ 351)$ to capture the target object's size. Finally, the masks origin is placed at $\mathbf{x}$ and the intensity value at $\mathbf{x}$ is subtracted from the marked pixel intensities, resulting in our F-dimensional feature vector $\mathbf{f}_i^k(\mathbf{x})$.

Boostrapping is used to train the regression trees in a discriminative fashion by iteratively growing a set $\mathcal{O}_i^k \subseteq \mathbb{R}^F \times \mathbb{R}$ of feature vectors and corresponding target values over all training images. We start out by collecting "positive" samples for each training image by computing feature vectors $\mathbf{f}_i^k(\mathbf{x})$ for all $M = 317$ pixels within a circle with radius $R = 10$ (corresponding to the localization criterion) around the respective annotated landmark position $\mathbf{x}_i^*$. We allow for some ambiguity by introducing a Gaussian distribution $\mathcal{N}_i\left(\mathbf{x}_i^*, \frac{1}{9}R^2\left(\begin{smallmatrix} 1 & 0 \\ 0 & 1 \end{smallmatrix}\right)\right)$ around $\mathbf{x}_i^*$ and use the density values computed at position $\mathbf{x}$ as regression targets. All "positive" samples are added to the set $\mathcal{O}_i^k$ and an intermediate tree is trained on them. After that, "negative" samples are generated by iterating over all training images and applying the intermediate tree to the training image in order to find the most offending responses. NMS is used to select the M pixels with the largest pseudo probabilities outside the circle located at $\mathbf{x}_i^*$. For those M "negative" pixels, feature vectors are computed and added – with a target regression value 0 – to the growing set of samples $\mathcal{O}_i^k$. After each iteration, a new intermediate and more discriminative tree is trained on the larger set of samples $\mathcal{O}_i^k$ and used in the next iteration. The final tree is then added to the ensemble.

All parameters of the regression tree ensemble have been optimized on a previous task [14] and were adapted to the current one. Some parameters (like the sampling mask) were intuitively chosen to match the dataset, while others (e.g., the number of trees) were chosen to match the hardware constraints.

3.2   CRF with Pool of Potential Functions and "Missing" Label

To compensate for incorrect first best localization hypotheses $\hat{\mathbf{x}}_{i,1}$ for arbitrary landmarks i, we use a CRF to model geometric relationships between landmarks. For notational simplicity, we introduce an index $s_i \in \{0, 1, \ldots, n\}$ for each landmark i to denote the "missing" label $s_i = 0$ and the selection $s_i > 0$ of one of the localization hypotheses $\hat{\mathcal{X}}_i$. For instance, $s_i = 2$ means that the second localization hypothesis $\hat{\mathbf{x}}_{i,2}$ is assigned to the i-th landmark in the CRF. We apply an energy-based formulation [13], where a low energy $E(\mathbf{S})$ of a configuration $\mathbf{S} = (s_1, \ldots, s_N)$ of localization hypotheses over all landmarks implies a large posterior probability. The energy $E(\mathbf{S})$ of the CRF is parameterized by a set of T potential functions $\Phi = \{\phi_1(\cdot), \ldots, \phi_T(\cdot)\}$ (of arbitrary arity) with corresponding weights $\mathbf{\Lambda} = (\lambda_1, \ldots, \lambda_T)$ scaling each term, and missing potential values $\boldsymbol{\beta} = (\beta_1, \ldots, \beta_T)$:

$$E(\mathbf{S}) = \sum_{j=1}^{T} \lambda_j \cdot \begin{cases} \beta_j & \text{if } s_i = 0 \text{ for any } i \in \text{Scope}(\phi_j) \\ \phi_j(\mathbf{S}) & \text{else} \end{cases} . \tag{1}$$

The explicit inclusion of the missing potential values $\boldsymbol{\beta}$ is necessary to allow computation of $E(\mathbf{S})$ in case of missing landmarks and to automatically learn their values. In inference, the task is to find the selection $\hat{\mathbf{S}}$ amongst all $(n+1)^N$ possible selections $\mathcal{S}$ that minimizes the energy from Eq. (1):

$$\hat{\mathbf{S}} = \arg \min_{\mathbf{S} \in \mathcal{S}} E(\mathbf{S}).   \tag{2}$$

The search problem depicted in Eq. (2) becomes intractable very fast with a growing number of states and landmarks, which might require the usage of approximate inference. However, in our case we can still use exact inference in form of the A* search algorithm by Bergtholdt et al. [1], which uses an admissible heuristic to find the global optimum.

The idea of our approach is to define a "pool" Φ of potential functions $\phi_j(\mathbf{S})$ (motivated clinically, anatomically, by geometric considerations or by "helpful" image features) and to automatically learn their weights λ_j w.r.t. the detection and localization criterion. Potentials with a low weight can then be removed. To illustrate this principle, we define one unary potential for each landmark and three – in this work purely geometrically motivated – binary potentials per landmark pair in Φ.

Unary Localizer Potential. Let $\mathbf{U}_i = (u_{i,1}, \ldots, u_{i,n})$ be the regressed scores for the localization hypotheses $\hat{\mathcal{X}}_i$. We define the unary localizer potential for the i-th landmark as

$$\phi_i^{\text{loc}}(\mathbf{S}) = -\log(u_{i,o_i}).   \tag{3}$$

Binary Distance Potential. The first binary potential uses a Gaussian distribution to model the distance between two landmarks i and j. Assuming we estimated the empirical mean $\mu_{i,j}^{\text{dist}}$ and variance $\sigma_{i,j}^2$ of distances on training annotations, and that $f(\cdot)$ is the probability density function of a normal distribution, we define the binary distance potential as

$$\phi_{i,j}^{\text{dist}}(\mathbf{S}) = -\log\left(f(\|\hat{\mathbf{x}}_{i,s_i} - \hat{\mathbf{x}}_{j,s_j}\| \mid \mu_{i,j}^{\text{dist}}, \sigma_{i,j}^2) \right).   \tag{4}$$

Binary Angle Potential. The second binary potential uses a von Mises distribution to model the angle of the line spanned between two landmarks i and j in relation to the x-axis. Similar to the previous distribution, we estimated the distribution's parameters $\mu_{i,j}^{\text{ang}}$ and $\kappa_{i,j}$ using training annotations. Finally, with $g(\cdot)$ being the distribution's probability density function and $\alpha(\mathbf{x})$ a function computing the angle between the vector $\mathbf{x}$ and the x-axis, we define the potential as

$$\phi_{i,j}^{\text{ang}}(\mathbf{S}) = -\log\left(g(\alpha(\hat{\mathbf{x}}_{i,s_i} - \hat{\mathbf{x}}_{j,s_j}) \mid \mu_{i,j}^{\text{ang}}, \kappa_{i,j}) \right).   \tag{5}$$

Binary Vector Potential. For the third binary potential, we use a multivariate Gaussian distribution to model the vector between two landmarks i and j. This includes distance and orientation. However, the vector potential is neither scaling nor rotation invariant, whereas the distance and angle potentials are rotation and scaling invariant, respectively. We include the vector potential to illustrate the concept of a "pool" of potential functions. Again, we estimate the necessary parameters $\boldsymbol{\mu}_{i,j}^{\text{vec}}$ and $\boldsymbol{\Sigma}_{i,j}$ on training annotations. Finally, with $h(\cdot)$ being the probability density function of a multivariate normal distribution, we define this potential as

$$\phi_{i,j}^{\text{vec}}(\mathbf{S}) = -\log\left(h(\hat{\mathbf{x}}_{i,s_i} - \hat{\mathbf{x}}_{j,s_j} \mid \boldsymbol{\mu}_{i,j}^{\text{vec}}, \boldsymbol{\Sigma}_{i,j})\right). \tag{6}$$

Pool of Potentials. With these definitions, we define our pool of potential functions for a fully connected graph as

$$\begin{aligned}\Phi =&\{\phi_i^{\text{loc}}(\cdot) \mid i = 1..N\} \cup \\ &\{\phi_{i,j}^{\text{dist}}(\cdot), \phi_{i,j}^{\text{ang}}(\cdot), \phi_{i,j}^{\text{vec}}(\cdot) \mid i = 1..N, \ j = i+1..N\}.\end{aligned} \tag{7}$$

The remaining tasks are to weight each potential ($\boldsymbol{\Lambda}$), estimate the energies when an involved landmark is missing ($\boldsymbol{\beta}$) and to remove unnecessary potentials. Note that in principle our approach works with potentials of arbitrary arity.

3.3   Learning of Parameters and Removing Potentials

There exist heuristics [2] to estimate the potential weights as well as the missing energies, but a more common approach is to learn those parameters from data. We follow the latter path by defining an appropriate loss function over data $\mathcal{D}$ and use a gradient descent scheme to optimize it. The probabilistic approach is to use maximum likelihood, which has the drawbacks that one must compute the partition function, which gets intractable quickly, and that it stresses the influence of outliers. Thus, we follow a max-margin approach [12,13] and try to increase the margin between the correct selection $\mathbf{S}^*$ and the best (lowest energy) incorrect selection $\mathbf{S}^-$. This requires appropriate inference for which we again use the A* algorithm.

A well known loss function is the hinge loss, which tries to increase the energy gap between $\mathbf{S}^*$ and $\mathbf{S}^-$ until a certain margin $m = 1$ is satisfied. The intuition is that a margin m improves generalization and that only samples not satisfying the margin continue to contribute to the parameter updates. Let our loss function be defined as

$$L(\boldsymbol{\Lambda}, \boldsymbol{\beta}) = \frac{1}{K}\sum_{k=1}^{K}\max\left(0, m + E(\mathbf{S}_k^*) - E(\mathbf{S}_k^-)\right) + \theta\cdot\sum_{j=1}^{T}|\lambda_j|. \tag{8}$$

In addition to the data term over all K training samples, we added a θ-weighted L1 regularization term w.r.t. $\boldsymbol{\Lambda}$ to further accelerate the sparsification of terms. I.e., instead of defining a topology and manually selecting appropriate potential functions, our idea is to start with a fully connected graph and a pool of different potentials Φ and to learn which of those potentials are meaningful.

Once we optimized Λ, we can simply remove all zero-weighted ($\lambda_j = 0$) potentials. This solves the problem of defining a topology as well as selecting meaningful potentials.

To optimize the loss function from Eq. (8), we apply a variant of stochastic gradient descent in form of the Adam algorithm by Kingma and Ba [11]. We use a global step-size of $\alpha = 0.01$ and leave all remaining parameters as proposed in [11]. Furthermore, we use a mini-batch size of $K = 40$ samples per iteration, which greatly improves the time until convergence, which is usually reached after $\sim$200 iterations. To improve generalization, we optimize the potential weights Λ and missing energies β on a different portion of training examples than used to train the potential functions themselves (i.e., probability distribution parameters, localizers, etc.). Once all parameters are estimated, we remove all unnecessary potentials where $\lambda_j = 0$ to reduce the runtime and complexity of the system.

4 Results

We evaluated the proposed approach on an in-house dataset of 660 images showing the lower extremities of 606 patients with an age in the range of 19 to 100 years. The task is to detect and localize (if present) up to 6 different landmarks, namely the femur, knee and ankle of both legs. A few sample images are shown in Fig. 1. We downsampled the images to an isotropic resolution of 1 mm/px to speed up the processing. Due to a restricted field of view and missing limbs in a subset of images, not all landmarks are present in all images. Only 73.4% of the images contain all landmarks, while 8, 78, 77, and 10 images only contain 5, 4, 3, and 2 landmarks, respectively. Hence, the task is to detect whether a landmark is present in conjunction with the task to localize it, if present. We consider two kinds of results to be correct. First, the landmark is missing and the algorithm predicted it to be missing. Second, the landmark is not missing and the algorithm detected it and predicted a position with an Euclidean distance to the true position below 10 mm. The tolerance of 10 mm has been chosen by Ruppertshofen et al. [17] and is illustrated in the third image in Fig. 3a.

We used patient-grouped 5-fold cross validation in our experiments, which provided us with, on average, 530 training images per fold. 30% of the training images of each fold were used to train the localizer (Sect. 3.1) and to estimate the parameters of the probability distributions (Sect. 3.2), while the remaining 70% were used to learn the weights and missing potential values (Sect. 3.3). Note that we exclusively used 15% of the latter training images as validation set to properly select a regressor weight θ. The final results over all folds in terms of correct detection and localization (as described above) are shown in Fig. 2a. The localizer itself, i.e., always using the first best localization hypothesis, shows mediocre performance with on average 81.2 %. First, it assumes a landmark is always present and thus the numbers are biased. Second, it performs significantly worse when the landmarks are close to the image's border, i.e., for the femur and

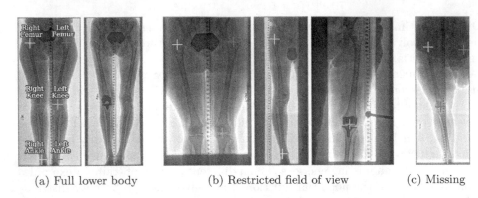

(a) Full lower body   (b) Restricted field of view   (c) Missing

Fig. 1. A few samples including annotations of the 660 images showing (a) full lower bodies, (b) a restricted field of view and (c) a full lower body with missing limbs. Note the two knee prostheses. The small circle annotations in the second image correspond to the area in which a localization is assumed correct.

ankle landmarks due to only partly available information. In contrast to previous works [6,14,18], we have to properly estimate the CRF weights. Without learning the parameters Λ and β, just setting them to 1, we obtain an accuracy of only 52.9%. In contrast, after learning all parameters we handle 2.8% of the samples correctly, averaged over the different landmarks. Furthermore, our approach is also very robust against altered target objects in form of prostheses. 97.5% of the 319 prostheses were properly detected and localized. The performance of our approach is broken down in Fig. 2b. We see that the detection task was solved on average in 82.5% TP + 10.3% TN + 5.3% mis-loc. = 98.1% of the images. The largest amount of errors is due to mis-localization with 5.3%, in contrast to mis-detection with only 0.7% FP + 1.3% FN = 2.0%.

Looking at resulting images (see examples in Fig. 3a), the localization tolerance of 10 mm appears to be quite strict, which is also illustrated in the second image in Fig. 1. This is addressed in Fig. 3b, where the amount of correct images w.r.t. a certain number of errors per image in relation to the localization tolerance is plotted. Increasing the tolerance from 10 mm to 20 mm, the percentage of images where all 6 landmarks are handled correctly increases by 12.3% points to 85.3%; the average detection and localization rate for a single landmark increases to 96.2%. Depending on the application, e.g., if the localization hypothesis is further refined by post-processing on a small crop of the image, a less strict localization tolerance might be sufficient.

A quantitative comparison to [16] is difficult due to different evaluation setups (cross-validation in our work and a single unknown training and test split in [16]) and a different objective (namely localization only, not detection). However, if we only consider cases where an existing landmark was detected (true positives), we can quantify the localization performance of our approach. Note, due to the above reasons we refrain from drawing any conclusions. Using the same tolerance of 10 mm as used by Ruppertshofen et al., we achieved to correctly localize

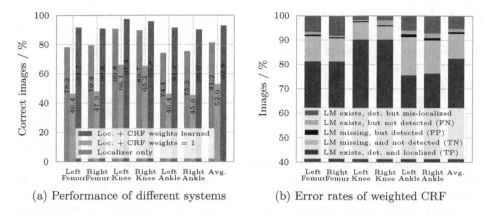

(a) Performance of different systems   (b) Error rates of weighted CRF

Fig. 2. (a) Amount of correct images in percent w.r.t. the different landmarks; 100% corresponds to 660 images. (b) Distribution of errors across detection and localization over all images in percent for the localizer with learned CRF weights. The two bottom-most bars correspond to the rates of our approach depicted in (a), followed by three bars for the three different sources of errors.

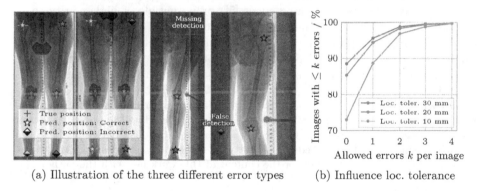

(a) Illustration of the three different error types   (b) Influence loc. tolerance

Fig. 3. (a) Illustration of the three different kinds of errors: The first two images illustrate mis-localization due to the error tolerance of 10 mm. However, note the accurate localization despite the prostheses. The third image shows a landmark (left femur) not being detected. The fourth image illustrates a falsely detected landmark. (b) Distribution function of landmark errors per image (between 0 and 6) for different localization tolerance levels.

91.7%, 98.1% and 92.0% of the femur, knee and ankle landmarks, respectively, averaged over both legs. In contrast, Ruppertshofen et al. achieved a respective performance of 73.9%, 93.7% and 86.6%.

By dropping all zero-weighted potentials, we were able to remove on average 45.5% of $6 + 3 \cdot \frac{6 \cdot 5}{2} = 51$ CRF potentials: All unary potentials remained, while 3, 7, and 13 of the angle, distance and vector potentials were removed, respectively. This reduced the inference time on average by 20.1%.

5   Discussion and Conclusions

In this paper, we proposed an automatic approach for learning the weights of potentials as well as the values of the potentials for missing landmarks in a conditional random field using a max-margin hinge loss and gradient descent. In particular, we suggested to define a pool of potential functions for the CRF, learn their weights and remove all potentials which were assigned a weight of 0 by employing an L1 sparsity prior. This allows to automatically select the most appropriate potential functions and to define the CRF graph topology, starting from a fully connected graph, in a single optimization framework. We investigated our approach to localize six landmarks of the lower extremities on a dataset of 660 X-ray images with significant fractions of missing landmarks due to restricted field of view. Although on average 45.5% of the CRF potentials have been removed, we detected and localized (within 10 mm) on average 92.8% of the different landmarks while being very robust against prostheses. Increasing the localization tolerance to 20 mm further improved the performance to 96.2%. Our approach can be extended to use different (and additional) landmark localizers (e.g., deep convolutional neural networks), further binary potentials (e.g., incorporating gray value profiles along edges [5]) or potentials of higher arity (e.g., the relative position of landmark triples), where higher order clique reduction techniques [10] seem promising. Also, a zooming approach [9] could be added to further refine the landmark positions. Since our approach is fairly general, we can apply it to different landmark localization tasks with limited manual effort.

Acknowledgements. The authors thank the Diagnosezentrum Urania, Vienna and the Dartmouth Hitchcock Medical Center, Lebanon for providing the radiographs that served as training and test sets; Gooßen [8] for the annotations. This work has been financially supported by the Federal Ministry of Education and Research under the grant 03FH013IX5. The liability for the content of this work lies with the authors.

References

1. Bergtholdt, M., Kappes, J.H., Schnörr, C.: Learning of graphical models and efficient inference for object class recognition. In: Franke, K., Müller, K.-R., Nickolay, B., Schäfer, R. (eds.) DAGM 2006. LNCS, vol. 4174, pp. 273–283. Springer,
Heidelberg (2006). doi:10.1007/11861898_28
2. Bergtholdt, M., et al.: A study of parts-based object class detection using complete graphs. IJCV **87**(1), 93–117 (2010)
3. Calonder, M., Lepetit, V., Strecha, C., Fua, P.: BRIEF: binary robust independent elementary features. In: Daniilidis, K., Maragos, P., Paragios, N. (eds.) ECCV 2010. LNCS, vol. 6314, pp. 778–792. Springer, Heidelberg (2010). doi:10.1007/978-3-642-15561-1_56
4. Criminisi, A., et al.: Regression forests for efficient anatomy detection and localization in computed tomography scans. Med. Image Anal. **17**(8), 1293–1303 (2013)
5. Donner, R., et al.: Sparse MRF appearance models for fast anatomical structure localisation. In: BMVC (2007)

6. Donner, R., et al.: Global localization of 3d anatomical structures by pre-filtered hough forests and discrete optimization. Med. Image Anal. **17**(8), 1304–1314 (2013)
7. Glocker, B., Zikic, D., Konukoglu, E., Haynor, D.R., Criminisi, A.: Vertebrae localization in pathological spine CT via dense classification from sparse annotations. In: Mori, K., Sakuma, I., Sato, Y., Barillot, C., Navab, N. (eds.) MICCAI 2013. LNCS, vol. 8150, pp. 262–270. Springer, Heidelberg (2013). doi:10.1007/978-3-642-40763-5_33
8. Gooßen, A.: Computational Imaging in Orthopaedic Radiography. BoD (2012)
9. Hahmann, F., et al.: Model interpolation for eye localization using the discriminative generalized hough transform. In: BIOSIG (2012)
10. Ishikawa, H.: Higher-order clique reduction in binary graph cut. In: CVPR, pp. 2993–3000. IEEE (2009)
11. Kingma, D., Ba, J.: Adam: A method for stochastic optimization. In: ICLR (2014)
12. Komodakis, N., Xiang, B., Paragios, N.: A framework for efficient structured max-margin learning of high-order mrf models. IEEE TPAMI **37**(7), 1425–1441 (2015)
13. LeCun, Y., Chopra, S., Hadsell, R.: A tutorial on energy-based learning. In: Predicting Structured Data (2006)
14. Mader, A.O., Schramm, H., Meyer, C.: Efficient epiphyses localization using regression tree ensembles and a conditional random field. Bildverarbeitung für die Medizin 2017. Informatik aktuell, pp. 179–184. Springer, Heidelberg (2017). doi:10.1007/978-3-662-54345-0_42
15. Payer, C., Štern, D., Bischof, H., Urschler, M.: Regressing heatmaps for multiple landmark localization using CNNs. In: Ourselin, S., Joskowicz, L., Sabuncu, M.R., Unal, G., Wells, W. (eds.) MICCAI 2016. LNCS, vol. 9901, pp. 230–238. Springer, Cham (2016). doi:10.1007/978-3-319-46723-8_27
16. Ruppertshofen, H., et al.: Discriminative generalized hough transform for localization of joints in the lower extremities. CSRD **26**(1), 97–105 (2011)
17. Ruppertshofen, H., et al.: Shape model training for concurrent localization of the left and right knee. In: SPIE Medical Imaging (2011)
18. Štern, D., Ebner, T., Urschler, M.: From local to global random regression forests: exploring anatomical landmark localization. In: Ourselin, S., Joskowicz, L., Sabuncu, M.R., Unal, G., Wells, W. (eds.) MICCAI 2016. LNCS, vol. 9901, pp. 221–229. Springer, Cham (2016). doi:10.1007/978-3-319-46723-8_26
19. Wang, C., Komodakis, N., Paragios, N.: Markov random field modeling, inference & learning in computer vision & image understanding: a survey. CVIU **117**, 1610–1627 (2013)

6th International Workshop on Mathematical Foundations of Computational Anatomy, MFCA 2017

Bridge Simulation and Metric Estimation on Landmark Manifolds

Stefan Sommer[1][(✉)], Alexis Arnaudon[2], Line Kuhnel[1], and Sarang Joshi[3]

[1] Department of Computer Science (DIKU),
University of Copenhagen, Copenhagen, Denmark
sommer@di.ku.dk
[2] Department of Mathematics, Imperial College London, London, UK
[3] Department of Bioengineering, Scientific Computing and Imaging Institute,
University of Utah, Salt Lake City, USA

Abstract. We present an inference algorithm and connected Monte Carlo based estimation procedures for metric estimation from landmark configurations distributed according to the transition distribution of a Riemannian Brownian motion arising from the Large Deformation Diffeomorphic Metric Mapping (LDDMM) metric. The distribution possesses properties similar to the regular Euclidean normal distribution but its transition density is governed by a high-dimensional PDE with no closed-form solution in the nonlinear case. We show how the density can be numerically approximated by Monte Carlo sampling of conditioned Brownian bridges, and we use this to estimate parameters of the LDDMM kernel and thus the metric structure by maximum likelihood.

Keywords: Landmarks · Brownian motion · Brownian bridges · MLE

1 Introduction

Finite dimensional landmark configurations are essential in shape analysis and computational anatomy, both for marking and following anatomically important areas in e.g. changing brain anatomies and discretely represented curve outlines, and in being among the simplest non-linear shape spaces. This simplicity, in particular the finite dimensionality, makes landmarks useful for theoretical investigations and for deriving algorithms that can subsequently be generalized to infinite dimensional shape spaces.

While probability distributions in Euclidean space can often be specified conveniently from their density function, e.g. the normal distribution with the density $p_{\mu,\Sigma}(x) \propto e^{-\frac{1}{2}(x-\mu)^T \Sigma^{-1}(x-\mu)}$, the non-linear nature of shape spaces often rules out closed form functions. Indeed, a density defined in coordinates will be dependent on the chosen coordinate chart and thus not geometrically intrinsic, and normalization factors can be inherently hard to compute. A different approach defines probability distributions as transition distributions of stochastic processes. Because stochastic differential equations (SDEs) can be

© Springer International Publishing AG 2017
M.J. Cardoso et al. (Eds.): GRAIL/MFCA/MICGen 2017, LNCS 10551, pp. 79–91, 2017.
DOI: 10.1007/978-3-319-67675-3_8

specified locally from their infinitesimal variations, it is natural to define them in geometric spaces. Belonging to this category, the present paper aligns with a range of recent research activities on nonlinear SDEs in shape analysis and geometric mechanics [3, 4, 14, 25, 26].

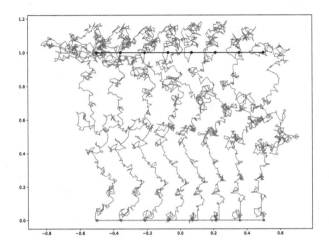

Fig. 1. A Brownian bridge connecting a configuration of 8 landmarks (blue points) to corresponding target landmarks (black points). Blue curves shows the stochastic trajectory of each landmark. The bridge arises from a Riemannian Brownian motion conditioned on hitting the target at time $T = 1$. The transition density p_T can be evaluated by taking expectation over such bridges. (Color figure online)

We consider here observations distributed according to the transition distribution of a Brownian motion, which is arguably one of the most direct generalizations of the Gaussian distribution to nonlinear geometries. For the Brownian motion, each infinitesimal step defining the SDE can be considered normally distributed with isotropic covariance with respect to the Riemannian metric of the space. Then, from observations, we aim to infer parameters of this metric. In the Large Deformation Diffeomorphic Metric Mapping (LDDMM) setting, this can be framed as inferring parameters of the kernel mapping K between the dual Lie algebra $\mathfrak{g}^*$ and the Lie algebra $\mathfrak{g} = \mathfrak{X}(\Omega)$ of the diffeomorphism group $\text{Diff}(\Omega)$ that acts on the domain Ω containing the landmarks. We achieve this by deriving a scheme for Monte Carlo simulation of Brownian landmark bridges conditioned on hitting the observed landmark configurations (Fig. 1). Based on the Euclidean diffusion bridge simulation scheme of Delyon and Hu [6], we can compute expectation over bridges using the correction factor of a guided diffusion process to obtain the transition density of the Brownian motion. From this, we can take derivatives to obtain an iterative optimization algorithm for the most likely parameters. The scheme applies to the situation when the landmark configurations are considered observed at a fixed positive time $t = T$. The time interval $[0, T]$ will generally be sufficiently large that many time discretization points are needed to accurately represent the stochastic process.

We begin in Sect. 2 with a short survey of LDDMM landmark geometry, metric estimation, large deformation stochastics, and uses of Brownian motion in shape analysis. In Sect. 3, we derive a scheme for simulating Brownian landmark bridges. We apply this scheme in Sect. 4 to derive an inference algorithm for estimating parameters of the metric. Numerical examples are presented in Sect. 5 before the paper ends with concluding remarks.

2   Landmarks Manifolds and Stochastic Landmark Dynamics

We start with a short survey of landmark geometry with the LDDMM framework as derived in papers including [5,7,11,24]. The framework applies to general shape spaces though we focus on configurations $\mathbf{q} = (q_1, \ldots, q_N)$ of N landmarks $q_i \in \Omega \subseteq \mathbb{R}^d$. We denote the resulting manifold Q. Two sets of shapes $\mathbf{q}^0, \mathbf{q}^1$ are in LDDMM matched by minimizing the energy functional

$$E(u_t) = \int_0^1 l(u_t)dt + \frac{1}{2\lambda^2}\|g_1.\mathbf{q}^0 - \mathbf{q}^1\|^2. \tag{1}$$

The parameter of E is a time-dependent vector field $u_t \in \mathfrak{X}(\Omega)$ that via a reconstruction equation

$$\partial_t g_t = u_t \circ g_t \tag{2}$$

generates a corresponding time-dependent flow of diffeomorphisms $g_t \in \mathrm{Diff}(\Omega)$. The endpoint diffeomorphism g_1 move the landmarks through the action $g.\mathbf{q} = (g(q_1), \ldots, g(q_N))$ of $\mathrm{Diff}(\Omega)$ on Q. The right-most term of (1) measures the dissimilarity between $g_1.\mathbf{q}^0$ and $\mathbf{q}^1$ weighted by a factor $\lambda > 0$. In the landmark case, the squared Euclidean distance when considering the landmarks elements of $\mathbb{R}^{Nd}$ is often used here.

The Lagrangian l on u is often in the form $l(u) = \langle u, Lu \rangle$ with the L^2-pairing and L being a differential operator. Because $\mathfrak{X}(\Omega)$ can formally be considered the Lie algebra $\mathfrak{g}$ of $\mathrm{Diff}(\Omega)$, l puts the dual Lie algebra $\mathfrak{g}^*$ into correspondence with $\mathfrak{g}$ by the mapping $\frac{1}{2}\frac{\delta l}{\delta u} : \mathfrak{g} \to \mathfrak{g}^*$, $u \mapsto Lu$. The inverse of the mapping arise from the Green's function of L, written as the kernel K. Such l defines a right-invariant inner product on the tangent bundle $T\,\mathrm{Diff}(\Omega)$ that descends to a Riemannian metric on Q. Because Q can be considered a subset of $\mathbb{R}^{Nd}$ using the representation above, the metric structure can be written directly as a cometric

$$\langle \xi, \eta \rangle_{\mathbf{q}} = \xi^T K(\mathbf{q}, \mathbf{q})\eta \tag{3}$$

using the kernel K evaluated on $\mathbf{q}$ for two covectors $\xi, \eta \in T_{\mathbf{q}}^* Q$. The kernel is often specified directly in the form $K(\mathbf{q}_1, \mathbf{q}_2) = \mathrm{Id}_d k(\|\mathbf{q}_1 - \mathbf{q}_2\|^2)$ for appropriate kernels k. One choice of k is the Gaussian kernel $k(x) = \alpha e^{-\frac{1}{2}x^T \Sigma^{-1} x}$ with matrix $\Sigma = \sigma\sigma^T$ specifying the spatial correlation structure, and $\alpha > 0$ a scaling of the general kernel amplitude.

Estimating parameters of K, with K as above α and the entries of Σ or σ, has to our knowledge previously only been treated for landmarks in the small-deformation setting [1]. While a linear vector space probability distribution is mapped to the manifold with small deformations, this paper concerns the situation when the probability distribution is constructed directly from the Riemannian metric on the nonlinear space Q. The approach has similarities with the estimation procedures derived in [20] where a metric on a finite dimensional Lie group is estimated to optimize likelihood of data on a homogeneous space arising as the quotient of the group by a closed subgroup. Though the landmark space can be represented as $\mathrm{Diff}(\Omega)/H$ with H the landmark isotropy subgroup [19], the approach of [20] can not directly be applied because of the infinite dimensionality of $\mathrm{Diff}(\Omega)$.

2.1 Brownian Motion

A diffusion processes $\mathbf{q}_t$ on a Riemannian manifold Q is said to be a Brownian motion if its generator is $\frac{1}{2}\Delta_g$ with Δ_g being the Laplace-Beltrami operator of the metric g. Such processes can be constructed in several ways, see e.g. [10]. By isometrically embedding Q in a Euclidean space $\mathbb{R}^p$, the process can be constructed as a process in $\mathbb{R}^p$ that will stay on Q a.s. The process can equivalently be characterized in coordinates as being solution to the Itô integral

$$dq_t^i = g^{kl}\Gamma(\mathbf{q}_t)_{kl}{}^i dt + \sqrt{g^*(\mathbf{q}_t)}^i dW_t \tag{4}$$

where $\sqrt{g^*}$ is a square root of the cometric tensor $[g^*]^{ij} = g^{ij}$, and the drift term arise from contraction of the Christoffel symbols $\Gamma_{kl}{}^i$ with the cometric. The noise term is infinitesimal increments dW of an $\mathbb{R}^{\dim(Q)}$-valued Brownian motion W_t. Equivalently, the Brownian motion can be constructed as a hypoelliptic diffusion processes in the orthonormal frame bundle OQ where a set of globally defined horizontal vector fields $H_1, \ldots, H_{\dim(Q)} \in TOQ$ gives the Stratonovich integral equation

$$du_t = H_i(u_t) \circ W_t^i . \tag{5}$$

Note the sum over the $\dim(Q)$ horizontal fields H_i. The process $\mathbf{q}_t = \pi(u_t)$ where $\pi : OQ \to Q$ is the bundle map is then a Brownian motion. This is known as the Eells-Elworthy-Malliavin construction of Brownian motion. The fields H_i evaluated at $u \in OQ$ model infinitesimal parallel transport of the vectors comprising the frame u in the direction of the ith frame vector, see e.g. [10].

While Brownian motion is per definition isotropic with equal variation in all directions, data with nontrivial covariance can be modeled by defining the SDE (5) in the larger frame bundle FQ [17,21] using nonorthonormal frames to model the square root of the local covariance structure. In this setup, the inference problem consists of finding the starting point of the diffusion and the square root covariance matrix. Estimators are defined via a Frechét mean-like minimization in FQ with square FQ distances used as proxy for the negative log-transition density. In this paper, we remove this proxy by approximating the actual transition density, but only in the isotropic Brownian motion case.

2.2 Large Deformation Stochastics

Several papers have recently derived models for Brownian motion [13] and stochastic dynamics in shape analysis and for landmark manifolds. [25, 26] considered stochastic shape evolution by adding finite and infinite dimensional noise in the momentum equation of the dynamics. In [14], noise is added to the momentum equation to make the landmark dynamics correspond to a type of heat bath appearing in statistical physics. In [3, 4] a stochastic model for shape evolution is derived that descends to the landmark space in the same fashion as the right-invariant LDDMM metric descends to Q. The fundamental structure is here the momentum map that is preserved by the introduction of right-invariant noise. The approach is linked to parametric SDEs in fluid dynamics [9] and stochastic coadjoint motion [2].

3 Brownian Bridge Simulation

Brownian motion can be numerically simulated on Q using the coordinate Itô form (4). With a standard Euler discretization, the scheme becomes

$$\mathbf{q}_{t_{k+1}} = \mathbf{q}_{t_k} + K(\mathbf{q}_{t_k}, \mathbf{q}_{t_k})^{kl} \Gamma(\mathbf{q}_t)_{kl} \Delta t + \sqrt{K(\mathbf{q}_{t_k}, \mathbf{q}_{t_k})}_j \Delta W_{t_k}^j \qquad (6)$$

with time discretization $t_1, \ldots, t_k$, $t_k - t_{k-1} = \Delta t$ and discrete noise $W_{t_1}, \ldots, W_{t_k} \in \mathbb{R}^{Nd}$, $\Delta W_{t_k} = \Delta W_{t_k} - \Delta W_{t_{k-1}}$. Alternatively, a Heun scheme for discrete integration of the Stratonovich Eq. (5) results in

$$v_{t_{k+1}} = H_i(u_{t_k}) \Delta W_{t_k}^i$$
$$u_{t_{k+1}} = u_{t_k} + \frac{v_{t_{k+1}} + H_i(u_{t_k} + v_{t_{k+1}}) \Delta W_{t_k}^i}{2}. \qquad (7)$$

Because the horizontal fields represent infinitesimal parallel transport, they can be expressed using the Christoffel symbols of g. The Christoffel symbols for the landmark metric are derived in [15] from which they can be directly implemented or implicitly retrieved from an automatic symbolic differentiation as done in the experiments in Sect. 5.

3.1 Bridge Sampling

The transition density $p_T(\mathbf{v})$ of a Brownian motion $\mathbf{q}_t$ evaluated at $\mathbf{v} \in Q$ at time $T > 0$ can be informally obtained by taking an expectation to get the "mass" of those of the sample paths hitting $\mathbf{v}$ at time T. We write $\mathbf{q}_t | \mathbf{v}$ for the process $\mathbf{q}_t$ conditioned on hitting $\mathbf{v}$ a.s. at $t = T$. Computing the expectation analytically is in nonlinear situations generally intractable. Instead, we wish to employ a Monte Carlo approach and thus derive a method for simulating from $\mathbf{q}_t | \mathbf{v}$. For this, we employ the bridge sampling scheme of Delyon and Hu [6]. We first describe the framework for a general diffusion process in Euclidean space before using it directly on the landmark manifold Q.

Let

$$dx_t = b(t, x_t)dt + \sigma(t, x_t)dW_t \qquad (8)$$

be an $\mathbb{R}^k$ valued Itô diffusion with invertible diffusion field σ. In order to sample from the conditioned process $x_t|v$, $v \in \mathbb{R}^k$, a modified processes is in [6] constructed by adding an extra drift term to the process giving the new process

$$dy_t = b(t, y_t)dt - \frac{y_t - v}{T - t}dt + \sigma(t, y_t)dW_t \ . \qquad (9)$$

As $t \to T$, the attraction term $-(y_t - v)/(T - t)dt$ becomes increasingly strong forcing the processes to hit y at $t = T$ a.s. It can be shown that the process y_t exists when b, σ and σ^{-1} are $C^{1,2}$ with bounded derivatives. The process is then absolutely continuous with respect to the conditioned process $x_t|v$. The Radon-Nikodym derivative between the laws $P_{x_t|v}$ and P_y is

$$\frac{dP_{x|v}}{dP_y}(y) = \frac{\varphi_T(y)}{E_y[\varphi_T]}$$

with $E_y[\cdot]$ denoting expectation with respect to P_y, and the correction factor $\varphi_T(y)$ defined as the $t \to T$ limit of

$$\varphi_t(y) = \exp\left(-\int_0^t \frac{\tilde{y}_s^T A(s, y_s)b(s, y_s)}{T - s}ds\right.$$
$$\left. -\frac{1}{2}\int_0^t \frac{\tilde{y}_s^T (dA(s, x_s))\tilde{y}_s + \sum_{i,j} d\langle A^{ij}(s, y_s), \tilde{y}_s^i \tilde{y}_s^j\rangle}{T - s}\right) \qquad (10)$$

Here $\tilde{y}_t = y_t - v$, $A = (\sigma\sigma^T)^{-1}$, and quadratic variation is denoted by $\langle .,.\rangle$. Then $E_x[f(x)|x_T = v] = E_{x|v}[f(x)] = E_y[f(y)\varphi_T(y)]/E_y[\varphi_T(y)]$ and

$$E[f(y)\varphi_t] = \frac{T^{k/2}e^{\frac{\|\sigma^{-1}(0, x_0)(x_0 - v)\|^2}{2T}}}{(T - t)^{k/2}}E\left[f(x)e^{-\frac{\|\sigma^{-1}(t, x_t)(x_t - v)\|^2}{2(T - t)}}\right]$$

for $t < T$. The fact that the diffusion field σ must be invertible for the scheme to work as outlined here can be seen explicitly from the use of the inverse of σ and A in these equations.

We can use the guided process (9) to take conditional expectation for general measurable functions on the Wiener space of paths $W(\mathbb{R}^k, [0, T])$ by sampling from y_t. Taking the particular choice of the constant function, the expression

$$p_T(v) = \sqrt{\frac{|A(T, v)|}{(2\pi T)^k}}e^{-\frac{\|\sigma(0, x_0)^{-1}(x_0 - v)\|^2}{2T}}E_y[\varphi_T(y)] \qquad (11)$$

for the transition density of x_t arise as shown in [16]. Note that both the leading factors and the correction factor φ_T are dependent on the diffusion field σ, the starting point x_0 of the diffusion, and the drift b. Again, we can approximate the expectation in (11) by sampling from y_t.

3.2 Landmark Bridge Simulation

Because the landmark manifold has a global chart on $\mathbb{R}^{Nd}$ from the standard representation of each landmark position in $\mathbb{R}^d$, we can conveniently apply the bridge construction of [6]. Writing the Itô coordinate form of the Brownian motion $\mathbf{q}_t$ (4) in the form (8), we have $b(t, \mathbf{q}) = K(\mathbf{q}, \mathbf{q})^{kl} \Gamma(\mathbf{q})_{kl}$ and $\sigma(t, \mathbf{q}) = \sqrt{K(\mathbf{q}, \mathbf{q})}$ giving the guided SDE

$$dy_t = K(\mathbf{y}_{t_k}, \mathbf{y}_{t_k})^{kl} \Gamma(\mathbf{y}_t)_{kl} dt - \frac{\mathbf{y}_t - \mathbf{v}}{T - t} dt + \sqrt{K(\mathbf{y}_{t_k}, \mathbf{y}_{t_k})} dW_t \qquad (12)$$

The attraction term $-(\mathbf{y}_t - \mathbf{v})/(T - t)dt$ is the difference between the current landmark configuration $\mathbf{y}_t$ and the target configuration $\mathbf{v}$. The transition density becomes

$$p_{T,\theta}(\mathbf{v}) = \frac{1}{\sqrt{|K(\mathbf{v}, \mathbf{v})|(2\pi T)^{Nd}}} e^{-\frac{\|(\mathbf{q}_0 - \mathbf{v})^T K(\mathbf{q}_0, \mathbf{q}_0)^{-1}(\mathbf{q}_0 - \mathbf{v})\|^2)}{2T}} E_{\mathbf{y}_\theta}[\varphi_{\theta,T}(\mathbf{y})] \qquad (13)$$

where we use the subscript θ to emphasize the dependence on the parameters $\mathbf{q}_0$ and the kernel K. As above, the expectation $E_{\mathbf{y}_\theta}[\varphi_{\theta,T}(\mathbf{y})]$ can be approximated by drawing samples from $\mathbf{y}_\theta$ and evaluating $\varphi_{\theta,T}(\mathbf{y})$.

Remark 1. A similar scheme is used for the bridge simulation of the stochastic coadjoint processes of [3,4]. In these cases, the flow is hypoelliptic in the phase space $(\mathbf{q}, \mathbf{p})$ and observations are partial in that only the landmark positions $\mathbf{q}$ are observed. The momenta $\mathbf{p}$ are unobserved. In addition, the fact that the landmarks can carry a large initial momentum necessitates a more general form of the guidance term $-(\mathbf{y}_t - \mathbf{v})/(T - t)dt$ that takes into account the expected value of $E_{\mathbf{y}}[\mathbf{y}_T | (\mathbf{q}_t, \mathbf{p}_t)]$ of the process at time T given the current time t position and momentum of the process.

4 Inference Algorithm

Given a set of i.i.d. observations $\mathbf{q}^1, \ldots, \mathbf{q}^N$ of landmark configurations, we assume the configurations $\mathbf{q}^i$ are distributed according to the time $t = T$ transition distribution $\mathbf{q}_T$ of a Brownian motion on Q started at $\mathbf{q}_0$. We now intend to infer parameters θ of the model. With the metric structure on Q given by (3) and kernel of the form $K(\mathbf{q}_1, \mathbf{q}_2) = \mathrm{Id}_d k(\|\mathbf{q}_1 - \mathbf{q}_2\|^2)$, $k(x) = \alpha e^{-\frac{1}{2} x^T \Sigma x}$, parameters are the starting position $\mathbf{q}_0$, α, and $\Sigma = \sigma \sigma^T$, i.e. $\theta = (\mathbf{q}_0, \alpha, \sigma)$.

The likelihood of the model given the data with respect to the Lebesgue measure on $\mathbb{R}^{Nd}$ is

$$\mathcal{L}_\theta(\mathbf{q}^1, \ldots, \mathbf{q}^N) = \prod_{i=1}^N p_{T,\theta}(\mathbf{q}^i). \qquad (14)$$

Using our ability to approximate (13) by bridge sampling, we aim to find a maximum-likelihood estimate (MLE) $\hat{\theta} \in \mathrm{argmin}_\theta \mathcal{L}_\theta(\mathbf{q}^1, \ldots, \mathbf{q}^N)$. We do this by a gradient based optimization on θ, see Algorithm 1. Note that the likelihood and thus the MLE of θ are dependent on the chosen background measure, in this case coming from the canonical chart on $\mathbb{R}^{Nd}$.

Algorithm 1. Metric estimation: Inference of parameters θ from samples.

for $l = 1$ *until convergence* **do**
  for $i = 1$ *to* N **do**
    sample J paths from guided process $\mathbf{y}_{\theta_l}$ hitting $\mathbf{q}^i$
    compute correction factors $\varphi_{\theta_l,T}^{i,j}$
  end
  $\mathcal{L}_{\theta_l}(\mathbf{q}^1,\ldots,\mathbf{q}^N) \leftarrow$
  $\prod_{i=1}^{N} \frac{1}{\sqrt{|K(\mathbf{q}^i,\mathbf{q}^i)|(2\pi T)^{Nd}}} e^{-\frac{\|(\mathbf{q}_0-\mathbf{q}^i)^T K(\mathbf{q}_0,\mathbf{q}_0)^{-1}(\mathbf{q}_0-\mathbf{q}^i)\|^2)}{2T}} \frac{1}{J}\sum_{j=1}^{J} \varphi_{\theta_l,T}^{i,j}$
  $\theta_{l+1} = \theta_l + \epsilon\nabla_{\theta_l}\mathcal{L}_{\theta_l}(\mathbf{q}^1,\ldots,\mathbf{q}^N)$
end

Remark 2. The inference Algorithm 1 optimizes the likelihood $\mathcal{L}_\theta$ directly by stochastic gradient descent. A different but related approach is an Expectation-Maximization approach where the landmark trajectories between $t = 0$ and the observation time $t = T$ are considered missing data. The E-step of the EM algorithm would then involve the expectation $E_{\mathbf{x}|\mathbf{q}^i}[\log p(\mathbf{x})]$ of the landmark bridges conditioned on the data with $p(\mathbf{x})$ formally denoting a likelihood of an unconditioned sample path $\mathbf{x}$. This approach is used in e.g. [4]. While natural to formulate, the approach involves the likelihood $p(\mathbf{x})$ of a stochastic path which is only defined for finite time discretizations. In addition, the expected correction factor $E_{\mathbf{y}}[\varphi_T(\mathbf{y})]$ that arise when using the guided process $\mathbf{y}$ in the estimation appears as a normalization factor in the EM Q-function. This can potentially make the scheme sensitive to the stochasticity in the Monte Carlo sampling of the expected correction $E_{\mathbf{y}}[\varphi_T(\mathbf{y})]$. While the differences between these approaches needs further investigation, we hypothesize that direct optimization of the likelihood is superior in the present context.

Remark 3. Instead of taking expectations over $\mathbf{q}_T$, we can identify the most probable path of the conditioned process $\mathbf{q}_t|\mathbf{v}$. This results in the Onsager-Machlup functional [8]. In [18], a different definition is given that, in the isotropic Brownian motion situation, makes the set of Riemannian geodesics from $\mathbf{q}_0$ to $\mathbf{v}$ equal to the set of most probable paths of the conditioned process $\mathbf{q}_t|\mathbf{v}$. The sample Frechét mean

$$\operatorname{argmin}_{\mathbf{q}_0} \frac{1}{N}\sum_{i=1}^{N} d_g(\mathbf{q}_0,\mathbf{q}_i)^2 \tag{15}$$

is in that case formally also a minimizer of the negative log-probability of the most probable path to the data. Given that we are now able to approximate the density function of the Brownian motion, the MLE of the likelihood (14) with respect to $\mathbf{q}_0$ is equivalent to

$$\operatorname{argmin}_{\mathbf{q}_0} -\frac{2}{N}\sum_{i=1}^{N} \log p_{T,\mathbf{q}_0}(\mathbf{q}_i) \ . \tag{16}$$

Compared to (15), the negative log-probability of the data is here minimized instead of the squared geodesic distance. The estimator (16) can therefore be considered a transition density equivalent of the sample Frechét mean.

5   Numerical Experiments

We here present examples of the method on simulated landmark configurations, and an application of the method and algorithm to landmarks annotated on cardiac images of left ventricles. We aim for testing the ability of the algorithm to infer the parameters of the model given samples. We here take the first steps in this direction and leave a more extensive simulation study to future work.

For the simulated data, we compare the results against the true values used in the simulation. In addition, we do simple model checking for both experiments by simulating with the estimated parameters and comparing the per-landmark sample mean and covariance.

We use code based on the Theano library [23] for the implementation, in particular the symbolic expression and automatic derivative facilities of Theano. The code used for the experiments is available in the software package *Theano Geometry* http://bitbucket.org/stefansommer/theanogeometry. The implementation and the use of Theano for differential geometry applications including landmark manifolds is described in [12].

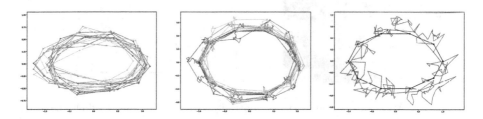

Fig. 2. (left) Samples from the transition distribution of a Brownian motion perturbing an ellipse configuration with 10 landmarks. (center) Subset of the samples shown together with trajectories of the stochastic landmark Brownian motion started at configuration q_0 (black points). (right) A guided bridge from q_0 (black points) to a sample (blue points). (Color figure online)

With 10 landmarks arranged in an ellipse configuration q_0, we sample 64 samples from the transition distribution at time $T = 1$ of a Brownian motion started at q_0, see Fig. 2. Parameters for the kernel are $\sigma = \text{diag}(\sigma_1, \sigma_2)$ with σ_1, σ_2 set to the average inter-point distance in q_0, and the amplitude parameter $\alpha = 0.01$.

We run Algorithm 1 with initial conditions for q_0 the pointwise mean of the samples. The parameter evolution trough the iterative optimization and the result of the inference can be seen in Fig. 3. The algorithm is able t estimate the

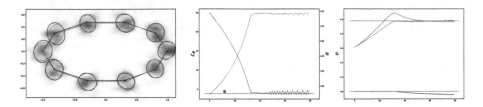

Fig. 3. (left) Result of the inference algorithm applied to the synthetic ellipse samples. The initial configuration $\mathbf{q}_0$ (black points) is showed along with the per-landmark sample covariance from the samples (black ellipses). The estimated initial configuration $\hat{\mathbf{q}}_0$ (blue points) is shown along with the per-landmark sample covariance from a new set of samples obtained with the inferred parameters (blue ellipses). (center) Evolution of likelihood (green) and α (blue) during the optimization. Horizontal axis shows number of iterations and red line is α ground truth. (right) Evolution of the entries of the kernel covariance σ (blue lines) during the optimization, red lines ground truth. (Color figure online)

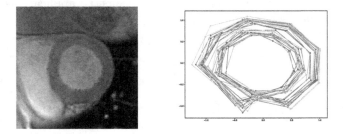

Fig. 4. (left) An image of a left cardiac ventricle with annotations. (right) The annotations from 14 cardiac images.

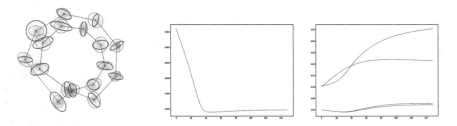

Fig. 5. Results of applying the inference algorithm to the cardiac data. Setup and subfigures as in Fig. 3.

initial configuration and the parameters of α and Σ with a reasonable precision. The sample per-landmark covariance as measured on a new set of simulated data with the estimated parameters is comparable to the per-landmark covariance of the original dataset.

5.1 Left Cardiac Ventricles

To exemplify the approach on real data, we here use a set of landmarks obtained from annotations of the left ventricle in 14 cardiac images [22]. Each ventricle is annotated with sets of landmarks from which we select 17 from each configuration for use in this experiment. Figure 4 shows an annotated image along with the sets of annotations for all images.

Figure 5 shows the results of the inference algorithm with setup equivalent to Fig. 3. While the parameters converges during the iterative optimization, we here have no ground-truth comparison. A subsequent sampling using the estimated parameters allows comparison of the per-landmark sample covariance. While the new sample covariance in magnitude and to some degree shape corresponds to the sample covariance from the original data, the fact that the Brownian motion is isotropic forces the covariance to be equivalent for all landmarks as measured by the Riemannian landmark metric. Including anisotropic covariance in the distribution or the right-invariant stochastics of [3,4] would allow the per-landmark covariance to vary and result in a closer fit.

6 Conclusion

In the paper, we have derived a method for maximum likelihood estimation of parameters for the starting point of landmark Brownian motions and for the Riemannian metric structure specified from the kernel K. Using the guided process scheme of [6] for sampling conditioned Brownian bridges, the transition density is approximated by Monte Carlo sampling. With this approximation of the data likelihood, we use a gradient based iterative scheme to optimize parameters. We show on synthetic and real data sets the ability of the method to infer the underlying parameters of the data distribution and hence the metric structure of the landmark manifold.

A direct extension of the method presented here is to generalize to the anisotropic normal distributions [17] defined via Brownian motions in the frame bundle FQ. This would allow differences in the per-landmark covariance and thus improve results on datasets such as the presented left ventricle annotations. Due to the hypoellipticity of the anisotropic flows that must be conditioned on hitting fibers in FQ above points $q \in Q$, further work is necessary to adapt the scheme presented here to the anisotropic case.

Acknowledgements. We are grateful for the use of the cardiac ventricle dataset provided by Jens Chr. Nilsson and Bjørn A. Grønning, Danish Research Centre for Magnetic Resonance (DRCMR).

References

1. Allassonnire, S., Amit, Y., Trouve, A.: Towards a coherent statistical framework for dense deformable template estimation. J. R. Stat. Soc. Ser. B (Stat. Methodol.) **69**(1), 3–29 (2007)
2. Arnaudon, A., Castro, A.L., Holm, D.D.: Noise and dissipation on coadjoint orbits. JNLS, arXiv:1601.02249 [math-ph, physics: nlin], January 2016
3. Arnaudon, A., Holm, D.D., Pai, A., Sommer, S.: A stochastic large deformation model for computational anatomy. In: Niethammer, M., Styner, M., Aylward, S., Zhu, H., Oguz, I., Yap, P.-T., Shen, D. (eds.) IPMI 2017. LNCS, vol. 10265, pp. 571–582. Springer, Cham (2017). doi:10.1007/978-3-319-59050-9_45
4. Arnaudon, A., Holm, D.D., Sommer, S.: A geometric framework for stochastic shape analysis. Submitted, arXiv:1703.09971 [cs, math], March 2017
5. Beg, M.F., Miller, M.I., Trouv, A., Younes, L.: Computing large deformation metric mappings via geodesic flows of diffeomorphisms. IJCV **61**(2), 139–157 (2005)
6. Delyon, B., Hu, Y.: Simulation of conditioned diffusion and application to parameter estimation. Stoch. Process. Appl. **116**(11), 1660–1675 (2006)
7. Dupuis, P., Grenander, U., Miller, M.I.: Variational problems on flows of diffeomorphisms for image matching. Q. Appl. Math. **56**(3), 587–600 (1998)
8. Fujita, T., Kotani, S.: The Onsager-Machlup function for diffusion processes. J. Math. Kyoto Univ. **22**(1), 115–130 (1982)
9. Holm, D.D.: Variational principles for stochastic fluid dynamics. Proc. Math. Phys. Eng. Sci. **471**(2176), 20140963 (2015). The Royal Society
10. Hsu, E.P.: Stochastic Analysis on Manifolds. American Mathematical Society, Providence (2002)
11. Joshi, S., Miller, M.: Landmark matching via large deformation diffeomorphisms. IEEE Trans. Image Process. **9**(8), 1357–1370 (2000)
12. Kuhnel, L., Sommer, S.: Computational anatomy in Theano. In: Mathematical Foundations of Computational Anatomy (MFCA) (2017)
13. Markussen, B.: Large deformation diffeomorphisms with application to optic flow. Comput. Vis. Image Underst. **106**(1), 97–105 (2007)
14. Marsland, S., Shardlow, T.: Langevin equations for landmark image registration with uncertainty. SIAM J. Imaging Sci. **10**(2), 782–807 (2017)
15. Micheli, M.: The differential geometry of landmark shape manifolds: metrics, geodesics, and curvature. Ph.D. thesis, Brown University, Providence, USA (2008)
16. Papaspiliopoulos, O., Roberts, G.O.: Importance sampling techniques for estimation of diffusion models. In: Statistical Methods for Stochastic Differential Equations. Chapman & Hall/CRC Press (2012)
17. Sommer, S.: Anisotropic distributions on manifolds: template estimation and most probable paths. In: Ourselin, S., Alexander, D.C., Westin, C.-F., Cardoso, M.J. (eds.) IPMI 2015. LNCS, vol. 9123, pp. 193–204. Springer, Cham (2015). doi:10.1007/978-3-319-19992-4_15
18. Sommer, S.: Anisotropically weighted and nonholonomically constrained evolutions on manifolds. Entropy **18**(12), 425 (2016)
19. Sommer, S., Jacobs, H.O.: Reduction by lie group symmetries in diffeomorphic image registration and deformation modelling. Symmetry **7**(2), 599–624 (2015)
20. Sommer, S., Joshi, S.: Brownian bridge simulation and metric estimation on lie groups and homogeneous spaces (2017, in preparation)
21. Sommer, S., Svane, A.M.: Modelling anisotropic covariance using stochastic development and sub-Riemannian frame bundle geometry. J. Geom. Mech. **9**(3), 391–410 (2017)

22. Stegmann, M.B., Fisker, R., Ersbll, B.K.: Extending and applying active appearance models for automated, high precision segmentation in different image modalities. In: Scandinavian Conference on Image Analysis, pp. 90–97 (2001)
23. Team, T.T.D.: Theano: a Python framework for fast computation of mathematical expressions. arXiv:1605.02688 [cs], May 2016
24. Trouve, A.: An infinite dimensional group approach for physics based models in patterns recognition (1995)
25. Trouve, A., Vialard, F.X.: Shape splines and stochastic shape evolutions: a second order point of view. Q. Appl. Math. **70**(2), 219–251 (2012)
26. Vialard, F.X.: Extension to infinite dimensions of a stochastic second-order model associated with shape splines. Stoch. Process. Appl. **123**(6), 2110–2157 (2013)

White Matter Fiber Segmentation Using Functional Varifolds

Kuldeep Kumar[1,2(✉)], Pietro Gori[2,4], Benjamin Charlier[2,5],
Stanley Durrleman[2], Olivier Colliot[2,3], and Christian Desrosiers[1]

[1] LIVIA, École de technologie supérieure (ÉTS), Montreal, Canada
kkumar@livia.etsmtl.ca, kuldeepkumar.iitkgp@gmail.com
[2] Aramis Project-team, Inria Paris, Sorbonne Universités, UPMC Univ Paris 06,
Inserm, CNRS, Institut du cerveau et la moelle (ICM), Hôpital Pitié-Salpêtrière,
Boulevard de l'hôpital, 75013 Paris, France
[3] AP-HP, Departments of Neurology and Neuroradiology, Hôpital Pitié-Salpêtrière,
75013 Paris, France
[4] LTCI Lab - IMAGES Group, Télécom ParisTech, Paris, France
[5] Université de Montpellier, Montpellier, France

Abstract. The extraction of fibers from dMRI data typically produces a
large number of fibers, it is common to group fibers into bundles. To this
end, many specialized distance measures, such as MCP, have been used
for fiber similarity. However, these distance based approaches require
point-wise correspondence and focus only on the geometry of the fibers.
Recent publications have highlighted that using microstructure measures
along fibers improves tractography analysis. Also, many neurodegenerative diseases impacting white matter require the study of microstructure
measures as well as the white matter geometry. Motivated by these, we
propose to use a novel computational model for fibers, called functional
varifolds, characterized by a metric that considers both the geometry
and microstructure measure (e.g. GFA) along the fiber pathway. We use
it to cluster fibers with a dictionary learning and sparse coding-based
framework, and present a preliminary analysis using HCP data.

1 Introduction

Recent advances in diffusion magnetic resonance imaging (dMRI) analysis have
led to the development of powerful techniques for the non-invasive investigation
of white matter connectivity in the human brain. By measuring the diffusion
of water molecules along white matter fibers, dMRI can help identify connection pathways in the brain and better understand neurological diseases related
to white matter [6]. Since the extraction of fibers from dMRI data, known as
tractography, typically produces a large number of fibers, it is common to group
these fibers into larger clusters called *bundles*. Clustering fibers is also essential
for the creation of white matter atlases, visualization, and statistical analysis of
microstructure measures along tracts [12].

Most fiber clustering methods use specialized distance measures, such as
Mean Closest Points (MCP) distance [4,11]. However, these distance-based

© Springer International Publishing AG 2017
M.J. Cardoso et al. (Eds.): GRAIL/MFCA/MICGen 2017, LNCS 10551, pp. 92–100, 2017.
DOI: 10.1007/978-3-319-67675-3_9

approaches require point-wise correspondence between fibers and only consider fiber geometry. Another important aspect for white matter characterization is the statistical analysis of microstructure measures. As highlighted in recent publications, using microstructure measures along fibers improves tractographic analysis [3, 10, 12, 15–17]. Motivated by these, we propose to use a novel computational model for fibers, called functional varifolds, characterized by a metric that considers both the geometry and microstructure measure (e.g. generalized fractional anisotropy) along fiber pathways.

Motivation for this work comes from the fact that the integrity of white matter is an important factor underlying many cognitive and neurological disorders. In vivo, tissue properties may vary along each tract for several reasons: different populations of axons enter and exit the tract, and disease can strike at local positions within the tract. Hence, understanding diffusion measures along each fiber tract (i.e., tract profile) may reveal new insights into white matter organization, function, and disease that are not obvious from mean measures of that tract or from the tract geometry alone [3, 17]. Recently, many approaches have been proposed for tract based morphometry [12], which perform statistical analysis of microstructure measures along major tracts after establishing fiber correspondences. While studies highlight the importance of microstructure measures, most approaches either consider the geometry or signal along tracts, but not both. The intuitive approach would be to consider microstructure signal during clustering also. However, this has been elusive due to lack of appropriate framework.

As a potential solution, we explore a novel computational model for fibers, called functional varifolds [1], which is a generalization of the varifolds framework [2]. The advantages of using functional varifolds are as follows. First, functional varifolds can model the fiber geometry as well as signal along the fibers. Also, it does not require pointwise correspondences between fibers. Lastly, fibers do not need to have the same orientation as in the framework of currents [5]. We test the impact of this new computational model on a fiber clustering task, and compare its performance against existing approaches for this task.

As clustering method, we reformulate the dictionary learning and sparse coding based framework proposed in [7–9]. This choice of framework is driven by its ability to describe the entire data-set of fibers in a compact dictionary of prototypes. Bundles are encoded as sparse non-negative combinations of multiple dictionary prototypes. This alleviates the need for explicit representation of a bundle centroid, which may not be defined or may not represent an actual object. Also, sparse coding allows assigning single fibers to multiple bundles, thus providing a soft clustering.

The contributions of this paper are threefold: (1) a novel computational model for modeling both fiber geometry and signal along fibers, (2) a generalized clustering framework, based on dictionary learning and sparse coding, adapted to the computational models, and (3) a comprehensive comparison of fully-unsupervised models for clustering fibers.

2   White Matter Fiber Segmentation Using Functional Varifolds

2.1   Modeling Fibers Using Functional Varifolds

In the framework of functional varifolds [1,2], a fiber X is assumed to be a polygonal line of P segments described by their center point $x_p \in \mathbb{R}^3$ and tangent vector $\boldsymbol{\beta_p} \in \mathbb{R}^3$ centered at x_p and of length c_p (respectively, $y_q \in \mathbb{R}^3$, $\boldsymbol{\gamma_q} \in \mathbb{R}^3$ and d_q for a fiber Y with Q segments). Let f_p and g_p be the signal values at center points x_p and y_q respectively, and ω the vector field belonging to a reproducing kernel Hilbert space (RKHS) W^*. Then the fibers X and Y can be modeled based on functional varifolds as: $V_{(X,f)}(\omega) \approx \sum_{p=1}^{P} \omega(x_p, \boldsymbol{\beta_p}, f_p)c_p$ and $V_{(Y,g)}(\omega) \approx \sum_{q=1}^{Q} \omega(y_q, \boldsymbol{\gamma_q}, g_p)d_q$. More details can be found in [1].

The inner product metric between X and Y is defined as:

$$\langle V_{(X,f)}, V_{(Y,g)} \rangle_{W^*} = \sum_{p=1}^{P} \sum_{q=1}^{Q} \kappa_f(f_p, g_q)\kappa_x(x_p, y_q)\kappa_\beta(\boldsymbol{\beta_p}, \boldsymbol{\gamma_q})c_p d_q \tag{1}$$

where κ_f and κ_x are Gaussian kernels and κ_β is a Cauchy-Binet kernel. This can be re-written as:

$$\langle V_{(X,f)}, V_{(Y,g)} \rangle_{W^*} = \sum_{p=1}^{P} \sum_{q=1}^{Q} \exp\left(\frac{-\|f_p - g_q\|^2}{\lambda_M^2}\right) \exp\left(\frac{-\|x_p - y_q\|^2}{\lambda_W^2}\right) \left(\frac{\boldsymbol{\beta_p}^T \boldsymbol{\gamma_q}}{c_p d_q}\right)^2 c_p d_q \tag{2}$$

where λ_M and λ_W are kernel bandwidth parameters. For varifolds [2], a computational model using only fiber geometry and used for comparison in the experiments, we drop the signal values at center points. Thus, the varifolds-based representation of fibers will be: $V_X(\omega) \approx \sum_{p=1}^{P} \omega(x_p, \boldsymbol{\beta_p})c_p$ and $V_Y(\omega) \approx \sum_{q=1}^{Q} \omega(y_q, \boldsymbol{\gamma_q})d_q$. Hence, the inner product is defined as:

$$\langle V_X, V_Y \rangle_{W^*} = \sum_{p=1}^{P} \sum_{q=1}^{Q} \exp\left(\frac{-\|x_p - y_q\|^2}{\lambda_W^2}\right) \left(\frac{\boldsymbol{\beta_p}^T \boldsymbol{\gamma_q}}{c_p d_q}\right)^2 c_p d_q. \tag{3}$$

2.2   Fiber Clustering Using Dictionary Learning and Sparse Coding

For fiber clustering, we extend the dictionary learning and sparse coding based framework presented in [7–9]. Let V_T be the set of n fibers modeled using functional varifolds, $A \in \mathbb{R}_+^{n \times m}$ be the atom matrix representing the dictionary coefficients for each fiber belonging to one of the m bundles, and $W \in \mathbb{R}_+^{m \times n}$ be the cluster membership matrix containing the sparse codes for each fiber. Instead of explicitly representing bundle prototypes, each bundle is expressed as a linear combination of all fibers. The dictionary is then defined as $D = V_T A$. Since this operation is linear, it is defined for functional varifolds.

The problem of dictionary learning using sparse coding [7,8] can be expressed as finding the matrix A of m bundle prototypes and the fiber-to-bundle assignment matrix W that minimize the following cost function:

$$\underset{A,W}{\arg\min} \quad \frac{1}{2}\|V_T - V_T AW\|_{W^*}^2, \quad \text{subject to: } \|\boldsymbol{w}_i\|_0 \leq S_{\max}. \tag{4}$$

Parameter $S_{\max}$ defines the maximum number of non-zero elements in $\boldsymbol{w}_i$ (i.e., the sparsity level), and is provided by the user as input to the clustering method.

An important advantage of using the above formulation is that the reconstruction error term only requires inner product between the varifolds. Let $Q \in \mathbb{R}^{n \times n}$ be the Gram matrix denoting inner product between all pairs of training fibers, i.e., $Q_{ij} = \langle V_{X_i, f_i}, V_{X_j, f_j} \rangle_{W^*}$. Matrix Q can be calculated once and stored for further computations. The problem then reduces to linear algebra operations involving matrix multiplications. The solution of Eq. (4) is obtained by alternating between sparse coding and dictionary update [8]. The sparse codes of each fiber can be updated independently by solving the following sub-problem:

$$\underset{\boldsymbol{w}_i \in \mathbb{R}_+^m}{\arg\min} \quad \frac{1}{2}\|V_{X_i} - V_T A\boldsymbol{w}_i\|_{W^*}^2, \quad \text{subject to: } \|\boldsymbol{w}_i\|_0 \leq S_{\max}. \tag{5}$$

which can be re-written as:

$$\underset{\boldsymbol{w}_i \in \mathbb{R}_+^m}{\arg\min} \quad \frac{1}{2}\left(Q(i,i) + \boldsymbol{w}_i^\top A^\top QA\boldsymbol{w}_i - 2Q(i,:)A\boldsymbol{w}_i\right), \quad \text{s.t.: } \|\boldsymbol{w}_i\|_0 \leq S_{\max}. \tag{6}$$

The non-negative weights $\boldsymbol{w}_i$ can be obtained using the kernelized Orthogonal Matching Pursuit (kOMP) approach proposed in [8], where the most *positively* correlated atom is selected at each iteration, and the sparse weights $\boldsymbol{w}_s$ are obtained by solving a non-negative regression problem. Note that, since the size of $\boldsymbol{w}_s$ is bounded by $S_{\max}$, it can be otained rapidly. Also, in case of a large number of fibers, the Nystrom method can be used for approximating the Gram matrix [7]. For dictionary update, A is recomputed by applying the following update scheme, until convergence:

$$A_{ij} \leftarrow A_{ij} \frac{(QW^\top)_{ij}}{(QAWW^\top)_{ij}}, \quad i = 1, \ldots, n, \quad j = 1, \ldots, m. \tag{7}$$

3   Experiments

Data: We evaluate different computational models on the dMRI data of 10 unrelated subjects (6 females and 4 males, age 22–35) from the Human Connectome Project (HCP) [14]. DSI Studio [18] was used for the signal reconstruction (in MNI space, 1 mm), and streamline tracking employed to generate 50,000 fibers per subject (minimum length 50 mm, maximum length 300 mm). Generalized Fractional Anisotropy (GFA), which extends standard fractional anisotropy to orientation distribution functions, was considered as along-tract measure of microstructure. While we report results obtained with GFA, any other along-tract measure may have been used.

Parameter impact: We performed k-means clustering and manually selected pairs of fibers from clusters most similar to major bundles. We then modeled these fibers using different computational models, and analyzed the impact of varying the kernel bandwidth parameters. The range of these parameters were estimated by observing the values of distance between centers of fiber segments and difference between along tract GFA values for selected multiple pairs of fibers. Figure 1 (top left) shows GFA color-coded fibers for 3 pairs corresponding to (a) right Corticospinal tract – CST (R), (b) Corpus Callosum – CC, and (c) right Inferior Fronto-Occipital Fasciculus – IFOF (R). Cosine similarity (in degrees) is reported for the fiber pairs modeled using varifolds (Var) and functional varifolds (fVar), for $\lambda_W = 7$ mm and $\lambda_M = 0.01$.

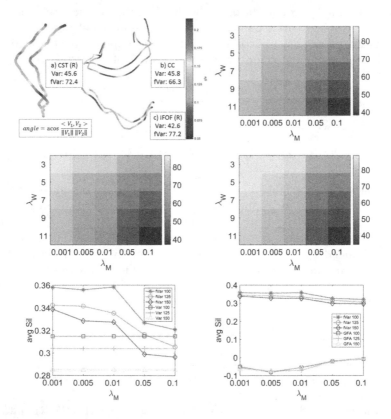

Fig. 1. Along-fiber GFA visualization and cosine similarity between pairs of fibers from three prominent bundles: (a) CST (R), (b) CC, (c) IFOF (R), using framework of varifolds (Var) and functional varifolds (fVar) (top left), and Comparing variation of cosine similarity for the select fiber pairs over kernel bandwidth parameters λ_W and λ_M for the framework of functional varifolds (top right: CST (R), middle left: CC, middle right: IFOF (R)); Impact of λ_M on clustering consistency (measured using Average Silhouette) for $m = 100, 125, 150$ for functional Varifolds vs Varifolds (bottom left), and functional Varifolds vs GFA only (bottom right) (Color figure online)

Figure 1 (top left) shows GFA color-coded fiber pairs. The color-coded visualization reflect the variation of fiber geometry, microstructure measure (i.e. GFA) along fiber, and difference in GFA along fiber for the select fiber pairs. This visualization of variation and difference in GFA values along fibers support our hypothesis that modeling along tract signal along with geometry provides additional information. The change in cosine similarity for CC from 45.8° (using varifolds) to 66.3° (using functional varifolds) while for CST (R) from 45.6° to 72.4°, reflect more drop in cosine similarity if along tract signal profiles are not similar. This shows that functional varifolds imposes penalty for different along fiber signal profiles.

Figure 1 also compares the impact of varying the kernel bandwidth parameters for functional varifolds using similarity angle between pairs of these selected fibers (top right: CST (R), bottom left: CC, bottom right: IFOF (R)). We show variation over $\lambda_W = 3$, 5, 7, 9 and 11 (mm) and $\lambda_M = 0.001$, 0.005, 0.01, 0.05, and 0.1.

Comparing the parameter variation images in Fig. 1 we observe that the cosine similarity values over the parameter space show similar trends for all 3 pairs of fibers. This observation allows us to select a single pair of parameter values for our experiments. We have used $\lambda_W = 7$ mm and $\lambda_M = 0.01$ for our experiments based on the cosine similarity values in Fig. 1. The smaller values for λ_W (<7 mm) and λ_M (<0.01 mm) will make the current fiber pairs orthogonal while for larger values we lose the discriminative power as all fiber pairs will have very high similarity.

Quantitative analysis: We report a quantitative evaluation of clusterings obtained using as functional varifolds (fVar), varifolds (var), MCP and GFA computational model. The same dictionary learning and sparse coding framework is applied for all computational models. For each of the 10 HCP subjects, we compute the Gramian matrix using 5,000 fibers randomly sampled over the full brain for 3 seed values. The MCP distance d_{ij} is calculated between each fiber pair (i, j), as described in [4], and the Gramian matrix obtained using a radial basis function (RBF) kernel: $k_{ij} = \exp\left(-\gamma \cdot d_{ij}^2\right)$. Parameter γ was set empirically to 0.007 in our experiments.

Model	$m{=}100$	$m{=}125$	$m{=}150$
fVar	**0.3624**	**0.3451**	**0.3314**
Var	0.3356	0.3089	0.2905
GFA	-0.0579	-0.0584	-0.0610
MCP	0.3240	0.2888	0.2619

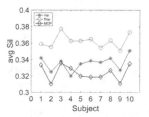

Fig. 2. Mean silhouette obtained with Varifolds, Varifolds, GFA, and MCP, computed for varying a number of clusters, over 10 subjects and 3 seed values *(left)*. Detailed results obtained for 10 subjects using $m = 100$ *(right)*.

Since our evaluation is performed in an unsupervised setting, we use the silhouette measure [11,13] to assess and comparing clustering consistency. Silhouette values, which range from -1 to 1, measure how similar an object is to its own cluster (cohesion) compared to other clusters (separation). Figure 1 (bottom row) shows impact of λ_M on clustering consistency for functional Varifolds w.r.t Varifolds and GFA only. Figure 2 (right) gives the average silhouette for $m = 100$, 125, and 150 clusters, computed over 10 subjects and 3 seed values. The impact of using both geometry and microstructure measures along fibers is evaluated quantitatively by comparing clusterings based on functional varifolds with those obtained using only geometry (i.e., varifolds, MCP), and only along-fiber signal (i.e., GFA). As can be seen, using GFA alone leads to poor clusterings, as reflected by the negative silhouette values. Comparing functional varifolds with varifolds and GFA, we observe a consistently improved performance for different numbers of clusters. To further validate this hypothesis, we also report the average silhouette (over 3 seed values) obtained for 10 subjects using $m = 100$. These

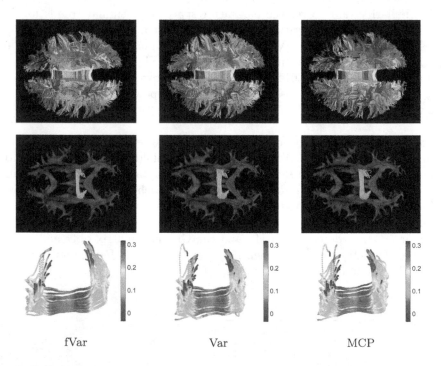

Fig. 3. Full clustering visualization ($m = 100$, top row), single cluster visualization (mid row), and GFA based color coded visualization of the selected single cluster (bottom row). Using following computational models for fibers: functional varifolds (left column), varifolds (middle column), and MCP distance (right column). Superior axial views. Note: (top row) each figure has a unique color code. (Color figure online)

results demonstrate that functional varifolds give consistently better clustering, compared to other computational models using the same framework[1].

Qualitative visualization: Figure 3 (top row) shows the dictionary learned for a single subject ($m = 100$) using functional varifolds (fVar), varifolds (Var), and MCP distance. For visualization purposes, each fiber is assigned to a single cluster, which is represented using a unique color. The second and third rows of the figure depict a specific cluster and its corresponding GFA color-coded profiles. We observe that all three computational models produce plausible clusterings. From the GFA profiles of the selected cluster (with correspondence across computational models), we observe that functional varifolds enforce both geometric *as well as* along-tract signal profile similarity. Moreover, the clustering produced with varifolds or MCP (i.e., using only geometric properties of fibers), are similar to one another and noticeably different from that of functional varifolds.

4 Conclusion

A novel computational model, called functional varifolds, was proposed to model both geometry and microstructure measure along fibers. We considered the task of fiber clustering and integrated our functional varifolds model within framework based on dictionary learning and sparse coding. The driving hypothesis that combining along-fiber signal with fiber geometry helps tractography analysis was validated quantitatively and qualitatively using data from Human Connectome Project. Results show functional varifolds to yield more consistent clusterings than GFA, varifolds and MCP. While this study considered a fully unsupervised setting, further investigation would be required to assess whether functional varifolds augment or aid the reproducibility of results.

Acknowledgements. Data were provided by the Human Connectome Project.

References

1. Charlier, B., Charon, N., Trouvé, A.: The fshape framework for the variability analysis of functional shapes. Found. Comput. Math. **17**, 1–71 (2014)
2. Charon, N., Trouvé, A.: The varifold representation of nonoriented shapes for diffeomorphic registration. SIAM J. Imaging Sci. **6**(4), 2547–2580 (2013)
3. Colby, J.B., Soderberg, L., Lebel, C., Dinov, I.D., Thompson, P.M., Sowell, E.R.: Along-tract statistics allow for enhanced tractography analysis. Neuroimage **59**(4), 3227–3242 (2012)
4. Corouge, I., Gouttard, S., Gerig, G.: Towards a shape model of white matter fiber bundles using diffusion tensor MRI. In: ISBI 2004, pp. 344–347. IEEE (2004)
5. Gori, P., et al.: A prototype representation to approximate white matter bundles with weighted currents. In: Golland, P., Hata, N., Barillot, C., Hornegger, J., Howe, R. (eds.) MICCAI 2014. LNCS, vol. 8675, pp. 289–296. Springer, Cham (2014). doi:10.1007/978-3-319-10443-0_37

---

[1] Silhouette analyzes only clustering consistency, not the along-fiber signal profile.

6. Hagmann, P., Jonasson, L., Maeder, P., Thiran, J.P., Wedeen, V.J., Meuli, R.: Understanding diffusion mr imaging techniques: from scalar diffusion-weighted imaging to diffusion tensor imaging and beyond. Radiographics **26**(suppl-1), S205–S223 (2006)

7. Kumar, K., Desrosiers, C.: A sparse coding approach for the efficient representation and segmentation of white matter fibers. In: ISBI 2016, pp. 915–919. IEEE (2016)

8. Kumar, K., Desrosiers, C., Siddiqi, K.: Brain fiber clustering using non-negative kernelized matching pursuit. In: Zhou, L., Wang, L., Wang, Q., Shi, Y. (eds.) MLMI 2015. LNCS, vol. 9352, pp. 144–152. Springer, Cham (2015). doi:10.1007/978-3-319-24888-2_18

9. Kumar, K., Desrosiers, C., Siddiqi, K., Colliot, O., Toews, M.: Fiberprint: a subject fingerprint based on sparse code pooling for white matter fiber analysis. NeuroImage **158**, 242–259 (2017)

10. Maddah, M., Grimson, W.E.L., Warfield, S.K., Wells, W.M.: A unified framework for clustering and quantitative analysis of white matter fiber tracts. Med. Image Anal. **12**(2), 191–202 (2008)

11. Moberts, B., Vilanova, A., van Wijk, J.J.: Evaluation of fiber clustering methods for diffusion tensor imaging. In: VIS 2005, pp. 65–72. IEEE (2005)

12. O'Donnell, L.J., Westin, C.F., Golby, A.J.: Tract-based morphometry for white matter group analysis. Neuroimage **45**(3), 832–844 (2009)

13. Siless, V., Medina, S., Varoquaux, G., Thirion, B.: A comparison of metrics and algorithms for fiber clustering. In: PRNI 2013, pp. 190–193. IEEE (2013)

14. Van Essen, D.C., Smith, S.M., Barch, D.M., Behrens, T.E., Yacoub, E., Ugurbil, K., Consortium, W.M.H.: The WU-Minn human connectome project: an overview. Neuroimage **80**, 62–79 (2013)

15. Wang, Q., Yap, P.T., Wu, G., Shen, D.: Application of neuroanatomical features to tractography clustering. Hum. Brain Mapp. **34**(9), 2089–2102 (2013)

16. Wassermann, D., Bloy, L., Kanterakis, E., Verma, R., Deriche, R.: Unsupervised white matter fiber clustering and tract probability map generation: applications of a Gaussian process framework for white matter fibers. NeuroImage **51**(1), 228–241 (2010)

17. Yeatman, J.D., Dougherty, R.F., Myall, N.J., Wandell, B.A., Feldman, H.M.: Tract profiles of white matter properties: automating fiber-tract quantification. PloS One **7**(11), e49790 (2012)

18. Yeh, F.C., Tseng, W.Y.I.: NTU-90: a high angular resolution brain atlas constructed by q-space diffeomorphic reconstruction. Neuroimage **58**(1), 91–99 (2011)

Prediction of the Progression of Subcortical Brain Structures in Alzheimer's Disease from Baseline

Alexandre Bône[1,2(✉)], Maxime Louis[1,2], Alexandre Routier[1,2],
Jorge Samper[1,2], Michael Bacci[1,2], Benjamin Charlier[2,3], Olivier Colliot[1,2],
Stanley Durrleman[1,2], and the Alzheimer's Disease Neuroimaging Initiative

[1] Sorbonne Universités, UPMC Université Paris 06,
Inserm, CNRS, Institut du Cerveau et de la Moelle (ICM) -
Hôpital Pitié-Salpêtrière, 75013 Paris, France
alexandre.bone@icm-institute.org
[2] Aramis Project-team, Inria Paris, 75013 Paris, France
[3] Université de Montpellier, Montpellier, France

Abstract. We propose a method to predict the subject-specific longitudinal progression of brain structures extracted from baseline MRI, and evaluate its performance on Alzheimer's disease data. The disease progression is modeled as a trajectory on a group of diffeomorphisms in the context of large deformation diffeomorphic metric mapping (LDDMM). We first exhibit the limited predictive abilities of geodesic regression extrapolation on this group. Building on the recent concept of parallel curves in shape manifolds, we then introduce a second predictive protocol which personalizes previously learned trajectories to new subjects, and investigate the relative performances of two parallel shifting paradigms. This design only requires the baseline imaging data. Finally, coefficients encoding the disease dynamics are obtained from longitudinal cognitive measurements for each subject, and exploited to refine our methodology which is demonstrated to successfully predict the follow-up visits.

1 Introduction

The primary pathological developments of a neurodegenerative disease such as Alzheimer's are believed to spring long before the first symptoms of cognitive decline. Subtle gradual structural alterations of the brain arise and develop along the disease course, in particular in the hippocampi regions, whose volumes are classical biomarkers in clinical trials. Among other factors, those transformations ultimately result in the decline of cognitive functions, which can be assessed through standardized tests. Being able to track and predict future structural changes in the brain is therefore key to estimate the individual stage of disease progression, to select patients and provide endpoints in clinical trials.

A. Bône and M. Louis—Equal contributions.

© Springer International Publishing AG 2017
M.J. Cardoso et al. (Eds.): GRAIL/MFCA/MICGen 2017, LNCS 10551, pp. 101–113, 2017.
DOI: 10.1007/978-3-319-67675-3_10

To this end, our work settles down to predict the future shape of brain structures segmented from MRIs. We propose a methodology based on three building blocks: extrapolate from the past of a subject; transfer the progression of a reference subject observed over a longer time period to new subjects; and refine this transfer with information about the relative disease dynamics extracted from cognitive evaluations. Instead of limiting ourselves to specific features such as volumes, we propose to see each observation of a patient at a given time-point as an image or a segmented surface mesh in a shape space.

In computational anatomy, shape spaces are usually defined via the action of a group of diffeomorphisms [1,16,17]. In this framework, one may estimate a flow of diffeomorphisms such that a shape continuously deformed by this flow best fits repeated observations of the same subject over time, thus leading to a subject-specific spatiotemporal trajectory of shape changes [8,12]. If the flow is geodesic in the sense of a shortest path in the group of diffeomorphisms, this problem is called geodesic regression [4,5,8,12] and may be thought of as the extension to Riemannian manifolds of the linear regression concept. It is tempting then to use such regression to infer the future evolution of the shape given several past observations. To the best of our knowledge, the predictive power of such a method has not yet been extensively assessed. We will demonstrate that satisfying results can only be obtained when large numbers of data points over extensive periods of time are available, and that poor ones should be expected in the more interesting use-case scenario of a couple of observations.

In such situations, an appealing workaround would be to transfer previously acquired knowledge from another patient observed over a longer period of time. This idea requires the definition of a spatiotemporal matching method to transport the trajectory of shape changes into a different subject space. Several techniques have been proposed to register image time series of different subjects [11,18]. They often require time series to have the same number of images, or to have correspondences between images across time series, and are therefore unfit for prognosis purposes. Parallel transport in groups of diffeomorphisms has been recently introduced to infer deformation of follow-up images from baseline matching [10,15]. Such paradigms have been used mostly to transport spatiotemporal trajectories to the same anatomical space for hypothesis testing [6,13]. Two main methodologies have emerged: either by parallel-transporting the time series along the baseline matching as in [5], or by parallel-transporting the baseline matching along the time series as in [14]. We evaluate both in this paper.

In any case, these approaches require to match the baseline shape with one in the reference time series. Ideally, we should match observations corresponding to the same disease stage, which is unknown. We propose to complement such approaches with estimates of the patient stage and pace of progression using repeated neuropsychological assessments in the spirit of [14]. These estimates are used to adjust the dynamics of shape changes of the reference subject to the test one, according to the dynamical differences observed in the cognitive tests.

Among the main contributions of this papers are: the first quantitative study of the predictive power of geodesic regression; a new methodology for the prediction of shape progression from baseline; the evaluation of its accuracy for two different parallel shifting protocols; new evidence of the utter importance of capturing the individual dynamics in Alzheimer's disease models.

Section 2 sets the theoretical background and incrementally describes our methodology. Section 3 presents and discusses the resulting performances.

2   Method

Let $(y_j)_{j=1,..,n_i}$ be a time series of segmented surface meshes for a given subject $i \in \{1, ..., N\}$, obtained at the ages $(t_j)_{j=1,..,n_i}$. We build a group of diffeomorphisms of the ambient space which act on the segmented meshes, following the procedure described in [3]. Flows of diffeomorphisms of $\mathbb{R}^3$ are generated by integrating time-varying vector fields of the form $v(t,x) = \sum_{k=1}^{n_{cp}} K[x, c_k(t)]\beta_k(t)$ where K is a Gaussian kernel, $c(t) = [c_k(t)]_{k=1,..,n_{cp}}$ and $\beta(t) = [\beta_k(t)]_{k=1,..,n_{cp}}$ are respectively the control points and the momenta of the deformation.

We endow the space of diffeomorphisms with a norm which measures the cost of the deformation. In the following, we only consider geodesic flows of diffeomorphisms i.e. flows of minimal norm connecting the identity to a given diffeomorphism. Such flows are uniquely parametrized by their initial control points and momenta $c^0 = c(0)$, $\beta^0 = \beta(0)$. Under the action of the flow of diffeomorphisms, an initial template shape T is continuously deformed and describes a trajectory in the shape space, which we will note $t \rightarrow \gamma_{(c^0, \beta^0)}(T, t)$. Simultaneously, we endow the surface meshes with a varifold norm $\| \cdot \|$ which allows to measure a data attachment term between meshes without point correspondence [3].

2.1   Geodesic Regression

In the spirit of linear regression, one can perform geodesic regression in the shape space by estimating the intercept T and the slope (c^0, β^0) such that $\gamma_{(c^0, \beta^0)}(T, \cdot)$ minimizes the following functional :

$$\inf_{c^0, \beta^0, T} \sum_{j=1}^{n_i} \|\gamma_{(c^0, \beta^0)}(T, t_j) - y_j\|^2 + R(c^0, \beta^0) \tag{1}$$

where R is a regularization term which penalizes the kinetic energy of the deformation. We estimate a solution of Eq. (1) with a Nesterov gradient descent as implemented in the software Deformetrica (www.deformetrica.org), where the gradient with respect to the control points, the momenta and the template is computed with a backward integration of the data attachment term along the geodesic [2].

Once an optimum is found, we obtain a description of the progression of the brain structures which lies in the tangent space at the identity of the group of diffeomorphisms. It is natural to attempt to extrapolate from the obtained geodesic to obtain a prediction of the progression of the structures.

2.2 Two Methods to Transport Spatiotemporal Trajectories of Shapes

As it will be demonstrated in Sect. 3, geodesic regression extrapolation produces an accurate prediction only if data over a long time span is available for the subject, which is not compatible with the goal of early prognosis.

As proposed in [10,19], given a reference geodesic, we use the Riemannian parallel transport to generate a new trajectory. We first perform a baseline matching between the reference subject and the new subject, which can be described as a vector in the tangent space of the group of diffeomorphisms. Two paradigms are available to obtain a parallel trajectory. [15] advises to transport the reference regression along the matching and then shoot. In the shape space, this generates a geodesic starting at the baseline shape; for this reason, we call this solution *geodesic parallelization*, and is illustrated on Figure (A1). On the other hand, [14] advocates to transport the matching vector along the reference geodesic and then build a trajectory with this transported vector from every point of the reference geodesic, as described on Figure (B1). We will call this procedure *exp-parallelization*.

In such a high-dimensional setting, the computation of parallel transport classically relies on the Schild's ladder scheme [9]. However, in our case the computation of the Riemannian logarithm may only be computed by solving a shape matching problem, resulting not only in an computationally expensive algorithm but also in an uncontrolled approximation of the scheme. To implement these parallel shifting methods, we use the algorithm suggested in [19], which relies on an approximation of the transport to nearby points by a well-chosen Jacobi field, with a sharp control on the computational complexity. The same rate of convergence as Schild's ladder is obtained at a reduced cost.

2.3 Cognitive Scores Dynamics

The protocol described in the previous section has two main drawbacks. First, the choice of the matching time in the reference trajectory is arbitrary: the baseline is purely a convenience choice and ideally the matching should be performed at similar stages of the disease. Second, it does not take into account the pace of progression of the subject. In [14], the authors propose a statistical model allowing to learn, in an unsupervised manner, dynamical parameters of the subjects from ADAS-cog test results, a standardized cognitive test designed for disease progression tracking. More specifically, they suppose that each patient follows a parallel to a mean trajectory, with a time reparametrization:

$$\psi(t) = \alpha(t - t_0 - \tau) + t_0 \qquad (2)$$

which maps the subject time to a normalized time frame, where $\alpha > 0$ and τ are scalar parameters. A high (resp. low) α hence corresponds to a fast (resp. slow) progression of the scores, when a negative (resp. positive) τ corresponds to an early decay (resp. late decay) of those scores. In the dataset introduced below, the acceleration factors $(\alpha_i)_i$ range from 0.15 to 6.01 and the time-shifts $(\tau_i)_i$ from -20.6 to 22.8, thus showing a tremendous variability in the individual dynamics of the disease, which must be taken into account.

With these dynamic parameters, the shape evolution can be adjusted by reparametrizing the parallel trajectory with the same formula (2), as illustrated on Figures (A2) and (B2).

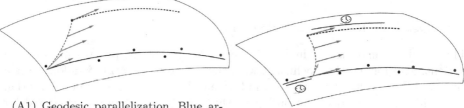

(A1) Geodesic parallelization. Blue arrow: baseline matching. Red arrows: transported regression. Black dotted line : exponentiation of the transported regression.

(A2) Reparametrized geodesic parallelization. Matching time and exp-parallel trajectory are reparametrized.

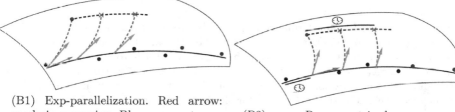

(B1) Exp-parallelization. Red arrow: geodesic regression. Blue arrows: transported baseline matching. Black dotted line : exp-parallelization of the reference geodesic for the given subject.

(B2)   Reparametrized   exp-parallelization. Matching time and exp-parallel trajectory are reparametrized.

3   Results

3.1   Data, Preprocessing, Parameters and Performance Metric

MRIs are extracted from the ADNI database, where only MCI converters with 7 visits or more are kept, for a total of $N=74$ subjects and 634 visits. Subjects are observed for a period of time ranging from 4 to 9 years (5.9 on average), with 12 visits at most. The 634 MRIs are segmented using the FreeSurfer software. The extracted brain masks are then affinely registered towards the Colin 27 Average Brain using the FSL software. The estimated transformations are finally applied to the pairs of caudates, hippocampi and putamina subcortical structures.

All diffeomorphic operations i.e. matching, geodesic regression estimation, shooting, exp-parallelization and geodesic parallelization are performed thanks to the Deformetrica software previously mentioned. A varifold distance with Gaussian kernel width of 3 mm for each structure and a deformation kernel width of 5 mm are chosen. The time discretization resolution is set to 2 months.

The chosen performance metric between two sets of meshes is the Dice coefficient, that is the sum of the volumes of the intersections of the corresponding meshes, divided by the total sum of the volumes. We only measure the volume of the intersection between corresponding structures. The Dice coefficient is comprised between 0 and 1: it equals 1 for a perfect match, and 0 for disjoint structures.

3.2   Geodesic Regression Extrapolation

The acceleration factor α in Eq. (2) encodes the rate of progression of each patient. Multiplying this coefficient with the actual observation window gives a notion of the absolute observation window length, in the disease time referential. Only the 22 first subjects according to this measure have been considered for this section: they are indeed expected to feature large structural alterations, making the geodesic regression procedure more accurate. The geodesic regression predictive performance is compared to a naive one consisting in leaving the last observed brain structures in the learning dataset unchanged.

Table 1. Averaged Dice performance measures between predictions and observations for varying extents of learning datasets and extrapolation. The [reg] tag indicates the regression-based prediction, and [naive] the naive one. Each row corresponds to an increasingly large learning dataset, patients being observed for widening periods of time. Each column corresponds to an increasingly remote predicted visit from baseline. Significance levels [.05, .01, .001, .0001] for the Mann-Whitney test.

Learning period (months)	Method	Predicted follow-up visit					
		M12 N=22	M24 N=21	M36 N=19	M48 N=18	M72 N=16	M96 N=5
6	[reg]	.878	.800	.737	.624	.509	.483
	[naive]	.888	.850	.803	.708	.626	.602
12	[reg]	-	.839	.769	.658	.523	.465
	[naive]	-	.875	.832	.735	.644	.608
18	[reg]	-	.885	.823	.738	.611	.579
	[naive]	-	.890	.851	.764	.661	.627
24	[reg]	-	-	.864	.778	.681	**.657**
	[naive]	-	-	.869	.779	.689	.653
max - 1	[reg]	**.807**	Prediction at the most remote possible time				
~60 months	[naive]	.797	point (~76 months) for all subjects (N=22).				

Table 1 presents the results obtained for varying learning dataset and extrapolation extents. We perform a Mann-Whitney test with the null hypothesis that the observed Dice coefficients distributions are the same to obtain the statistical significance levels. The extrapolated meshes are satisfying only in the case where all but one data points are used to perform the geodesic regression, achieving a high Dice index and outperforming the naive one, by a small margin though and failing to reach the significance level ($p = 0.25$). When the window of observation becomes narrower, the prediction accuracy decreases and becomes worse than the naive one. Indeed, the lack of robustness of the – although standard – segmentation pipeline imposes a high noise level, which seems to translate into a too low signal-to-noise ratio after extrapolation from only a few observations.

Figure 1 displays an extrapolated geodesic regression for a specific subject, with a large learning period of 72 months, and a prediction at 108 months from the baseline (Dice performance of 0.74 versus 0.65 with the naive approach).

3.3 Non Reparametrized Transport

Among the 22 subjects whose regression-based predictive power has been evaluated in the previous section, the two which performed best are chosen as references for the rest of this paper. Their progressions are transported onto the 73 other subjects with the two different parallel shifting methods.

Table 2. Averaged Dice performance measures between predictions and observations for two modes of transport, with or without refinement by the cognitive scores. In each cell, the first line corresponds to the exp-parallelization-based prediction [exp], the middle line to the geodesic parallelization-based one [geod], and the last line to the naive approach [naive]. Each column corresponds to an increasingly remote predicted visit from baseline. Significance levels for the Mann-Whitney test [.05, .01, .001, .0001].

Time reparam.	Method	Predicted follow-up visit					
		M12	M24	M36	M48	M72	M96
		N=144	N=138	N=130	N=129	N=76	N=11
Without reparam.	[exp]	.878	.841	.799	.744	.650	.647
	[geod]	.883	.847	.806	.753	.664	**.661**
	[naive]	.882	**.850**	.806	**.754**	**.682**	.611
		N=140	N=134	N=123	N=113	N=62	N=17
With reparam.	[exp]	.882	.852	.825	.796	.756	.730
	[geod]	**.888**	**.858**	**.831**	**.802**	**.762**	**.732**
	[naive]	.884	.852	.809	.764	.706	.636

In more details, for each pair of reference and target subjects, the baseline target shape is first registered to the reference baseline. The reference geodesic regression is then either geodesically or exp-parallelized. Prediction performance is finally assessed: the Dice index between the prediction and the actual observation, for the two modes of transport, are computed and compared to the Dice

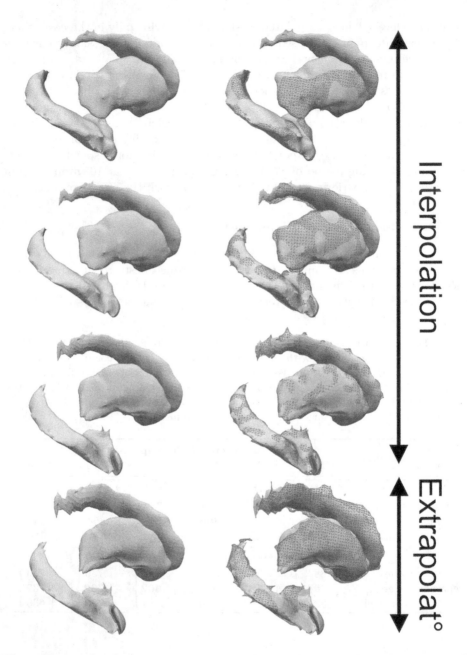

Fig. 1. Extrapolated geodesic regression for the subject s0671. Are only represented the right hippocampus, caudate and putamen brain structures in each subfigure. The three first rows present the interpolated brain structures, corresponding to ages 61.2, 64.2 and 67.2 (years). The last row presents the extrapolation result at age 70.2. On the right column are added the target brain structures (red wireframes), segmented from the original images. (Color figure online)

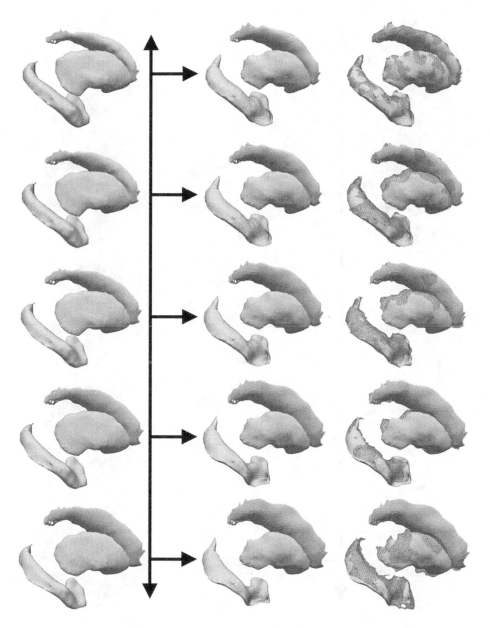

Fig. 2. Exp-parallelization of the reference subject s0906 (first column) towards the subject s1080 (second column), giving predictions for ages 81.6, 82.6, 83.6, 84.6 and 85.6 (years). On the third column are added the target brain structures (red wireframes), segmented from the original images. (Color figure online)

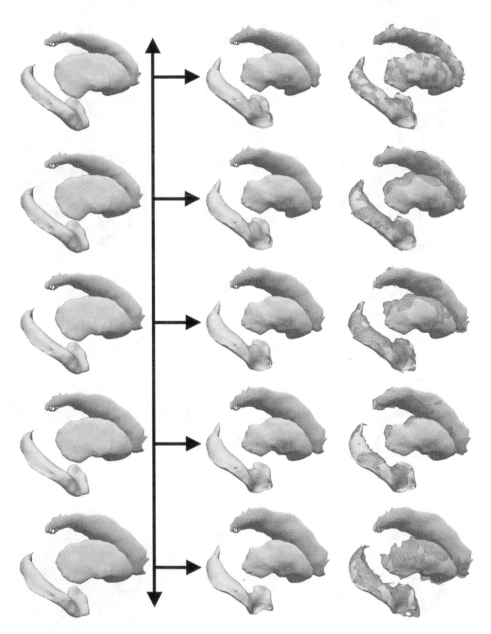

Fig. 3. Time-reparametrized exp-parallelization of the reference subject s0906 (first column) towards the subject s1080 (second column), giving predictions for ages 81.6, 82.6, 83.6, 84.6 and 85.6 (years). On the third column are added the target brain structures (red wireframes), segmented from the original images. (Color figure online)

index between the baseline meshes and the actual observation – the only available information in the absence of a predictive paradigm.

The upper part of Table 2 presents the results. In most cases, the obtained meshes by the proposed protocol are of lesser quality than the reference ones, according to the Dice performance metric. The two methods of transport are essentially similarly predictive, although geodesic parallelization slightly outperforms the exp-parallelization for the M12 prediction.

3.4 Refining with Cognitive Dynamical Parameters

The two reference progressions are transported through geodesic and exp-parallelization onto all remaining subjects. After time-reparametrization, the obtained parallel trajectories then deliver predictions for the brain structures.

Figure 3 displays a reference geodesic and an exp-parallelized curve. The predicted progression graphically matches the datapoints, and it can be noticed that the final prediction at age 85.6 (Dice 0.73) outperforms the corresponding one on Fig. 2, obtained without time-reparametrization (Dice 0.69).

Quantitative results are presented in the lower part of Table 2. At the exception of the M12 prediction, both protocols outperform the naive one. The M36, M48, M72 and M96 predictions are the most impressive ones, with p-values always lesser than 1%. This shows that the pace of cognitive score evolution is well correlated with the pace of structural brain changes, and therefore allows an enhanced prediction of follow-up shapes.

No conclusion can be drawn concerning the two parallel shifting methodologies, a single weak significance result being obtained only for the M12 prediction where the geodesic parallelization method slightly outperforms the exp-parallelization one with a Dice score of 0.888 versus 0.882.

4   Conclusion

We conducted a quantitative study of geodesic regression extrapolation, exhibiting its limited predictive abilities. We then proposed a method to transport a spatiotemporal trajectory into a different subject space with cognitive decline-derived time reparametrization, and demonstrated its potential for prognosis. The results show how crucial the dynamics are in disease modeling, and how cross-modality data can be exploited to improve a learning algorithm. The two main paradigms that have emerged for the transport of parallel trajectories were shown to perform equally well in this prediction task. Nonetheless, the exp-parallelization offers a methodological advantage in that the generated trajectories do not depend on a particular choice of point on the reference geodesic, in contrast with the trajectories obtained by geodesic parallelization. It takes full advantage of the isometric property of the parallel transport, and eases the combination with time-warp functions based on the individual disease dynamics.

In future work, more complex time reparametrization could be considered as in [7]. Finally, the robustness of the proposed protocol to the choice of reference subject has not been assessed. Such a choice could be avoided by constructing an average disease model as in [15], or by translating for shapes the method of [14]. We may also use this framework to estimate a joint image and cognitive model to better estimate individual dynamical parameters of disease progression.

Acknowledgments. This work has been partly funded by the European Research Council (ERC) under grant agreement No 678304, European Union's Horizon 2020 research and innovation program under grant agreement No 666992, and the program Investissements d'avenir ANR-10-IAIHU-06.

References

1. Beg, M., Miller, M., Trouvé, A., Younes, L.: Computing large deformation metric mappings via geodesic flows of diffeomorphisms. IJCV **61**(2), 139–157 (2005)
2. Durrleman, S., Allassonnière, S., Joshi, S.: Sparse adaptive parameterization of variability in image ensembles. IJCV **101**(1), 161–183 (2013)
3. Durrleman, S., Prastawa, M., Charon, N., Korenberg, J.R., Joshi, S., Gerig, G., Trouvé, A.: Morphometry of anatomical shape complexes with dense deformations and sparse parameters. NeuroImage **101**, 35–49 (2014)
4. Fishbaugh, J., Prastawa, M., Gerig, G., Durrleman, S.: Geodesic regression of image and shape data for improved modeling of 4D trajectories. In: Proceedings of the International Symposium on Biomedical Imaging (2014)
5. Fletcher, T.: Geodesic regression and the theory of least squares on riemannian manifolds. IJCV **105**(2), 171–185 (2013)
6. Hadj-Hamou, M., Lorenzi, M., Ayache, N., Pennec, X.: Longitudinal analysis of image time series with diffeomorphic deformations: A computational framework based on stationary velocity fields. Front. Neurosci. **10**, 236 (2016)
7. Hong, Y., Singh, N., Kwitt, R., Niethammer, M.: Time-warped geodesic regression. In: Golland, P., Hata, N., Barillot, C., Hornegger, J., Howe, R. (eds.) MICCAI 2014. LNCS, vol. 8674, pp. 105–112. Springer, Cham (2014). doi:10.1007/978-3-319-10470-6_14
8. Lorenzi, M., Ayache, N., Frisoni, G., Pennec, X.: 4D registration of serial brain MR images: a robust measure of changes applied to Alzheimer's disease. In: MICCAI, Spatio Temporal Image Analysis Workshop (STIA) (2010)
9. Lorenzi, M., Ayache, N., Pennec, X.: Schild's ladder for the parallel transport of deformations in time series of images. In: Székely, G., Hahn, H.K. (eds.) IPMI 2011. LNCS, vol. 6801, pp. 463–474. Springer, Heidelberg (2011). doi:10.1007/978-3-642-22092-0_38
10. Lorenzi, M., Pennec, X.: Geodesics, parallel transport & one-parameter subgroups for diffeomorphic image registration. IJCV **105**(2), 111–127 (2013)
11. Metz, C., Klein, S., Schaap, M., van Walsum, T., Niessen, W.: Nonrigid registration of dynamic medical imaging data using nD + t B-splines and a groupwise optimization approach. Med. Image Anal. **15**(2), 238–249 (2011)
12. Peyrat, J.-M., Delingette, H., Sermesant, M., Pennec, X., Xu, C., Ayache, N.: Registration of 4D time-series of cardiac images with multichannel diffeomorphic demons. In: Metaxas, D., Axel, L., Fichtinger, G., Székely, G. (eds.) MICCAI 2008. LNCS, vol. 5242, pp. 972–979. Springer, Heidelberg (2008). doi:10.1007/978-3-540-85990-1_117

13. Qiu, A., Younes, L., Miller, M.I., Csernansky, J.G.: Parallel transport in diffeomorphisms distinguishes the time-dependent pattern of hippocampal surface deformation due to healthy aging and the dementia of the Alzheimer's type. NeuroImage **40**(1), 68–76 (2008)
14. Schiratti, J.B., Allassonnière, S., Colliot, O., Durrleman, S.: Learning spatiotemporal trajectories from manifold-valued longitudinal data. In: NIPS, vol. 28 (2015)
15. Singh, N., Hinkle, J., Joshi, S., Fletcher, P.T.: Hierarchical geodesic models in diffeomorphisms. IJCV **117**(1), 70–92 (2016)
16. Vercauteren, T., Pennec, X., Perchant, A., Ayache, N.: Non-parametric diffeomorphic image registration with the demons algorithm. In: Ayache, N., Ourselin, S., Maeder, A. (eds.) MICCAI 2007. LNCS, vol. 4792, pp. 319–326. Springer, Heidelberg (2007). doi:10.1007/978-3-540-75759-7_39
17. Wang, L., Beg, F., Ratnanather, T., Ceritoglu, C., Younes, L., Morris, J.C., Csernansky, J.G., Miller, M.I.: Large deformation diffeomorphism and momentum based hippocampal shape discrimination in dementia of the Alzheimer type. IEEE Trans. Med. Imaging **26**(4), 462–470 (2007)
18. Wu, G., Wang, Q., Lian, J., Shen, D.: Estimating the 4D respiratory lung motion by spatiotemporal registration and building super-resolution image. In: Fichtinger, G., Martel, A., Peters, T. (eds.) MICCAI 2011. LNCS, vol. 6891, pp. 532–539. Springer, Heidelberg (2011). doi:10.1007/978-3-642-23623-5_67
19. Younes, L.: Jacobi fields in groups of diffeomorphisms and applications. Q. Appl. Math. **65**(1), 113–134 (2007)

A New Metric for Statistical Analysis of Rigid Transformations: Application to the Rib Cage

Baptiste Moreau[1,2(✉)], Benjamin Gilles[1], Erwan Jolivet[3], Philippe Petit[2], and Gérard Subsol[1]

[1] Research-Team ICAR, LIRMM,
University of Montpellier/CNRS, Montpellier, France
baptiste.moreau@lirmm.fr
[2] LAB, PSA Renault, Paris, France
[3] CEESAR, Nanterre, France

Abstract. Statistical analysis of an anatomical structure composed of multiple objects is useful for many computational anatomy tasks as registration or classification. As rigid transformations do not belong to an Euclidean space, conventional mean and covariance formulas could not be applied to study the movement of each object with respect to the others. Some tools from Riemannian geometry are used instead, requiring the definition of a metric. We show that common metrics are not intuitive in the case of an object with an elongated shape and we propose a new one based on displacements of all the points of the structure. We describe the method to study the pose variability of a multi-object structure with this new metric. It is then applied to the statistical analysis of the rib cage which is composed of 24 elongated bones.

Keywords: Computational anatomy · Rigid transformations · Metric · Statistical analysis · Rib cage

1 Introduction

Statistical Shape Models are widely used to study variations of shapes for 3D anatomical structures. A simple and generic model to represent shapes is to distribute a set of points across the surface of the anatomical structure. Cootes *et al.* [1] proposed a method called Point Distribution Model, which consists of extracting the mean shape and a set of orthogonal modes of variation from a collection of training samples. Those statistical models are built on point-to-point correspondences. The number of variables could reach several hundreds depending on the point density of the geometry description. Such a statistical model correctly describes the intrinsic shape of the anatomical structure, and they are used to improve the performances of segmentation and registration algorithms [2,3].

However, they cannot represent in an intuitive way an articulated anatomical structure which is composed of several substructures which can move relatively

© Springer International Publishing AG 2017
M.J. Cardoso et al. (Eds.): GRAIL/MFCA/MICGen 2017, LNCS 10551, pp. 114–124, 2017.
DOI: 10.1007/978-3-319-67675-3_11

to the others, as for example a rib cage which is built from independent 24 ribs. In this case, we would like to characterize the intrinsic shapes of each substructure (e.g. each rib) but also the rigid motion (also called the pose) of the substructure with respect to a general frame (e.g. fixed on the spine). Capturing the pose variation of the substructures will lead to a Statistical Shape Model which is much more intuitively interpretable.

In general, a Statistical Shape Model is composed of a mean description and an analysis of the covariance of the variability of the structure shape with regard to the mean description which is given as a set of ordered orthogonal variation modes. In the case of sets of points, we are in an Euclidean space and we can use Principal Component Analysis (PCA). But, if we want to study pose statistics, we face the difficulty that the space of rigid transformations is not an Euclidean space. Thus, it is not possible to compute the mean of 3D rotations by using the conventional definition of the mean, regardless of the chosen representation for rotation (rotation matrix, rotation axis, Euler angles or quaternions).

Nevertheless, the set of rigid transformations $SE(3)$ has the structure of a manifold. A Riemannian metric on a manifold allows one to measure distances and angles. By defining a distance function between two 3D rigid transformations, the manifold locally resembles an Euclidean space, called the tangent space. Pennec [4] gave basic tools for probabilities and statistics in this general framework of Riemannian manifold and applies it to the statistics of rigid transformations. Fletcher [5] used the Riemannian framework to define Principal Geodesic Analysis (PGA) for statistical analysis of 3D boundary representations based on medial atoms linked by rigid transformations.

PGA aims at finding a geodesic subspace that minimize the sum of square distance of the points to their projection. However, as it is generally computationally complex, it is often approximated by a tangent PCA (tPCA), which maximizes the explanation of the covariance matrix by unfolding the distribution around the mean and making a standard PCA in the tangent space. Nevertheless, maximizing the explained variance (tPCA) and minimizing the unexplained variance (PGA) lead to different results on manifolds [6].

A key-point is then to define an efficient metric which is adapted to the application. In the case of the rib cage, we have very elongated objects: a small rotation applied on a point located far from the axis of rotation induces a large displacement even if the rotation angle is small. In this paper, we propose a new metric which takes into account in a more intuitive way the application of 3D rigid transformations on elongated objects. Then we use it to build an articulated Statistical Shape Model of the rib cage.

2   Defining an Adapted Metric for Elongated Structures

2.1   Limits of the Current Metric

Defining a distance function between two rigid transformations H_1 and H_2 is based on a norm function N:

$$d(H_1, H_2) = N(H_2^{-1} \circ H_1). \tag{1}$$

Several previous studies have defined a metric to perform tPCA on articulated anatomical structures with rigid transformations. First, a representation for 3D rotations has to be set: rotation matrix components [3,7], rotation vector with the Rodrigues' formula [8,9] or quaternions [10].

The most common norm is based on the vector representation of rotations. For $H \in SE(3)$ a rigid transformation decomposed into a rotation vector $r = \omega.(n_x, n_y, n_z)^T$ and a translation $t = (t_x, t_y, t_z)^T$:

$$N_{rotv}(H)^2 = t^T.t + r^T.r. \tag{2}$$

It is important to control the relative magnitude between translation (usually given in mm) and rotation (usually in radians) by a normalization process. For example, Boisvert *et al.* [9] defined an empirical real number that controls the relative weight of the translation and rotation in the computation of the norm. Without this normalization process, the first modes would be translation modes as they account for most of the variance magnitude compared to the rotation which values in radians are generally quite low.

Another normalization consists of scaling the object geometry so that its mean radius is set to 1. The displacements of points on the unit sphere is then given by the rotation angle in radian units [7].

With λ a normalization factor, the norm function is then:

$$N_{rotv}(H)^2 = t^T.t + \lambda r^T.r. \tag{3}$$

Nevertheless, to the authors' knowledge, available normalization methods cannot tackle the issue for elongated shape described below, as the ones shown in Fig. 1.

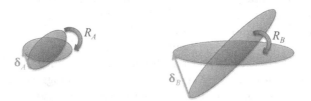

Fig. 1. Identical rotation applied on two objects: one compact and one elongated. The usual metric N_{rotv} is the same in both cases $[R_A = R_B \Rightarrow N_{rotv}(R_A) = N_{rotv}(R_B)]$ although displacements are different $[\delta_A < \delta_B]$.

This paper aims at providing a generic metric for $SE(3)$, relevant for all kind of shapes including elongated shapes, in order to apply a tPCA. The second contribution is of a more practical value and lies in applying this technique to the construction of an articulated statistical shape model of the rib cage.

2.2 A New Metric for Elongated Objects

For an object, a rigid transformation $H \in SE(3)$ induces a displacement field $\boldsymbol{\delta}(H)$. The object is sampled by points and the vector $\boldsymbol{\delta}(H)$ contains the displacements of these points. The norm function is now defined as follow:

$$N(H)^2 = \boldsymbol{\delta}(H)^T.\boldsymbol{\delta}(H). \tag{4}$$

This new norm can be compared with the common norm by introducing the moment of inertia.

The norm defined by rotation vector is commonly used [8], [9]. Let $\boldsymbol{r} \in SO(3)$ be a rotation vector. $\boldsymbol{r} = \omega.\boldsymbol{n}$ with ω the angle of rotation and $\boldsymbol{n}$ the unit vector of rotation. We have seen that the usual norm is:

$$N_{rotv}(\boldsymbol{r})^2 = \boldsymbol{r}^T.\boldsymbol{r} = \omega^2.\boldsymbol{n}^T.\boldsymbol{n}. \tag{5}$$

The inertia tensor of the object is $\overline{\overline{I}}$. The moment of inertia is defined for the rotation as follows:

$$I_C = \boldsymbol{n}^T.\overline{\overline{I}}.\boldsymbol{n}. \tag{6}$$

For a point $\boldsymbol{p_k} = (x, y, z)$ of the object, the displacement induced by the rotation $\boldsymbol{r}$ is $\boldsymbol{\delta_k} = \boldsymbol{r} \times \boldsymbol{p_k}$ with ω a small angle. With our metric:

$$N(\boldsymbol{r})^2 = \boldsymbol{\delta_k}^T.\boldsymbol{\delta_k},$$

$$= \omega^2.\boldsymbol{n}^T.(J_k^T.J_k).\boldsymbol{n} \text{ with } J_k = -\boldsymbol{p_k}\times = \begin{pmatrix} 0 & z & -y \\ -z & 0 & x \\ y & -x & 0 \end{pmatrix},$$

$$J_k^T.J_k = \begin{pmatrix} (y^2 + z^2) & -xy & -xz \\ -yx & (z^2 + x^2) & -yz \\ -zx & -zy & (x^2 + y^2) \end{pmatrix}.$$

Supposing that an object of mass m is homogeneous and uniformly sampled with points k, the inertia tensor is:

$$\overline{\overline{I}} = m \sum_k J_k^T.J_k. \tag{7}$$

Therefore, using the usual metric N_{rotv} makes the assumption that the inertia tensor is the identity matrix, and therefore that the shape is spherical. This usual norm is a good approximation when the object of interest is compact, but with elongated shape like ribs, the norm should take into account the specific geometry. For this purpose, our method uses the inertia tensor inertia tensor. We believed that using this metric, distances between pose of arbitrary shaped objects will be more appropriately measured as there is no more requirement for ad-hoc normalization between rotations and translations.

Under certain conditions (uniformly sampled object centered on its center of mass, undergoing a rigid motion), our distance has a physical interpretation: it is proportional to the kinetic energy necessary to move the object from one position to another.

3 Statistical Description of Rigid Transformations

3.1 Pose Variations

Some studies used a joint description to perform a tPCA [9,11]. They defined an anatomical frame for each object and the transformation between two connected objects was a joint. In particular, the joint method for tPCA is suitable for the spine as it describes physical articulations, but there are drawbacks for other structures. First, the connection graph must not contain any cycles as it is the case for the rib cage (Fig. 2). Indeed, a rib is articulated on both extremities with the spine and the sternum. Secondly, a fixed object as root of the tree must be determined. This can lead to numerical drift when an object is far from the fixed one. It is the same kind of issue than the elongated shape problem expressed previously.

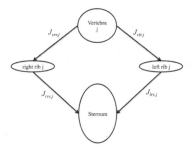

Fig. 2. Connection graph of the rib cage that shows the articulation loops.

To study pose variations of objects in the dataset, a generalized Procrustes analysis [12] is performed on each object separately. The rigid transformations (translation + rotation) applied to perform these multiple alignments as well as the mean shapes are used to study the pose variations (Fig. 3). With this method, we go beyond issues described for the joint description.

For an object j belonging to an instance i, $F_{i,j}$ is the coordinate vector of points. The mean shape of an object j among instances is $\overline{F_j}$ obtained from the multiple alignments. The rigid transformation $H_{i,j}$ is:

$$H_{i,j} = \underset{H \in SE(3)}{\arg\ \min} \| H(F_{i,j}) - \overline{F_j} \|. \tag{8}$$

The rigid transformations obtained from the multiple alignments revealed how instances differ rigidly from the mean shape of each object.

The mathematical space of rigid transformations is not an Euclidean space. Therefore, conventional statistics do not apply. However, tPCA concepts can be applied to generalize statistical notions like average and variance [5].

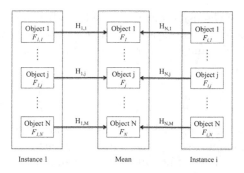

Fig. 3. The dataset contains instances composed of N objects described by point clouds $F_{i,j}$. $H_{i,j}$ is the rigid transformation that aligns the instance i on the mean shape.

3.2   Generalized Covariance

For a rigid transformation $H_{i,j} \in SE(3)$, $\delta_j(H_{i,j}) = H_{i,j}(\overline{F_j}) - \overline{F_j}$ is the displacement field induced by $H_{i,j}$ on the mean shape. The norm function was defined as follow:

$$N_j(H_{i,j})^2 = \delta_j(H_{i,j})^T . \delta_j(H_{i,j}). \tag{9}$$

The norm function is defined based on the mean shape, which means that only the mean shape inertia tensor is taken into account. This ensures that the norm does not change with the object being transformed.

With this definition of norm function, the distance between two rigid transformations, $H_{i_1,j}$ and $H_{i_2,j}$, from two different instances is:

$$d(H_{i_1,j}, H_{i_2,j}) = N_j(H_{i_2,j}^{-1} \circ H_{i_1,j}). \tag{10}$$

This distance is left-invariant as $d(H_3 \circ H_1, H_3 \circ H_2) = d(H_1, H_2)$.

Let us call *Log* the function that calculates the tangent description of a transformation according to the distance definition. The *Exp* function is the reverse of the *Log* function.

$$\boldsymbol{Log_{Id}}(H_{i,j}) = \delta_j(H_{i,j}),$$
$$\boldsymbol{Log_{H_{i_1,j}}}(H_{i_2,j}) = \boldsymbol{Log_{Id}}(H_{i_2,j}^{-1} \circ H_{i_1,j}).$$

$$Exp_{Id}(\boldsymbol{\delta_{i,j}}) = \underset{H \in SE(3)}{\arg\min}(N_j(H)^2),$$
$$Exp_{H_{i_1,j}}(\boldsymbol{\delta_{i_2,j}}) = H_{i_1,j} \circ Exp_{Id}(\boldsymbol{\delta_{i_2,j}}).$$

They correspond to the Riemannian *Exp/Log* for the left-invariant distance generated by the inertia tensor. This *Log* function is valid for small angles of rotation to get the property: $\boldsymbol{Log_{Id}}(H^{-1}) \approx -\boldsymbol{Log_{Id}}(H)$.

A generalization of the usual mean – called Fréchet mean – can be obtained by defining for an object j the mean as the rigid transformation μ_j that minimizes the sum of the distances with respect to the set of rigid transformations $H_{1,j}, \ldots, H_{N_i,j}$.

$$\mu_j = \arg\min_{H \in SE(3)} \left(\sum_{i=1}^{N_i} d(H, H_{i,j})^2 \right). \tag{11}$$

The Fréchet mean is computed by a simple gradient descent procedure [4]. This procedure is summarized by the following recurrent equation, with i an instance and N_i the number of instances in the sample.

$$\mu_{j,n+1} = Exp_{\mu_{j,n}} \left(\frac{1}{N_i} \sum_{i=1}^{N_i} \boldsymbol{Log}_{\mu_{j,n}}(H_{i,j}) \right). \tag{12}$$

In addition, a dispersion measure is needed to perform most tasks of practical interest. The covariance is usually defined as the expectation of the matrix product of the vectors from the mean. Thus, a similar definition for tPCA would be to compute the expectation in the tangent space of the mean using the Log function. Let j_1, j_2 be two objects with two mean shapes $\overline{F_{j_1}}, \overline{F_{j_2}}$, two sets of rigid transformations $set_{j_1} = \{H_{1,j_1}, \ldots, H_{N_i,j_1}\}, set_{j_2} = \{H_{1,j_2}, \ldots, H_{N_i,j_2}\}$ and two Fréchet means μ_{j_1}, μ_{j_2}, respectively. The definition of the covariance between these two objects is:

$$Cov(set_{j_1}, set_{j_2}) = \frac{1}{N_i - 1} \sum_{i=1}^{N_i} \boldsymbol{Log}_{\mu_{j_1}}(H_{i,j_1}).\boldsymbol{Log}_{\mu_{j_2}}(H_{i,j_2})^T. \tag{13}$$

The displacement $\boldsymbol{Log}_{\mu_j}(H_{i,j})$ is a vertical vector of size $3N_j$ with N_j the number of points of the object j.

Unlike the manifold itself, the tangent space is a vector space and its basis could be changed using a simple linear transformation. With the definition of covariance generalized, eigenvectors are computed with the tangent description, and the Exp function is applied to get principal components in terms of rigid transformations. This is the simplest generalization called tangent PCA (tPCA), which amounts to unfold the whole distribution in the tangent space at the mean, and to compute the principal components of the covariance matrix in the tangent space. tPCA is good for analyzing data which are sufficiently centered around a central value [13].

For an object j, the r first principal displacements $\boldsymbol{\delta_{tPCA_1,j}}, \ldots, \boldsymbol{\delta_{tPCA_r,j}}$ are obtained by tPCA. Associated scores $\alpha_{tPCA_1,i,j}, \ldots, \alpha_{tPCA_r,i,j}$ are describing the i-instance position along the principal displacements, with dataset variances (eigenvalues) $\lambda_{tPCA_1,j}, \ldots, \lambda_{tPCA_r,j}$. The following equation is used to re-create an instance's object with a reduced number of modes:

$$H_{tPCA,i,j} = Exp_{\mu_j} \left(\sum_{k=1}^{r} \alpha_{tPCA_k,i,j}.\boldsymbol{\delta_{tPCA_k,j}} \right),$$

$$\boldsymbol{F_{tPCA,i,j}} = H_{tPCA,i,j}(\overline{\boldsymbol{F_j}}).$$

3.3   Application to the Rib Cage

The dataset of rib cage meshes was obtained from 3D CT images. The 26 subjects were males, around 70 years old (73.3 ± 11) with a standard morphology (70 ± 9.8 kg in weight; 172 ± 5.5 cm in height). Meshes were obtained by using a model-based segmentation described in [14]. This also ensures point correspondences between all the meshes. The atlas mesh M_{ref} was constituted of 37 independent sub-meshes (1,570 nodes per mesh in average $\pm$ 314) representing the 12 vertebrae, 24 ribs and the sternum.

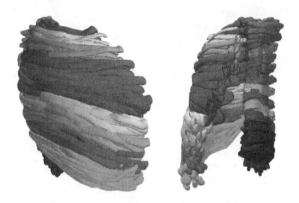

Fig. 4. Illustration of superposed right-side rib cages from the dataset with variations of pose and shape in lateral (left) and frontal views (right). The various colors enable to distinguish bones. (Color figure online)

We applied the proposed method to the rib cage dataset, instances were subjects and objects were bones. A pre-alignment was applied to superimpose subjects (Fig. 4). Multiple alignments were applied to compute rigid transformations used in tPCA and mean shapes used to define the norm.

To illustrate (Fig. 5) the different orthogonal modes retrieved using the proposed method, three models were reconstructed for each of the first three principal modes. Those models were reconstructed by setting α_m to $-3\sqrt{\lambda_m}, 0, 3\sqrt{\lambda_m}$ for $m = 1, 2, 3$ in the formula:

$$H_{tPCA_m,j} = Exp_{\mu_j}(\alpha_m.\delta_{tPCA_m,j}),$$
$$F_{tPCA_m,j} = H_{tPCA_m,j}(\overline{F_j}).$$

As expected, a relatively small number of modes accounted for most of the pose variability in the dataset. The accuracy of the model was evaluated by reconstructing subjects from a reduced number of components and comparing them with true geometries. The reconstruction errors were calculated as mean Euclidean distances.

The method to study pose variations was compared with the method using rotation vector description as tangent space [8,9]. The reconstruction distances

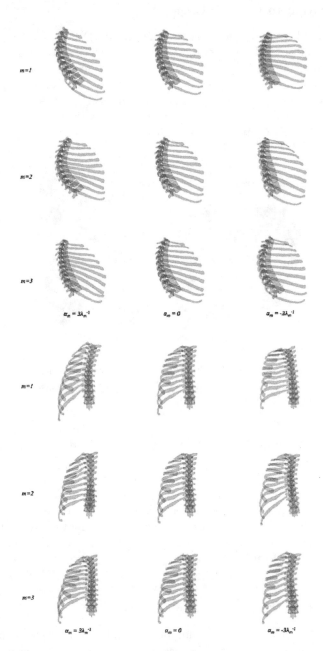

Fig. 5. First ($m = 1$), second ($m = 2$) and third ($m = 3$) principal modes of the rib cages dataset in lateral view and frontal view. The right side fo the rib cage models was rendered for -3, 0, 3 times the standard deviation explained by the corresponding mode. The middle column is the mean shape.

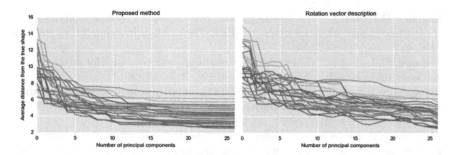

Fig. 6. Subject reconstruction error with respect to the number of principal modes after a tPCA. Each color refers to a subject. Left, principal modes were computed with the new metric. Right, principal modes were obtained with the standard rotation metric. (Color figure online)

were better in average for a reduced number of tPCA modes with the method presented in this study. We can see in Fig. 6 on the left graph that for a small number of modes, the error is much lower. The proposed metric facilitated lower reconstruction error for given number of components retained. About 4 components are needed for a similar reconstruction error obtained with 10 components of the standard metric. This shows that the new method is adapted to study articulated elongated bones like ribs.

4   Conclusion

In this paper, we introduced a new metric to perform statistical analysis on rigid transformations. Unlike previous metric, this one takes into account the shape of the object by integrating the inertia matrix. A tPCA was performed with this new metric on a dataset of rib cages. As the rib is an elongated anisotropic structure which is very elongated, it highlights the interest of this metric. In particular, the principal modes we obtained appear more suitable to reconstruct a subject with a reduced number of parameters.

References

1. Cootes, T.F., Taylor, C.J., Cooper, D.H., Graham, J.: Active shape models-their training and application. Comput. Vis. Image Underst. **61**(1), 38–59 (1995)
2. Zheng, G., Gollmer, S., Schumann, S., Dong, X., Feilkas, T., Ballester, M.A.G.: A 2D/3D correspondence building method for reconstruction of a patient-specific 3d bone surface model using point distribution models and calibrated X-ray images. Med. Image Anal. **13**(6), 883–899 (2009)
3. Rasoulian, A., Rohling, R., Abolmaesumi, P.: Lumbar spine segmentation using a statistical multi-vertebrae anatomical shape+pose model. IEEE Trans. Med. Imaging **32**(10), 1890–1900 (2013)
4. Pennec, X.: Intrinsic statistics on Riemannian manifolds: basic tools for geometric measurements. J. Math. Imaging Vis. **25**(1), 127–154 (2006)

5. Fletcher, P.T., Lu, C., Pizer, S.M., Joshi, S.: Principal geodesic analysis for the study of nonlinear statistics of shape. IEEE Trans. Med. Imaging **23**(8), 995–1005 (2004)
6. Sommer, S., Lauze, F., Nielsen, M.: Optimization over geodesics for exact principal geodesic analysis. Adv. Comput. Math. **40**(2), 283–313 (2014)
7. Bossa, M.N., Olmos, S.: Statistical model of similarity transformations: building a multi-object pose. In: 2006 Conference on Computer Vision and Pattern Recognition Workshop (CVPRW 2006), pp. 59–59. IEEE (2006)
8. Anas, E.M.A., Rasoulian, A., John, P.S., Pichora, D., Rohling, R., Abolmaesumi, P.: A statistical shape+ pose model for segmentation of wrist CT images. In: SPIE Medical Imaging, International Society for Optics and Photonics, pp. 90340T–90340T (2014)
9. Boisvert, J., Cheriet, F., Pennec, X., Labelle, H., Ayache, N.: Geometric variability of the scoliotic spine using statistics on articulated shape models. IEEE Trans. Med. Imaging **27**(4), 557–568 (2008)
10. Said, S., Courty, N., Le Bihan, N., Sangwine, S.J.: Exact principal geodesic analysis for data on SO (3). In: Signal Processing Conference, 2007 15th European, pp. 1701–1705. IEEE (2007)
11. Bindernagel, M., Kainmueller, D., Seim, H., Lamecker, H., Zachow, S., Hege, H.C.: An articulated statistical shape model of the human knee. In: Handels, H., Ehrhardt, J., Deserno, T., Meinzer, H.P., Tolxdorff, T. (eds.) Bildverarbeitung für die Medizin 2011, pp. 59–63. Springer, Heidelberg (2011)
12. Goodall, C.: Procrustes methods in the statistical analysis of shape. J. Roy. Stat. Soc. Ser. B (Methodol.) **53**, 285–339 (1991)
13. Pennec, X.: Barycentric subspaces and affine spans in manifolds. In: Nielsen, F., Barbaresco, F. (eds.) GSI 2015. LNCS, vol. 9389, pp. 12–21. Springer, Cham (2015). doi:10.1007/978-3-319-25040-3_2
14. Gilles, B., Revéret, L., Pai, D.K.: Creating and animating subject-specific anatomical models. Comput. Graph. Forum **29**(8), 2340–2351 (2010)

Unbiased Diffeomorphic Mapping of Longitudinal Data with Simultaneous Subject Specific Template Estimation

Daniel Tward[1,2(✉)], Michael Miller[1,2,3],
and the Alzheimer's Disease Neuroimaging Initiative

[1] Center for Imaging Science, Johns Hopkins University,
Baltimore, MD 21218, USA
dtward@cis.jhu.edu
[2] Kavli Neuroscience Discovery Institute, Johns Hopkins University,
Baltimore, MD 21218, USA
[3] Department of Biomedical Engineering, Johns Hopkins University,
Baltimore, MD 21218, USA

Abstract. Longitudinal mapping techniques for neuroimage analysis in computational anatomy have an important potential for bias associated to the order of input scans. Geodesic trajectories which pass from a template onto a baseline image and then through each follow up image have been shown to overestimate atrophy rate in the entorhinal cortex, while the reverse is true for trajectories pass through the data in the opposite order. We propose a method to remove this source of bias by inserting a patient specific template into a time series at a specific point to be estimated from the data, and simultaneously producing a time varying mapping connecting each image in the series. We demonstrate the efficacy of this method using segmentations of the entorhinal and surrounding cortex in subjects with early Alzheimer's disease.

1 Introduction

Longitudinal techniques for shape analysis in neuroimaging are now becoming widespread, allowing researches to explicitly model anatomical changes over time. In computational anatomy [9] biological form is described by the action of the diffeomorphism group on a particular example, diffeomorphisms being generated by a time dependent flow of smooth vector fields. It is natural to develop longitudinal techniques by associating this flow parameter to a physical time of

---

Alzheimer's Disease Neuroimaging Initiative—Data used in preparation of this article were obtained from the Alzheimer's Disease Neuroimaging Initiative (ADNI) database (adni.loni.usc.edu). As such, the investigators within the ADNI contributed to the design and implementation of ADNI and/or provided data but did not participate in analysis or writing of this report. A complete listing of ADNI investigators can be found at: http://adni.loni.usc.edu/wp-content/uploads/how_to_apply/ ADNI_Acknowledgement_List.pdf.

M.J. Cardoso et al. (Eds.): GRAIL/MFCA/MICGen 2017, LNCS 10551, pp. 125–136, 2017.
DOI: 10.1007/978-3-319-67675-3_12

imagery being examined, such as a patient's age. In [5], methods have been developed for working with longitudinal datasets, including registering one timeseries to another. In [7], a framework is developed for working with geodesic flows, a natural analogue to linear regression. These methods have been extended to include more complex hierarchical models [21,22] of entire populations, or joint modeling of shape and image intensity [8]. Other types of flows are explored in [17], including piecewise geodesic, geodesic, or spline based.

Our work involves studying neuroimaging biomarkers to quantify the progression of mild cognitive impairment (MCI), an early stage of Alzheimer's disease [18]. We focus on the entorhinal and surrounding cortex in the medial temporal lobe, the site of some of the earliest pathological changes due to the disease as measured in well characterized brains at autopsy [1]. One of the largest sources of variability in our data are inconsistencies between manual segmentations in the same subject over time, and we have been developing geodesic diffeomorphic mapping procedures to filter out this source of noise. Following the approach described in [24], we use a parameterization of the diffeomorphism group based on the bounding surfaces of our structures of interest, and perform matching by deforming a segmentation image template to match manual segmentation image targets. We have previously demonstrated the success of this method in reducing this source of variability [27].

With the adoption of longitudinal mapping methods, an understanding of their potential pitfalls needs to be developed. A potential for bias exists due to the order of the scans being examined. Methods that build flows of diffeomorphism to pass through the baseline scan first, and then through each follow up scan are susceptible. Longitudinal Freesurfer [6,20] removes this source of bias by constructing a subject specific initialization first, followed by independent analysis of each point in the timeseries. In this work we develop a method for addressing the issue which remains in the geodesic regression framework, preserving the desirable noise-reduction properties. Our approach is to insert the template into the timeseries at a specific time which is estimated from the data (not the baseline scan in general). The result is a subject specific template, as well as a geodesic flow through the longitudinal dataset.

We demonstrate the performance of this method visually through an example, and show how it removes bias in atrophy rate measurements on a population of entorhinal and transentorhinal cortex segmentations.

2   Methods

2.1   Diffeomorphisms and Geodesics

Diffeomorphisms, $\varphi : \Omega \subset \mathbb{R}^3 \to \Omega$, are generated from flows of smooth velocity fields $v : \Omega \to \mathbb{R}^3$ [9]

$$\dot{\varphi} = v(\varphi), \quad \varphi_0 = \text{Identity}. \tag{1}$$

To ensure sufficient smoothness, velocity fields are embedded in a Hilbert space of smooth functions V, with inner product given by $\langle u, v \rangle_V = \langle Lu, Lv \rangle_{L^2} =$

$\int_\Omega (L^*Lu)^T(x)v(x)dx$, where L is a differential operator and L^* its adjoint [3]. In this work we choose L implicitly by specifying the Green's kernel of L^*L as $K(x, x') = \exp\left(-\frac{1}{2\sigma_V^2}|x - x'|^2\right)$ with $\sigma_V = 6\,\mathrm{mm}$. We define the quantity $p = L^*Lv$ called the *momentum*, and also write $v = K \cdot p$. Further, we write the norm $\|v\|_V^2 = \langle v, v \rangle_V$ or equivalently $\|p\|_{V^*}^2 = \|K \cdot p\|_V^2$.

We perform regression using straight lines, or goedesics, through this space of diffeomorphisms. These are expressed through the equation (see [16], Eq. 49, referred to as "landmark transport")

$$\dot{p} = -Dv^T(\varphi)p \ . \tag{2}$$

We use the Riemannian exponential notation to express a geodesic flow with initial condition v_0

$$\varphi_t = \exp(v_0 t) \ . \tag{3}$$

2.2   Sparse Parameterization

Because diffeomorphisms are infinite dimensional objects, working with an appropriate low dimensional parametrization is critical for computational performance as well as for handling multiple comparison corrections in statistical hypothesis testing. Landmark based sparse parameterizations were first developed in [12], and expanded to more general cost functions in [4]. Sparsity in a basis determined through principal component analysis has been investigated in [19,26], as well as a Fourier basis in [28], or a surface harmonic basis in [24].

Our approach [24] uses the idea that neuroimages are typically well represented as piecewise constant functions. It has been shown [16] that in this situation, optimal momenta fields are singular with support on surfaces contouring these boundaries. We model these surfaces explicitly within our region of interest through a function $f : U \subset \mathbb{R}^2 \to \mathbb{R}^3$, defining our velocity fields parametrically as

$$v = \int_U K(\cdot, f(u))p(u)du$$

We use the familiar form of the Riemann integral, but more generally U can be considered a measure space, allowing us to include closed surfaces, unions of several surfaces, or discrete surfaces.

2.3   Group Actions and Notation

In this work we consider two geodesic trajectories, one mapping a template into our time series, and one passing through the time series. We use the superscripts 0 and 1 to refer to these two flows, and reserve subscripts for the time indexing a position within the geodesic flow. We write the diffeomorphisms, which are geodesic flows specified by some initial velocity (to be determined), as

$$\varphi_s^0, \ s \in [0, 1], \qquad \varphi_t^1, \ t \in \text{elapsed time measured in years} \ . \tag{4}$$

We write the deforming surface in terms of advection

$$f_s^0 = \varphi_s^0 \cdot f_0^0 = \varphi_s^0(f_0^0), \qquad f_t^1 = \varphi_t^1 \cdot f_1^0 = \varphi_t^1(f_1^0), \tag{5}$$

which is expressed using the differential equation

$$\dot{f}_s^0 = v_s^0(f_s^0), \qquad \dot{f}_t^1 = v_t^1(f_t^1) \tag{6}$$

for a fixed template f_0^0 and appropriate boundary conditions connecting the two flows (described below).

We also consider images, as functions $I : \Omega \to \mathbb{R}^C$ for a C channel image. This could refer to C different binary segmentation labels, or to C different modalities (e.g. diffusion weighted, fractional anisotropy, etc.). To avoid a double superscript, we write the inverse of each diffeomorphism φ^i as ψ^i (rather than φ^{i-1} for example). We write the deforming images in terms of optical flow

$$I_s^0 = \varphi_s^0 \cdot I_0^0 = I(\psi_s^0), \qquad I_t^1 = \varphi_t^1 \cdot I_1^0 = I_1^0(\psi_t^1) \tag{7}$$

which is expressed using the differential equation

$$\dot{I}_s^0 = -DI_s^0 v_s^0, \qquad \dot{I}_t^1 = -DI_t^1 v_t^1 \tag{8}$$

where DI is a $C \times 3$ matrix with each channel down a column, and each spatial derivative across a row. Here I_0^0 is a fixed template and appropriate boundary conditions connect the two flows (described below). These equations hold when diffeomorphisms and velocity fields are linked by (1).

2.4   Cost Function for Timeseries Mapping

Our goal will be to construct two geodesic trajectories to map our atlas image I_0^0 onto a series of target images J^i sampled at times t_i (for example age in years) for $i \in \{1, \ldots, N\}$. Originally [27] we proposed the following cost function

$$E = \frac{1}{2\sigma_{p^0}^2}\|p_0^0\|_{V^*}^2 + \frac{1}{2\tilde{\sigma}_{p^1}^2}\|p_0^1(t_N - t_1)\|_{V^*}^2 + \sum_{i=1}^{N} \frac{1}{2\sigma_I^2}\|I_{t_i}^1 - J^i\|_{L_2}^2 \tag{9}$$

with $I_{t_i}^1 = \exp(v_0^1(t_i - t_1)) \cdot \exp(v_0^0) \cdot I_0^0$. The two flows are connected by $I_{t_1}^1 = I_1^0$ and $f_{t_1}^1 = f_1^0$. The first two terms are regularization terms, with p_0^1 multiplied by the scalar factor $(t_N - t_1)$ so the term reflects the length of the entire geodesic curve. This is optimized over p_0^0 and p_0^1, defining one geodesic trajectory from a template to the baseline image (determined by the initial momentum p_0^0), and a second geodesic trajectory from the baseline image through the entire time series (determined by the initial momentum p_0^1). Here the σ are parameters controlling the relative weighting between regularization and fidelity terms. In this work they are set to 1. An illustration of this setup is shown in Fig. 1 (left).

This approach has a processing bias, where the result depends on the order of the scans. This bias can be evaluated by reversing the order of the scans

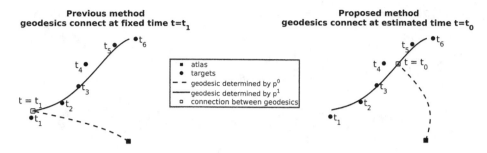

Fig. 1. Cartoon illustration of our mapping procedure (right), contrasted with the previous method (9) (left).

and comparing results. For example, when measuring volumetric atrophy in the entorhinal and transentorhinal cortex, we found a bias of about 1% volume loss per year.

In order to remedy this situation, we draw our motivation from template estimation [13,14], where one geodesic trajectory is defined from a template to a population average, and one is defined from the population average to each target:

$$E = \sum_{i=1}^{N} \frac{1}{2N\sigma_{p^0}^2} \|p_0^0\|_{V^*}^2 + \frac{1}{2\sigma_{p^1}^2} \|p_0^i\|_{V^*}^2 + \frac{1}{2\sigma_I^2} \|I_{t_i}^1 - J^i\|_{L_2}^2 \ . \tag{10}$$

We modify this by imposing the single geodesic time series model

$$p_0^i = p_0^1 (t_i - t_0) \ . \tag{11}$$

with $I_{t_i}^1 = \exp(v_0^1(t_i - t_0)) \cdot \exp(v_0^0) \cdot I_0^0$. The two flows are connected by $I_{t_0}^1 = I_1^0$ and $f_{t_0}^1 = f_1^0$. In addition to optimizing over p_0^0 and p_0^1, we also optimize over t_0. The result at time $t = t_0$ can be considered a patient specific template. Note that for a fixed $t_0 = t_1$, the two cost functions (9) and (10) are identical with appropriate choice of constants $\sigma_{p^1}, \tilde{\sigma}_{p^1}$. An illustration of this setup is shown in Fig. 1 (right).

We have also incorporated the first regularization term into the summation, so that the cost can be written as a sum of separate terms for each target in the time series. The gradient with respect to each parameter can be computed separately for each term, enabling distributed computing such as discussed in [11].

A specific example of our framework is illustrated in Fig. 2, where the target images J^i are shown in the top row, and the deforming template surface f_t^1 is shown in the second row. The initial template f_0^0 is shown in the bottom row, positioned at its estimated time t_0.

To summarize our setup, we use images for our matching cost, while we use surfaces contouring structures of interest to parameterize their deformation, a representation that is sparse in $\mathbb{R}^3$. In the application described here, where images are binary, our surface representation differs from the image gradient by providing smoothness and well defined normals.

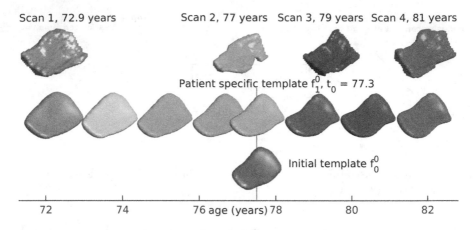

Fig. 2. Illustration of our mapping procedure applied to one entorhinal cortex time-series. Target images J^i are shown in the top row. Several snapshots of the template surface f_t^1, deforming as a function of age, are shown in the second row. The patient specific template is included in cyan. The initial template f_0^0 is shown in the bottom row, positioned at its estimated time t_0.

2.5   Optimization Algorithm

We use a gradient descent based optimization strategy. We enforce dynamics (6), (8), (2) through the Lagrange multipliers, $\lambda^{I^i}, \lambda^{f^i}, \lambda^{p^i}$ for $i \in \{0, 1\}$, augmenting the cost function to

$$
\begin{aligned}
L = E &+ \int_0^1 \int_\Omega \lambda_s^{I^0 T}(x)(\dot{I}_s^0(x) + DI_s^0(x)v_s^0(x))dx \\
&+ \int_U \lambda_s^{f^0 T}(u)(\dot{f}_s^0(u) - v_s^0(f_s^0(u))) + \lambda_s^{p^0 T}(u)(\dot{p}_s^0(u) + Dv_s^{0T}(f_s^0(u)))duds \\
&+ \int_{t_1}^{t_N} \int_\Omega \lambda_t^{I^1 T}(x)(\dot{I}_t^1(x) + DI_t^1(x)v_t^1(x))dx \\
&+ \int_U \lambda_t^{f^1 T}(u)(\dot{f}_t^1(u) - v_t^1(f_t^1(u))) + \lambda_t^{p^1 T}(u)(\dot{p}_t^1(u) + Dv_t^{1T}(f_t^1(u)))dudt
\end{aligned}
\tag{12}
$$

Optimization proceeds by flowing the system forward in time to the i-th target using the current guess of parameters, initializing the Lagrange multipliers at the endpoint of the flow with the derivative of the cost function,

$$
\lambda_{t_i}^{I^1} = -\frac{1}{\sigma_I^2}(I_{t_i} - J^i), \qquad \lambda_{t_i}^{f^1} = 0, \qquad \lambda_{t_i}^{p^1} = 0
\tag{13}
$$

and then flowing this error backward according to a dual dynamical system for each λ. This procedure is called an adjoint method, similar to backpropogation, and specific equations for the λ dynamics can be found in [24]. The derivative with respect to p^i is then

$$\frac{dE}{dp^i} = \frac{1}{\sigma_{p^1}^2} K \cdot p_0^i - \lambda_0^{p^1} \ . \tag{14}$$

Applying the chain rule, we see that the gradient with respect to p^1 is

$$\frac{dE}{dp^1} = \sum_{i=1}^{N} \frac{dE}{dp^i} \frac{dp^i}{dp^1} = \sum_{i=1}^{N} \frac{dE}{dp^i} (t_i - t_0) \ . \tag{15}$$

That for t_0 is

$$\frac{dE}{dt_0} = \sum_{i=1}^{N} \int \frac{dE}{dp^i}(u) \frac{dp^i}{dt_0}(u) du = - \sum_{i=1}^{N} \int \frac{dE}{dp^i}(u) p^1(u) du \ . \tag{16}$$

This is essentially projection of the gradient with respect to each p^i onto p^1, with a negative sign. In other words, if making p^i bigger will reduce the cost, then this can be achieved by increasing p^i or by decreasing t_0. If there were no error in our matching ($\lambda^{I^1} = 0$), we could explicitly calculate $t_0 = \frac{1}{N} \sum_{i=1}^{N} t_i$, a simple average. In general, t_0 is weighted toward timepoints with more error.

The above algorithm was implemented on the GPU using OpenCL as described in [25].

2.6   Atrophy in the Medial Temporal Lobe

We demonstrate the efficacy of our algorithm using data from the Alzheimer's Disease Neuroimaging Initiative[1] as well as the BIOCARD study (http://www.alzresearch.org/biocard.cfm, see [15] for an overview of this dataset) to quantify the atrophy of the entorhinal and surrounding cortex in early Alzheimer's disease. Medial temporal lobe segmentations were performed manually using the protocol discussed in [2,10].

We show an example mapping onto a timeseries of entorhinal cortex segmentations, demonstrating the estimate of the parameter t_0 and resulting patient specific template. Further, we demonstrate the removal of processing bias due to the scan order with this procedure using nonparametric permutation testing.

---

[1] Data used in the preparation of this article were obtained from the Alzheimer's Disease Neuroimaging Initiative (ADNI) database (adni.loni.usc.edu). The ADNI was launched in 2003 as a public-private partnership, led by Principal Investigator Michael W. Weiner, MD. The primary goal of ADNI has been to test whether serial magnetic resonance imaging (MRI), positron emission tomography (PET), other biological markers, and clinical and neuropsychological assessment can be combined to measure the progression of mild cognitive impairment (MCI) and early Alzheimer's disease (AD). For up-to-date information, see www.adni-info.org.

3 Results

3.1 Template Estimation and Longitudinal Mapping

We illustrate the performance of this algorithm with an example. The manual segmentations of the entorhinal cortex of a single subject over time are shown in Fig. 3 right, after being rigidly aligned using corresponding T1 images as shown in Fig. 3 left. Notice the variability in size, shape, orientation, and anterior-posterior extent. Differences in segmentations of even 1 slice, can be a significant source of noise when quantifying changes in such a small structure.

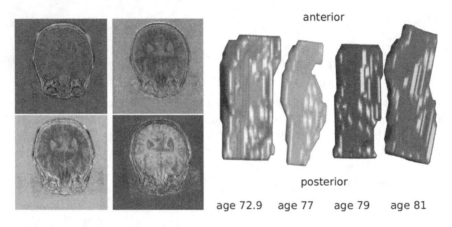

Fig. 3. Left: Accuracy of rigid alignment of T1 images is demonstrated by visualizing the difference between each image and average of the other three. Right: Manual segmentation of a left entorhinal cortex from a single subject over time demonstrating variability in manual segmentations.

We use the timeseries mapping procedure described above to filter out this variability, and simultaneously estimate patient specific template. The result of this mapping is show in Fig. 2.

We illustrate the estimation of the template time t_0 as a function of gradient descent iterations in Fig. 4. Two examples are shown. In the first case t_0 is initialized to t_1, whereas in the second case t_0 is initialized to t_4. In both cases our estimate converges to a value slightly less than the average scan time. Counter intuitively, the time t_0 begins by moving in the wrong direction. The reason is that early in the optimization process, much of the error is accounted for by $p_0^1(t - t_0)$ being too small. It can be made larger by simply decreasing t_0 in the case where t_0 starts at t_1 (the opposite is true when t_0 is set initially to t_4).

3.2 Processing Bias

We evaluate the removal of processing bias using a population of 40 left entorhinal and transentorhinal cortex segmentations from the ADNI dataset, scanned

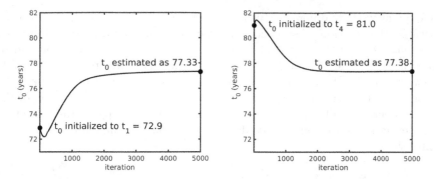

Fig. 4. Illustration of the estimation of template time t_0 as a function of gradient descent iteration during optimization. At left we initialize t_0 with the age of the patient at their baseline scan. At right we initialize t_0 with the age of the patient at their last follow up scan. The two converge to very similar values.

up to 5 times over 2 years. Volumetric atrophy rate was measured using a log linear fit to the volume of J^i for manual segmentations, or $I_{t_i}^1$ for "forward" maps ($t_0 = t_1$ fixed), for "unbiased" maps (t_0 estimated), and for "backward" maps ($t_0 = t_N$ fixed). A density estimate of these values is shown in Fig. 5 left. Notice that the peak (or mode) of the "forward" maps is shifted to the right, and the "backward" maps is shifted to the left relative to the manual segmentations. This difference of 3.1% per year indicates a substantial source of bias. The peak for the "unbiased" method is close to but higher than that for manual segmentations, showing a reduction in noise we have investigated previously [27].

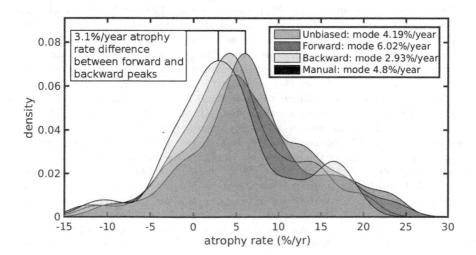

Fig. 5. Density estimate of atrophy rate measurements for subjects with Alzheimer's disease. The atrophy rate at the peak (or mode) of each distribution is indicated.

We quantify these differences using permutation testing. We choose as a test statistic T the fraction of subjects for which the "unbiased" method shows a value of atrophy in between the backwards method and the forwards method (in all but one case, the "forward" method shows a higher atrophy rate than the "backward" method). If there were no natural ordering, we would expect this fraction to be $1/6$, but the observed proportion is 0.61. The distribution of this statistic under the null hypotheses was determined through permutation testing. The ordering is seen to be preserved with a p value less than 1 in 100000 total permutations.

4   Conclusion

As longitudinal mapping procedures are becoming more widely adopted, the important potential for bias associated to the order of scans needs to be addressed. The procedure developed here overcomes it while preserving the filtering properties of geodesic regression that can reduce inconsistencies in anatomical definitions over time, as well as constructing a patient specific template. The optimization algorithm is formulated in a manner that can benefit from distributed computing resources. The separability of the cost function into each scan the timeseries provides the additional possibility for optimization to benefit from a stochastic gradient descent, an avenue that will be investigated in the future.

Acknowledgements. This work was supported by the Kavli Foundation. This work was supported by NIH grant R01EB020062-01A1. The imaging core of the BIOCARD project is supported by NIH grant U19AG033655-09. This work used the Extreme Science and Engineering Discovery Environment (XSEDE) [23], which is supported by National Science Foundation grant number ACI-1053575.

Data collection and sharing for this project was funded by the Alzheimer's Disease Neuroimaging Initiative (ADNI) (National Institutes of Health Grant U01 AG024904) and DOD ADNI (Department of Defense award number W81XWH-12-2-0012). ADNI is funded by the National Institute on Aging, the National Institute of Biomedical Imaging and Bioengineering, and through generous contributions from the following: AbbVie, Alzheimer's Association; Alzheimer's Drug Discovery Foundation; Araclon Biotech; BioClinica, Inc.; Biogen; Bristol-Myers Squibb Company; CereSpir, Inc.; Cogstate; Eisai Inc.; Elan Pharmaceuticals, Inc.; Eli Lilly and Company; EuroImmun; F. Hoffmann-La Roche Ltd and its affiliated company Genentech, Inc.; Fujirebio; GE Healthcare; IXICO Ltd.; Janssen Alzheimer Immunotherapy Research & Development, LLC.; Johnson & Johnson Pharmaceutical Research & Development LLC.; Lumosity; Lundbeck; Merck & Co., Inc.; Meso Scale Diagnostics, LLC.; NeuroRx Research; Neurotrack Technologies; Novartis Pharmaceuticals Corporation; Pfizer Inc.; Piramal Imaging; Servier; Takeda Pharmaceutical Company; and Transition Therapeutics. The Canadian Institutes of Health Research is providing funds to support ADNI clinical sites in Canada. Private sector contributions are facilitated by the Foundation for the National Institutes of Health (www.fnih.org). The grantee organization is the Northern California Institute for Research and Education, and the study is coordinated by the Alzheimer's Therapeutic Research Institute at the University of Southern California. ADNI data are disseminated by the Laboratory for Neuro Imaging at the University of Southern California.

References

1. Braak, H., Braak, E.: Neuropathological stageing of alzheimer-related changes. Acta Neuropathol. **82**, 239–259 (1991). doi:10.1007/BF00308809
2. Ding, S.L., Van Hoesen, G.W.: Borders, extent, and topography of human perirhinal cortex as revealed using multiple modern neuroanatomical and pathological markers. Hum. Brain Mapp. **31**(9), 1359–1379 (2010)
3. Dupuis, P., Grenander, U., Miller, M.I.: Variational problems on flows of diffeomorphisms for image matching. Q. Appl. Math. **56**, 587–600 (1998)
4. Durrleman, S., Allassonnière, S., Joshi, S.: Sparse adaptive parameterization of variability in image ensembles. Int. J. Comput. Vis. **101**(1), 161–183 (2013). doi:10.1007/s11263-012-0556-1
5. Durrleman, S., Pennec, X., Trouvé, A., Braga, J., Gerig, G., Ayache, N.: Toward a comprehensive framework for the spatiotemporal statistical analysis of longitudinal shape data. Int. J. Comput. Vis. **103**(1), 22–59 (2013)
6. Fischl, B.: Freesurfer. Neuroimage **62**(2), 774–781 (2012)
7. Fletcher, P.T.: Geodesic regression and the theory of least squares on riemannian manifolds. Int. J. Comput. Vis. **105**(2), 171–185 (2013)
8. Gao, Y., Zhang, M., Grewen, K., Fletcher, P.T., Gerig, G.: Image registration and segmentation in longitudinal mri using temporal appearance modeling. In: 2016 IEEE 13th International Symposium on Biomedical Imaging (ISBI), pp. 629–632. IEEE (2016)
9. Grenander, U., Miller, M.I.: Computational anatomy: an emerging discipline. Q. Appl. Math. **56**(4), 617–694 (1998)
10. Insausti, R., Juottonen, K., Soininen, H., Insausti, A.M., Partanen, K., Vainio, P., Laakso, M.P., Pitkänen, A.: MR volumetric analysis of the human entorhinal, perirhinal, and temporopolar cortices. Am. J. Neuroradiol. **19**(4), 659–671 (1998)
11. Jain, S., Tward, D.J., Lee, D.S., Kolasny, A., Brown, T., Ratnanather, J.T., Miller, M.I., Younes, L.: Computational anatomy gateway: leveraging xsede computational resources for shape analysis. In: Proceedings of the 2014 Annual Conference on Extreme Science and Engineering Discovery Environment, p. 54. ACM (2014)
12. Joshi, S., Miller, M.: Landmark matching via large deformation diffeomorphisms. IEEE Trans. Image Process. **9**(8), 1357–70 (2000)
13. Ma, J., Miller, M.I., Trouvé, A., Younes, L.: Bayesian template estimation in computational anatomy. NeuroImage **42**(1), 252–261 (2008)
14. Ma, J., Miller, M.I., Younes, L.: A bayesian generative model for surface template estimation. J. Biomed. Imaging **2010**, 16 (2010)
15. Miller, M.I., Ratnanather, J.T., Tward, D.J., Brown, T., Lee, D.S., Ketcha, M., Mori, K., Wang, M.C., Mori, S., Albert, M.S., et al.: Network neurodegeneration in alzheimer's disease via mri based shape diffeomorphometry and high-field atlasing. Front. Bioeng. Biotechnol. **3**, 54 (2015)
16. Miller, M.I., Trouvé, A., Younes, L.: Geodesic shooting for computational anatomy. J. Math. Imaging Vis. **24**(2), 209–228 (2006)
17. Miller, M.I., Trouvé, A., Younes, L.: Hamiltonian systems and optimal control in computational anatomy: 100 years since d'arcy thompson. Ann. Rev. Biomed. Eng. **17**, 447–509 (2015)
18. Petersen, R.C.: Mild cognitive impairment as a diagnostic entity. J. Intern. Med. **256**(3), 183–194 (2004)
19. Qiu, A., Younes, L., Miller, M.: Principal component based diffeomorphic surface mapping. IEEE Trans. Med. Imaging **31**(2), 302–311 (2012)

20. Reuter, M., Schmansky, N.J., Rosas, H.D., Fischl, B.: Within-subject template estimation for unbiased longitudinal image analysis. Neuroimage **61**(4), 1402–1418 (2012)
21. Schiratti, J.B., Allassonniere, S., Colliot, O., Durrleman, S.: Learning spatiotemporal trajectories from manifold-valued longitudinal data. In: Advances in Neural Information Processing Systems, pp. 2404–2412 (2015)
22. Singh, N., Hinkle, J., Joshi, S., Fletcher, P.T.: Hierarchical geodesic models in diffeomorphisms. Int. J. Comput. Vis. **117**(1), 70–92 (2016)
23. Towns, J., Cockerill, T., Dahan, M., Foster, I., Gaither, K., Grimshaw, A., Hazlewood, V., Lathrop, S., Lifka, D., Peterson, G.D., et al.: Xsede: accelerating scientific discovery. Comput. Sci. Eng. **16**(5), 62–74 (2014)
24. Tward, D., Miller, M., Trouve, A., Younes, L.: Parametric surface diffeomorphometry for low dimensional embeddings of dense segmentations and imagery. IEEE Trans. Pattern Anal. Mach. Intell. **39**, 1195–1208 (2016)
25. Tward, D.J., Kolasny, A., Sicat, C.S., Brown, T., Miller, M.I.: Tools for studying populations and timeseries of neuroanatomy enabled through gpu acceleration in the computational anatomy gateway. In: Proceedings of the XSEDE16 Conference on Diversity, Big Data, and Science at Scale, p. 15. ACM (2016)
26. Tward, D.J., Ma, J., Miller, M.I., Younes, L.: Robust diffeomorphic mapping via geodesically controlled active shapes. Int. J. Biomed. Imaging **2013**, 1–19 (2013)
27. Tward, D.J., Sicat, C.S., Brown, T., Bakker, A., Miller, M.I.: Reducing variability in anatomical definitions over time using longitudinal diffeomorphic mapping. In: Reuter, M., Wachinger, C., Lombaert, H. (eds.) SeSAMI 2016. LNCS, vol. 10126, pp. 51–62. Springer, Cham (2016). doi:10.1007/978-3-319-51237-2_5
28. Zhang, M., Wells, W.M., Golland, P.: Low-dimensional statistics of anatomical variability via compact representation of image deformations. In: Ourselin, S., Joskowicz, L., Sabuncu, M.R., Unal, G., Wells, W. (eds.) MICCAI 2016. LNCS, vol. 9902, pp. 166–173. Springer, Cham (2016). doi:10.1007/978-3-319-46726-9_20

Exact Function Alignment Under Elastic Riemannian Metric

Daniel Robinson[1], Adam Duncan[2(✉)], Anuj Srivastava[2], and Eric Klassen[3]

[1] Amazon.com, Inc., Seattle, USA
[2] Department of Statistics, Florida State University, Tallahassee, USA
a.duncan@stat.fsu.edu
[3] Department of Mathematics, Florida State University, Tallahassee, USA

Abstract. The problem of nonlinear alignment of functions is both fundamental and extremely important in pattern recognition. Most common approaches for alignment, including dynamic time warping (DTW), use penalized-$\mathbb{L}^2$ minimization that has significant shortcomings, including asymmetry. A recent mathematical framework, based on an elastic Riemannian metric and square-root velocity functions, overcomes these shortcomings. The time warping problem is currently solved using a dynamic programming algorithm (DPA) which relies heavily on dense sampling of functions and can be computationally expensive. Here we present a novel theory (and algorithms) for finding the exact pairwise alignment between functions, which uses an efficient sampling of functions, restricted to their change points. In many cases, the computational cost for matching is reduced by orders of magnitude. We demonstrate the superiority of this method over the DPA using several simulated and real datasets.

1 Introduction

Functional data analysis (FDA) [10] is a growing area of statistical research, which studies data objects that are real- or vector-valued functions on arbitrary domains. The simplest case is that of $\mathbb{R}$-valued functions on a unit interval, but functional data appears in many other forms. The spread of wearable sensors, smart phones, personalized monitors, and portable computing has resulted in abundance of biodata associated with humans – their health, activities, and daily routines – in function form. The goal in FDA is to develop statistical models and algorithms for inferences involving such functional data. These functions are considered as elements of a Hilbert space and typical procedures include deriving statistical summaries, capturing essential patterns, discovering modes of variations, and defining probability distributions. The Hilbert structure can be used to perform principal component analysis (PCA) and to deduce dominant

Electronic supplementary material The online version of this chapter (doi:10. 1007/978-3-319-67675-3_13) contains supplementary material, which is available to authorized users.

M.J. Cardoso et al. (Eds.): GRAIL/MFCA/MICGen 2017, LNCS 10551, pp. 137–151, 2017.
DOI: 10.1007/978-3-319-67675-3_13

modes of variation in the observed data. These tools are important in activity recognition, shape analysis, clinical diagnosis of biosignals, medical image registration, analysis of biological growth curves, utilization of educational learning curves, and so on. In this paper we focus on the real-valued functions on a fixed interval as the data objects of interest.

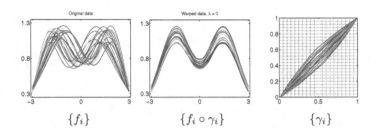

Fig. 1. Illustration of nonlinear alignment of multiple functions.

An important challenge in functional data analysis is the *registration* or *alignment* problem. The problem stems from the fact that observed functions exhibit random variations not only in their values (heights) but also in their domains (horizontal axis). This could be due to, for example, variability in the rate at speech is delivered and recorded [8], different growth rates for subjects, or different execution rates for activities [17–19]. The horizontal variability, if not accounted for, appears as a vertical variability and can destroy the underlying structure or pattern of given functional data. As an example, if we take the cross-sectional average of functions shown in left panel (unaligned) of Fig. 1, we will not get a bimodal curve, even though each individual function is bimodal. In contrast, the corresponding average for the middle panel (aligned) will preserve that structure. The same issues are relevant to cross-sectional variance, which can compromise methods such as ANOVA, PCA, etc.

A more precise statement of the problem is as follows: Given a set of functions, $\{f_i : [0, 1] \rightarrow \mathbb{R} | i = 1, 2, \ldots, r\}$, we seek warping functions $\{\gamma_i | i = 1, 2, \ldots, r\}$ such that the warped functions $\{f_i \circ \gamma_i\}$ are considered aligned. Figure 1 shows an illustration of this alignment.

This problem has been studied across many scientific communities for more than two decades and several methods have been presented. The most commonly used framework in almost all of image, signal, and FDA is based on minimizing the following objective function:

$$\|f_1 - f_2 \circ \gamma\|^2 + \lambda \mathcal{R}(\gamma) \,, \tag{1}$$

Here, $\| \cdot \|$ denotes the $\mathbb{L}^2$ norm and $\mathcal{R}$ denotes a roughness penalty on γ. This idea has been used in dynamic time warping (DTW) [4,11], curve alignment [12], previous FDA [7,9], and almost all image registration methods [1,16]. Despite its popularity this method some potential drawbacks. The solution is not inverse symmetric, i.e. the registration of f_1 to f_2 can be different from the registration of f_2 to f_1. As a consequence, the objective function in Eq. 1 is not a proper metric, so it cannot be used in some widely-used methods of analysis such as PCA. As a solution, several papers [14,15] have developed a mathematically elegant and intuitive technique for these alignments using a Riemannian approach. They defined a new mathematical representation of the given functions, termed square-root velocity function (SRVF) (presented later), which leads to a new alignment formulation and it addresses the three issues mentioned above. Naturally, it also requires an optimization step that has been performed using either the Dynamic Programming Algorithm (DPA) [2] or a gradient-based minimization [3,14]. These optimizations are problematic because of:

1. **Discretization**: The DPA is based on a discrete grid on the graph space of γ resulting from a sampling, uniform or otherwise, of the domain $[0,1]$. In the case the sampling is not fine enough, one can miss a feature (e.g. sharp peak or valley) of f_1, f_2 completely and, consequently, the resulting alignment takes a completely different form.
2. **Computational Cost**: If the domain of a function is sampled at k points, then the computational cost of solving for optimal γ on the chosen grid is order $O(k^4)$. There is a possibility of restricting the search space of instantaneous slopes to only m values, with $m << k$, and the cost goes down to $O(m^2 k^2)$. Still, this cost can be very high in situations where k is very large.

As an alternative, we propose a procedure that offers an *exact* solution to the pairwise matching problem and is often orders of magnitude cheaper in computational cost. It is based on the fact that most functions can be warped into a piecewise linear form, with junctions denoting the original change points (points where the slope changes signs). For piecewise linear functions, the alignments (or registrations) are relatively easier: similar slopes are aligned and opposite slopes are eliminated. The method is similar to the one proposed in [6], which registers curves, $f : [0,1] \rightarrow \mathbb{R}^n$, in the SRVF framework. The major difference is that the method proposed here uses an algorithm that applies specifically to the one-dimensional case.

The proposed algorithm has $O(n_1^2 n_2^2)$ running time, where n_1, n_2 are the numbers of change points of f_1, f_2 respectively. When n_1, n_2 are much smaller than k, this can give a drastic improvement in running time. In the more difficult case where there are a larger number of change points – such as functions with additive Gaussian noise – the time gains over the conventional DPA will disappear, but one will still have the assurance of having exact solutions rather than approximations.

The rest of this paper is as follows. We briefly summarize the mathematical setup for the optimization problem of interest. Section 3 describes the theory behind our solution for the pairwise matching problem with the corresponding algorithms derived in Sect. 4. Section 5 extends the solution to multiple functions and Sect. 6 presents experimental results on a variety of simulated and real datasets.

2   Mathematical Background

The proposed approach is based on an elastic Riemmanian framework [14] that allows nonlinear matching of curves by a combination of stretching and bending, thus allowing for better matching of geometrical features across curves. While the original elastic metric is a complicated one, an important idea that facilitates practical use of this framework is the introduction of the *square-root velocity function* (SRVF). As described in [14], the change of variables from the original curves to SRVFs helps flatten the curved elastic metric into the Euclidean metric. Due to this flattening, more standard tools for Hilbert spaces can be applied and nonlinear geometries are avoided. The SRVF for a real-valued function is defined as follows: Given a function $f : [0,1] \to \mathbb{R}$ that is absolutely continuous, the associated SRVF $q : [0,1] \to \mathbb{R}$ is defined as $q(t) = \text{sign}(\dot{f}(t))\sqrt{|\dot{f}(t)|}$, if $\dot{f}(t)$ exists and is nonzero. Otherwise, it is set to zero. For all t, we have $|q(t)| = \sqrt{|\dot{f}(t)|}$, which is the reason for the name *square root velocity function*. Given $q \in \mathbb{L}^2$, we can recover f (up to a vertical translation) via the formula $f(t) = \int_0^t q(s)|q(s)|ds$.

For an absolutely continuous real-valued function, $f : [0,1] \to \mathbb{R}$ its SRVFs is in an element of $\mathbb{L}^2$. In fact, the SRVF mapping between the set of all absolutely continuous functions and $\mathbb{L}^2$ forms a bijection up to vertical translation. That is, curves have the same representative SRVF in $\mathbb{L}^2$ if and only if they differ by vertical translation. For any two SRVFs $q_1, q_2 \in \mathbb{L}^2$, the distance between the two is given by $\|q_1 - q_2\|$, denoting the $\mathbb{L}^2$ norm of their difference. The curves that have the same shape – but whose corresponding features occur at different locations in the domain – will have different representatives in $\mathbb{L}^2$. To capture this horizontal component, we will use the warping functions to extract and represent the horizontal variability.

Let Γ denote the semigroup of weakly-increasing, absolutely continuous functions on $[0,1]$ that preserve the two boundaries. Elements of this set play the role of nonlinear warping functions as follows. For a given function, $f : [0,1] \to \mathbb{R}$ and a warping $\gamma \in \Gamma$, the warped f is simply the composition, $f \circ \gamma$. In the SRVF-space, this becomes a right-action of Γ on $\mathbb{L}^2$. If q is the SRVF of this f, then the action at this point is written $q * \gamma = \sqrt{\dot{\gamma}}(q \circ \gamma)$. This group action has the useful *isometry* property that distance is preserved with respect to identical warping. For any $q_1, q_2 \in \mathbb{L}^2$ and $\gamma \in \Gamma$. we have $\|q_1 * \gamma - q_2 * \gamma\|^2 = \|q_1 - q_2\|^2$. We also define an orbit $[q] = \{\sqrt{\dot{\gamma}}(q \circ \gamma)|\gamma \in \Gamma\}$ as the set of all possible warpings of an SRVF; one can verify that memberships of these orbits defines an equivalence relation on $\mathbb{L}^2$. (To result in closed orbits, the definition of $[q]$ involves first expressing q as $w * \gamma$, where w has constant absolute value for a $\gamma \in \Gamma$ and then setting $[q] = [w]$, but we skip the technical details.)

3   Pairwise Alignment Theory

Now we return to the problem of pairwise alignment of functional data. For any two given functions f_1, f_2 and their corresponding SRVFs q_1, q_2, the registration problem is given by:

$$\inf_{\gamma_1, \gamma_2 \in \Gamma} \|(q_1 * \gamma_2) - (q_2 * \gamma_2)\|$$

$$= \inf_{\gamma_1, \gamma_2 \in \Gamma} \|\sqrt{\dot{\gamma}_1}(q_1 \circ \gamma_1) - \sqrt{\dot{\gamma}_2}(q_2 \circ \gamma_2)\| . \qquad (2)$$

In view of the isometry property, one can also pose this as maximization of the inner-product $\langle (q_1 * \gamma_1), (q_2 * \gamma_2) \rangle$ over γ_1, γ_2. In practice, any function is represented in data as a finite sequence of sample values $\{(t_i, f(t_i)\}$. We can think of this as a piecewise-linear (PL) function defined by line segments between each pair of consecutive indices. It is important to note that any absolutely continuous function f, with the property that we can subdivide $[0, 1]$ into a finite union of intervals on each of which f is weakly monotone, is a warping away from a PL function [6]. Furthermore, SRVFs of PL functions are step functions and step functions are dense in $\mathbb{L}^2$. Together, this implies that every equivalence class, $[q]$, contains step functions, so this type of data is sufficient to solve any pairwise matching problem. We can further choose initial representation of a function as arc-length parameterized. Any such function will have an SRVF which only takes on the values 1 and -1, which will greatly simplify analysis.

Now we establish necessary conditions for an optimal match, which will eventually leave us with a finite search space. Let q_1 be a step function with change-point partition $0 = t_0^1 < t_1^1 < t_2^1 < \ldots < t_{n_1}^1$, and let q_2 be a step function with change-point partition $0 = t_0^2 < t_1^2 < t_2^2 < \ldots < t_{n_2}^2$. The change points are those points where the slope of a function changes sign. Let $0 = t_0 < t_1 < \ldots < t_n$ be the union of the partitions for q_1 and q_2, so that on each subinterval of this new partition, both functions are constant. We now introduce a notational convention to describe the form of the matching between q_1 and q_2. For $i = 1, 2$ and $j = 1, 2, \ldots, n$, we let

$$s_j^i = \begin{cases} \text{`U'} & \text{if } q_i > 0 \text{ on } (t_{j-1}, t_j) \\ \text{`0'} & \text{if } q_i = 0 \text{ on } (t_{j-1}, t_j) \\ \text{`D'} & \text{if } q_i < 0 \text{ on } (t_{j-1}, t_j) \end{cases}$$

Then, the structure of the matching can be represented by the $2 \times n$ matrix with top row (s^1) and bottom row (s^2). Each column of this matrix represents the type of the matching between q_1 and q_2 on the corresponding subinterval. The following definition establishes some terminology for describing a matching in terms of this matrix representation.

Definition 1. *An **up-segment** in a matching is a pattern consisting of $[U, U^T]$, followed by zero or more instances of $[0U, DU]^T$ or $[DU, 0U]^T$. A **down-segment** in a matching is a pattern consisting of $[D, D]^T$, followed by zero or more instances of $[0D, UD]^T$ or $[UD, 0D]^T$.*

It is shown in [6] that if any two functions f_1 and f_2 are PL, then a matching that is optimal in the sense of Eq. 2 exists. The following theorem gives constraints on the overall structure of an optimal matching.

Theorem 1. *Any optimal matching consists of the following components, in the following order:*

1. *Optionally, one column of the form* $[U, \ 0]^T$, $[0, \ U]^T$, $[D, \ 0]^T$, *or* $[0, \ D]^T$, *then*
2. *An alternating sequence of zero or more up-segments and down-segments, and finally*
3. *Optionally one column of the form* $[U, \ 0]^T$, $[0, \ U]^T$, $[D, \ 0]^T$, *or* $[0, \ D]^T$

This is a consequence of Theorem 6 in [6], which applies to the more general case of curves in $\mathbb{R}^N$. Within each up- or down-segment, the matching is constrained by the following lemma, which we state without proof due to space constraints.

Lemma 1. *Let* q_1 *and* q_2 *be step functions representing an optimal matching between their respective orbits, and assume that* q_1 *and* q_2 *have a common change point partition* $0 = t_1 < t_2 < \ldots < t_n = 1$. *Suppose the matching from* t_a *to* t_b *forms an up-segment, so that* $b - a$ *is odd, and the matching form is*

- $[U, \ U]^T$ *on* (t_a, t_{a+1}), (t_{a+2}, t_{a+3}), ..., *and* (t_{b-1}, t_b), *and*
- $[D, \ 0]^T$ *or* $[0, \ D]^T$ *on* (t_{a+1}, t_{a+2}), (t_{a+3}, t_{a+4}), ..., *and* (t_{b-2}, t_{b-1}).

Then, the ratio $q_2(t)/q_1(t)$ *is the same for all intervals on which both* q_1 *and* q_2 *are positive. Similarly, in a down-segment, the ratio* $q_2(t)/q_1(t)$ *must be the same for all intervals on which both* q_1 *and* q_2 *are negative.*

4   The Matching Algorithm

In the previous section, we deduced several properties of an optimal matching between piecewise constant SRVFs. Now we will shift our focus to actually finding optimal matching. We will start with two functions f_1, f_2 that are arc-length parameterized and have finitely-many change points. The corresponding SRVFs $q_1, q_2 \in \mathbb{L}^2$ are unit-speed step functions (i.e. taking only values 1 and -1). We seek warpings $\gamma_1, \gamma_2 \in \Gamma$ which solve Eq. 2, or equivalently maximize the inner product $\langle q_1 * \gamma_1, q_2 * \gamma_2 \rangle$.

The key idea is that for any up- or down-segment the corresponding contribution to the inner product between the warped SRVFs can be easily determined, as can the corresponding portions of γ_1 and γ_2 that realize the matching. Once we have an alternating sequence of up- and down-segments, the rest of the matching is determined (up to a common warping of both functions). Therefore, our matching problem boils down to an optimization over all possible alternating sequences of peak-to-peak and valley-to-valley matchings, and we will solve this using the dynamic programming. Before presenting the algorithm, we need to do one last bit of preliminary work.

4.1   The Contribution of an Up- or Down-Segment

Suppose that $\tilde{q}_1 = q_1 * \gamma_1$ and $\tilde{q}_2 = q_2 * \gamma_2$ are warped SRVFs constituting an optimal matching, and suppose that $\tilde{q}_1$ and $\tilde{q}_2$ are step functions sharing the common change point partition $t_0 = 0 < t_1 < \ldots < t_n = 1$. Suppose that $\tilde{q}_1$ and $\tilde{q}_2$ form an up-segment on the interval (t_a, t_{a+l}) for some odd integer $l \geq 1$, and let $\tilde{A}$ be the union of the intervals on which both functions are positive:

$$\tilde{A} = (t_a, t_{a+1}) \cup (t_{a+2}, t_{a+3}) \cup \ldots \cup (t_{a+l-1}, t_{a+l})$$

Let $A_1 = \gamma_1(\tilde{A})$ and let $A_2 = \gamma_2(\tilde{A})$, and note that these are the sets in the up-segment on which q_1 and q_2 are positive. Further, since q_1 and q_2 are unit-speed SRVFs, it is easy to see that the measures $|A_1|$ and $|A_2|$ of these sets are equal to the total rise of f_1 and f_2 (respectively) for the up-segment. Now, using the Cauchy-Schwarz inequality and a simple change of variable, we get the following upper bound for the contribution of the up-segment to the overall inner product between the matched functions:

$$\int_{t_a}^{t_{a+l}} \tilde{q}_1(t)\tilde{q}_2(t)dt = \int_{\tilde{A}} \tilde{q}_1(t)\tilde{q}_2(t)dt \leq \sqrt{|A_1|}\sqrt{|A_2|} .$$

Similarly, for a down-segment, the maximum contribution to the overall inner product is equal to $\sqrt{|A_1|}\sqrt{|A_2|}$, where A_1 and A_2 are the sets on which q_1 and q_2 are negative, and $|A_1|$ and $|A_2|$ are the total fall in f_1 and f_2 in the down-segment. Next we provide an efficient algorithm for constructing functions γ_1 and γ_2 which achieve these bounds.

4.2 The Matching Graph

Our optimization problem can be naturally formulated as a maximum-weight path problem in a certain weighted, directed, bipartite graph. Recall that SRVFs q_1 and q_2 are step functions with values in $\{-1, 1\}$. A legal assignment between peaks and valleys can be represented by a sequence $(i_1, j_1), (i_2, j_2), \ldots, (i_m, j_m) \subseteq \{0, 1, \ldots, n_1\} \times \{0, 1, \ldots, n_2\}$ satisfying the following:

1. For $k = 2, 3, \ldots, m$, $i_k > i_{k-1}$ and $j_k > j_{k-1}$.
2. For $k = 1, 2, \ldots, m$, $t_{i_k}^1$ and $t_{j_k}^2$ both correspond to peaks, or they both correspond to valleys.
3. If $t_{i_k}^1$ and $t_{j_k}^2$ correspond to peaks, then the next pair will correspond to valleys, and vice versa.
4. For i_1 and j_1, one of the following is true: $i_1 = 0$ and $j_1 = 0$, or, $i_1 = 1$ and $j_1 = 0$, or, $i_1 = 0$ and $j_1 = 1$
5. For i_m and j_m, one of the following is true: $i_m = n_1$ and $j_m = n_2$, or, $i_m = n_1 - 1$ and $j_m = n_2$, or, $i_m = n_1$ and $j_m = n_2 - 1$

Conditions (4) and (5) reflect the fact that in an optimal matching, there is at most one leading half-zero column and at most one trailing half-zero column. The set of all possible sequences is naturally represented as a directed bipartite graph G with a vertex for each peak-to-peak match and a vertex for each valley-to-valley match. G will have a vertex for every pair of indices (i, j) such that

t_i^1 and t_j^2 are either both peaks, or both valleys. G has a directed edge from (i, j) to (k, l) iff $i < k$, $j < l$, and one of the vertices represents a peak-peak matching while the other represents a valley-valley matching. Therefore, the edges of G correspond exactly to the possible up- and down-segments in an optimal matching. We will also assign a weight to each edge, which is equal to the contribution of the corresponding up- or down-segment to the total inner product of the matching. Figure 2 show examples of legal paths through the matching graph, corresponding to an alternating sequence of up- and down-segments. The total inner product of the matching represented by a path is equal to the sum of the weights of the edges in the path.

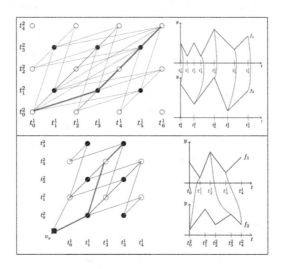

Fig. 2. Paths through matching graphs that represent correspondences between the peaks and valleys of two functions f_1 and f_2 (shown on right). Solid dots represent valley-to-valley matches, hollow circles represent peak-to-peak matches, and edges correspond to up- and down-segments. The red arcs indicate the peak-to-peak and valley-to-valley matchings.

In the top row of Fig. 2, both functions begin and end with peaks. Thus, all legal paths through the graph must start at the bottom-left vertex and end at the top-right vertex. However, if one function begins with a peak and the other begins with a valley, as in the bottom row of the figure, then the matching must begin with one of the half-zero forms: $[U, 0]^T, [0, U]^T, [D, 0]^T$, or $[0, D]^T$. In this case, paths can either start at the vertex $(0, 1)$ (corresponding to a matching beginning with $[0, U]^T$ or $[0, D]^T$), or at the vertex $(1, 0)$ (corresponding to a matching beginning with $[U, 0]^T$ or $[D, 0]^T$). Having two possible starting points is inconvenient, because our algorithm is basically a single-source shortest-path algorithm, and is handled by introducing a new vertex v_s to the graph (and adding zero-weight edges from v_s to $(0, 1)$ and from v_s to $(1, 0)$).

The algorithm for finding an optimal path through the matching graph (representing a sequence of peak-to-peak and valley-to-valley matchings yielding the highest possible inner product) is a straightforward application of dynamic programming. For each vertex v in our graph G, let $D[v]$ denote the weight of the path from the start vertex to v which has the highest total weight out of all such paths, and let $P[v]$ denote the predecessor of v along that path. The key idea that enables us to apply dynamic programming is that, since the total weight of a path is equal to the sum of the weights of its edges, the maximum-weight path problem has optimal substructure, and D can be given recursively by the following **dynamic programming functional equation** (DPFE): $D[v] = \max\limits_{p \in \mathrm{Preds}(v)} D[p] + W[p, v]$, where $\mathrm{Preds}(v)$ is the set of all vertices p from which there is a directed edge e_{pv} from p to v in the graph, and $W[p, v]$ is the weight of the edge from p to v. Recall that there will be an edge from $p = (i, j)$ to $v = (k, l)$ whenever $i < k$, $j < l$, and $k - i$ is odd (so that one vertex represents a peak-to-peak matching and the other represents a valley-to-valley matching). Therefore, when searching over the predecessors of v, we only need to consider vertices appearing strictly below and to the left of v in the grid. This predictable structure makes it possible for us to traverse the graph in a very simple way. We start by setting $D[(0, 0)] = 0$ (or $D[v_s] = 0$ if a dummy starting vertex was added), and then we compute the remaining values in a bottom-up flood-fill pattern. We work through the grid one row at a time, filling in the bottom row of the grid from left to right, then moving to the next row up, and so on. After D and P have been computed, we recover the path Π by starting at the top-right corner of the grid and tracing the path back to the starting vertex using P. See Algorithm 1 (supplementary material) for the details on computing D and P using dynamic programming, and Algorithm 2 (supplementary material) for details on recovering the optimal path Π given D and P.

4.3 Finding Optimal Matching γ_1 and γ_2

Now that we have a method for finding a maximum-weight path Π through the matching graph, we specify computation of functions $\gamma_1, \gamma_2 \in \Gamma$ which actually realize the optimal matching when applied to the unit-speed SRVFs q_1 and q_2. We should point out that there is not a unique solution to this problem: if $\gamma_1, \gamma_2 \in \Gamma$ is a pair of warpings realizing an optimal matching between our functions, then $\gamma_1 \circ \psi$ and $\gamma_2 \circ \psi$ also give us an optimal matching, for any PL $\psi \in \Gamma$. Suppose we have found a pair of optimal warpings $\gamma_1, \gamma_2 \in \Gamma$, so that the SRVFs comprising the optimal matching can be written as $\tilde{q}_1 = q_1 * \gamma_1$ and $\tilde{q}_2 = q_2 * \gamma_2$. Since q_1 and q_2 are unit-speed SRVFs, it follows that for any $t \in [0, 1]$, we have

$$|\tilde{q}_i(t)| = |(q_i * \gamma_i)(t)| = |\sqrt{\dot{\gamma}_i(t)} q_i(\gamma_i(t))| = \sqrt{\dot{\gamma}_i(t)}$$

for $i = 1, 2$. Since $\tilde{q}_1(t)$ and $\tilde{q}_2(t)$ are constant on each subinterval of the partition $\{t_i\}$, it follows that $\dot{\gamma}_1(t)$ and $\dot{\gamma}_2(t)$ are also constant on those subintervals.

Therefore, γ_1 and γ_2 are PL functions with $\{t_i\}$ as their common change point partition.

Above we noticed that choosing a different change point partition for $\tilde{q}_1$ and $\tilde{q}_2$ is equivalent to applying the same PL warping to both functions. Since the change points of $\tilde{q}_1$ and $\tilde{q}_2$ are also the change points of γ_1 and γ_2, this implies that *the change point parameters of γ_1 and γ_2 are completely arbitrary*. As we are building γ_1 and γ_2, we can choose any partition $\{t_i\}$ we like for the change point parameter values, so long as the partition has the correct number of points, and so long as we output the correct lists of function values $\{\gamma_1(t_i)\}$ and $\{\gamma_2(t_i)\}$. For lack of a "right" way to choose a change point partition, we simply use a uniformly-spaced partition of $[0, 1]$. For the most part we ignore the change point partition and focus on producing the lists of function values for γ_1 and γ_2. Let $\Pi = \{(i_1, j_1), (i_2, j_2), \ldots, (i_m, j_m)\}$ be the matching path produced by Algorithms 1 and 2. As above, let $\{t_i^1\}$ and $\{t_i^2\}$ denote the change point parameters of the original unit-speed SRVFs q_1 and q_2. Algorithm 3 (supplementary material) produces the lists of function values for γ_1 and γ_2.

We have described theory and algorithm for solving the optimization problem given in Eq. 2, resulting in two warping functions γ_1 and γ_2 that align f_1 and f_2. However, in some practical cases, it may be advantageous to fix one function, say f_1, and warping only f_2 to obtain optimal alignment. In fact, this is very useful in iterative alignment of multiple functions. We utilize a computational approximation that provides a single warping for approximating the exact dual-warping solution. To get there, we want to compose γ_2 with the inverse of γ_1 to obtain a single $\gamma^* = \gamma_2 \circ \gamma_1^{-1}$. Since Γ is a semigroup, γ_1 does not necessarily have an inverse, so we have to define a sort of pseudoinverse to approximate it. For each point, we take the largest value of its preimage: $\gamma_1^-(t) = \sup\left(\gamma_1^{-1}(\{t\})\right)$. Then, our alignment of f_2 to f_1 can be written as $\gamma^* = \gamma_2 \circ \gamma_1^-$. Because of the way γ_1^- is defined, it has jump discontinuities that correspond to intervals on which $\dot{\gamma}_1 = 0$. These jump discontinuities may seem, a priori, to be undesirable because they will cause $f_2 \circ \gamma$ to omit some segments of f_2. But the discontinuities correspond to flat segments of γ_1, and we know from Sect. 3 that such flat segments occur only where f_2 is increasing in a down-segment or decreasing in an up-segment. Thus γ^* will not remove any extrema of f_2 despite its discontinuities.

5   Multiple Function Alignment

Now we can address the problem of alignment of multiple functions – $f_1, f_2, \ldots, f_n$ with SRVFs $q_1, q_2, \ldots, q_n$ – using the pairwise solution derived above. We take an iterative approach where each iteration performs the following: (1) update a template function obtained using the cross-sectional mean of the currently aligned SRVFs $\mu_q = \frac{1}{n}\sum_{i=1}^{n}(q_i * \gamma_i)$, and (2) align each of the given SRVFs to this template μ_q in a pairwise fashion, i.e. find γ_i* that aligns q_i to μ_q. The latter step uses the single warping approximation discussed above. As described in earlier papers, μ_q represents the Karcher mean of given SRVFs and this algorithm corresponds to minimizing the error functional $H = \inf_{\mu_q}\left(\frac{1}{n}\sum_{i=1}^{n}\inf_{\gamma}\|\mu_q - (q_i * \gamma)\|^2\right)$.

6   Experimental Results

In this section we present a number of experimental results to demonstrate the efficiency and numerical accuracy of the proposed method. We will use two simulated and five real datasets of real-valued functions that have been used in the past to evaluate alignment performance. To evaluate alignment performance we use: (1) value of the objective function in Eq. 2 for pairwise alignment, (2) average computational cost, and (3) value of the error functional H for multiple function alignment.

We compare the proposed method only with the previous DPA since that (DPA + SRVF) is currently a state-of-the-art method for alignment of functions,

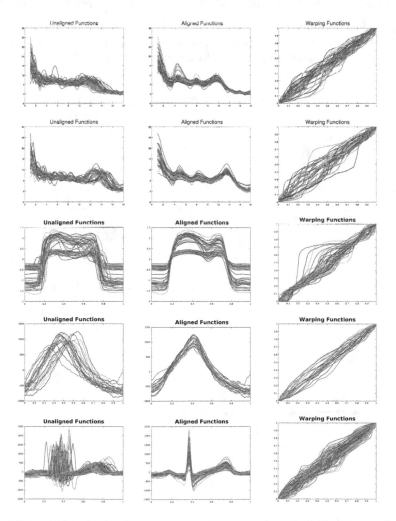

Fig. 3. Alignment results for datasets using the proposed method. From top to bottom, the datasets are: female growth, male growth, gait, respiration, and ECG datasets.

and the contribution here is to the algorithmic aspect of it. Comparisons between the SRVF framework and other mathematical frameworks can be found in other work related to the SRVF [13–15]. We also only make these comparisons on functions with relatively few change points, which is a case where the proposed method has an advantage. Noisy functions with many change points would present a more difficult challenge for the proposed method, and we do not deal with additive noise here. As justification, we point to an example dealing with additive noise in the SRVF framework in Chap. 4 of [13]. There, noise is dealt with by (1) smoothing the original noisy functions with a standard method, (2) registering the smooth functions, then (3) applying that warping registration to the original functions. Such a procedure would naturally reduce the number of change points and make the algorithm proposed in this paper more efficient.

Datasets: The two simulated datasets are made of functions with similar shapes but different in peak locations, as shown in the left column of Fig. 4. The first two real datasets we consider are growth velocity curves from the Berkeley Guidance

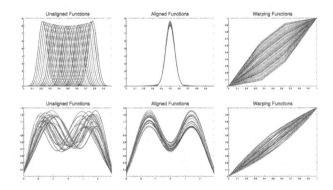

Fig. 4. Alignment of simulated data using the proposed method.

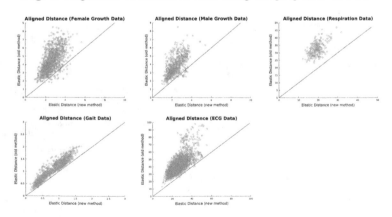

Fig. 5. Computed elastic distances between pairs of functions under DPA (Y axis) and new method (X axis).

Study. The heights of 54 female children and 39 male children were tracked between ages 1 and 18 and the rate of change in height was recorded as a function of time – the data we consider is the time derivative of the height functions. The remaining three real datasets are biosignal functions described in [5]. These signals are approximately periodic functions which are physical measurements of biological processes. We apply the proposed method to segmented cycles of these functions. The three signals are (1) respiration data, in which the function value is strain during respiration as measured by a pressure sensor on 24 subjects, (2) gait data, in which the function value represents the pressure under the foot of a person walking (50 subjects), and (3) ECG data, which consists of electrocardiogram cycles of 80 healthy control subjects. All of these real datasets are shown in the left column of Fig. 3.

Alignment Results. The alignment results for these different datasets are shown in are shown in Figs. 4 and 3. In each case, we display the original data $\{f_i\}$ – the smaller value implies a better performance, the aligned functions $\{f_i \circ \gamma_i\}$, and the warping functions $\{\gamma_i\}$. The high level of alignment is clearly discernible in these examples. Beyond visual evaluation, Fig. 5 plots the objective function in Eq. 2 computed by the two methods – ours and DPA – on a 2D graph with X coordinate being our method and Y coordinate being DPA. Since most of these points lie above the $X = Y$ line, we conclude that our method consistently obtained better optimization results in all the cases. Furthermore, Table 2 compares the computation costs (in seconds) of the two methods using the average time it takes to align two functions, for different datasets. These times are computed in MATLAB on a an Ubuntu laptop for both methods. The bottom row of this table provides the approximate gain in computational costs in using the new method over the DPA. We can see at least one order of magnitude improvement in all cases. Finally, we also quantify the level of alignment

Table 1. Multiple alignment performance evaluation using H, the average square distance of the aligned functions to the Karcher mean. In all datasets, H is smaller for the proposed method.

	Simu 1	Simu 2	Female	Male	Resp	Gait	ECG
DPA cost	0.058	0.009	10.323	7.559	368.0030	0.5499	823.4218
New cost	0.028	0.005	3.860	3.255	242.4702	0.4504	416.9259

Table 2. Average computation times (in seconds) to perform pairwise alignment and time gains by the new method over DPA.

Time(s)	Simu 1	Simu 2	Female	Male	Resp	Gait	ECG
DPA	11.9652	11.1796	4.2750	5.9494	8.0486	8.6609	10.3795
New	0.0061	0.0075	0.0970	0.1032	0.4207	0.0815	2.3494
Gain	1961	1491	44	57	19	106	4

using H, the average squared distance of each aligned SRVF $q_i * \gamma_i$ to the mean μ_q. These results are presented in Table 1. These values are found to be much smaller for our method than those for DPA, denoting a better alignment.

7   Conclusion

We have presented an efficient technique for registration of functional data that provides exact matching solutions in a fraction of time. While the past DPA algorithm needed a dense discretization of given functions, we exploit the fact that only the change points are relevant for matching. For functions with sparse change points, one can enumerate all potential matchings and use a dynamic programming, restricted to only these points, to select the best amongst them. In cases where the number of change points is much smaller than the discretization size, the gain in speed is tremendous. These results are demonstrated on several simulated and real datasets related to human biosignals.

References

1. Beg, M.F., Miller, M.I., Trouve, A., Younes, L.: Computing large deformation metric mappings via geodesic flows of diffeomorphisms. Int. J. Comput. Vis. **61**(2), 139–157 (2005)
2. Bertsekas, D.P.: Dynamic Programming and Optimal Control. Athena Scientific, Belmont (1995)
3. Huang, W., Gallivan, K.A., Srivastava, A., Absil, P.A.: Riemannian optimization for elastic shape analysis. In: The 21st International Symposium on Mathematical Theory of Networks and Systems (MTNS 2014) (2014)
4. Keogh, E., Ratanamahatana, C.A.: Exact indexing of dynamic time warping. Knowl. Inf. Syst. **7**, 358–386 (2005)
5. Kurtek, S., Wu, W., Christensen, G.E., Srivastava, A.: Segmentation, alignment and statistical analysis of biosignals with application to disease classification. J. Appl. Stat. **40**(6), 1270–1288 (2013)
6. Lahiri, S., Robinson, D., Klassen, E.: Precise matching of PL curves in $\mathbb{R}^N$ in the square root velocity framework (2015)
7. Liu, X., Muller, H.G.: Functional convex averaging and synchronization for time-warped random curves. J. Am. Stat. Assoc. **99**, 687–699 (2004)
8. Rabiner, L., Juang, B.H.: Fundamentals of Speech Recognition. Prentice-Hall Inc., Upper Saddle River (1993)
9. Ramsay, J.O., Li, X.: Curve registration. J. Roy. Stat. Soc. Ser. B **60**, 351–363 (1998)
10. Ramsay, J.O., Silverman, B.W.: Functional Data Analysis. Springer Series in Statistics, 2nd edn. Springer, New York (2005)
11. Sakoe, H., Chiba, S.: Dynamic programming algorithm optimization for spoken word recognition. IEEE Trans. Acoust. Speech Signal Process. **26**(1), 43–49 (1978)
12. Sebastian, T.B., Klein, P.N., Kimia, B.B.: On aligning curves. IEEE Trans. Pattern Anal. Mach. Intell. **25**(1), 116–125 (2003)
13. Srivastava, A., Klassen, E.: Functional and Shape Data Analysis. Springer Series in Statistics. Springer, New York (2016). https://books.google.com/books?id=0cMwDQAAQBAJ

14. Srivastava, A., Klassen, E., Joshi, S.H., Jermyn, I.H.: Shape analysis of elastic curves in Euclidean spaces. IEEE Trans. Pattern Anal. Mach. Intell. **33**(7), 1415–1428 (2011)
15. Srivastava, A., Wu, W., Kurtek, S., Klassen, E., Marron, J.S.: Registration of functional data using Fisher-Rao metric (2011). arXiv:1103.3817v2
16. Trouvé, A., Younes, L.: Diffeomorphic matching problems in one dimension: designing and minimizing matching functionals. In: Vernon, D. (ed.) ECCV 2000. LNCS, vol. 1842, pp. 573–587. Springer, Heidelberg (2000). doi:10.1007/3-540-45054-8_37
17. Veeraraghavan, A., Chellappa, R., Roy-Chowdhury, A.: The function space of an activity. In: IEEE Conference on Computer Vision and Pattern Recognition, vol. 1, pp. 959–968 (2006)
18. Veeraraghavan, A., Srivastava, A., Chowdhury, A.K.R., Chellappa, R.: Rate-invariant recognition of humans and their activities. IEEE Trans. Image Process. **18**(6), 1326–1339 (2009)
19. Zhou, F., Torre, F.: Canonical time warping for alignment of human behavior. In: Advances in Neural Information Processing Systems (2009)

Varifold-Based Matching of Curves via Sobolev-Type Riemannian Metrics

Martin Bauer[1], Martins Bruveris[2], Nicolas Charon[3],
and Jakob Møller-Andersen[1(✉)]

[1] Department of Mathematics, Florida State University, Tallahassee, USA
jmoeller@math.fsu.edu
[2] Department of Mathematics, Brunel University London, London, England
[3] CIS, Johns Hopkins University, Baltimore, USA

Abstract. Second order Sobolev metrics are a useful tool in the shape analysis of curves. In this paper we combine these metrics with varifold-based inexact matching to explore a new strategy of computing geodesics between unparametrized curves. We describe the numerical method used for solving the inexact matching problem, apply it to study the shape of mosquito wings and compare our method to curve matching in the LDDMM framework.

Keywords: Curve matching · Sobolev metrics · Riemannian shape analysis · Varifold distance · Minimizing geodesics · LDDMM

1 Introduction

Closed, unparametrized plane curves are used to represent the outline or shape of objects and as such they arise naturally in shape analysis and its applications [14]; these include medical imaging, computer animation, geometric morphometry and other fields. Analysis of shapes and their differences relies on the notion of distance between shapes. To define such a distance, we start from a Riemannian metric on the space of curves and compute its induced geodesic distance.

We consider in particular second order Sobolev metrics with constant coefficients. These are Riemannian metrics on $\mathrm{Imm}(S^1, \mathbb{R}^d)$, the space of regular, parametrized curves and they are invariant under the reparametrization group $\mathrm{Diff}(S^1)$. Hence they induce a Riemannian metric on the quotient space $\pi : \mathrm{Imm}(S^1, \mathbb{R}^d) \rightarrow \mathrm{Imm}(S^1, \mathbb{R}^d)/\mathrm{Diff}(S^1) \doteq B_i(S^1, \mathbb{R}^d)$ of unparametrized curves, whose elements are the shapes of objects one is interested in. To compute the geodesic distance between two shapes $\pi(c_0)$, $\pi(c_1)$ it is necessary to find minizing geodesics between the orbits $\pi(c_i) = c_i \circ \mathrm{Diff}(S^1)$.

In previous work [1] we achieved this by discretizing the diffeomorphism group $\mathrm{Diff}(S^1)$ and its action on curves to obtain a numerical representation of

M. Bauer, M. Bruveris, N. Charon, J. Møller-Andersen—All authors contributed equally to the article.

© Springer International Publishing AG 2017
M.J. Cardoso et al. (Eds.): GRAIL/MFCA/MICGen 2017, LNCS 10551, pp. 152–163, 2017.
DOI: 10.1007/978-3-319-67675-3_14

the orbit $c_1 \circ \mathrm{Diff}(S^1)$. Here we adopt a different approach. The varifold distance d^{Var} between curves, defined in Sect. 2.2, has reparametrizations in its kernel, meaning $d^{\mathrm{Var}}(c_0, c_1) = d^{\mathrm{Var}}(c_0, c_1 \circ \varphi)$ and hence we can check equivalence of shapes or unparametrized curves via

$$\pi(c_0) = \pi(c_1) \quad \Leftrightarrow \quad c_0 \in c_1 \circ \mathrm{Diff}(S^1) \quad \Leftrightarrow \quad d^{\mathrm{Var}}(c_0, c_1) = 0 \,.$$

Because the constraint $d^{\mathrm{Var}}(c_0, c_1) = 0$ is difficult to encode numerically we relax it and solve an inexact matching problem instead. Given two curves c_0, c_1, to find the geodesic between the shapes they represent, we minimize

$$E(c) + \lambda d^{\mathrm{Var}}(c(1), c_1) \,,$$

over all paths $c = c(t, \theta)$ with $c(0) = c_0$, where E is the Riemannian energy and λ a coupling constant; see Sect. 2.3 for details.

We describe the numerical implementation in Sect. 3 and then apply in Sect. 4 the proposed framework to analyse the shape of mosquito wings [13] and to classify fish outlines [7] using geodesic distances and spectral clustering. We also compare the behaviour of Sobolev metrics with curve matching in the LDDMM framework.

2 Mathematical Background

2.1 Sobolev Metrics on Shape Space of Curves

The space of smooth, regular curves with values in $\mathbb{R}^d$ is denoted by

$$\mathrm{Imm}(S^1, \mathbb{R}^d) = \{ c \in C^\infty(S^1, \mathbb{R}^d) \colon \forall \theta \in S^1, c'(\theta) \neq 0 \} \,, \tag{1}$$

where Imm stands for *immersions*. We call such curves parametrized, because as maps from the circle they carry with them a parametrization; we will define the space $B_{i,f}(S^1, \mathbb{R}^d)$ of unparametrized curves in (5). The space $\mathrm{Imm}(S^1, \mathbb{R}^d)$ is an open subset of the Fréchet space $C^\infty(S^1, \mathbb{R}^d)$ and therefore can be considered as a Fréchet manifold. Its tangent space $T_c \mathrm{Imm}(S^1, \mathbb{R}^d)$ at any curve c is the vector space $C^\infty(S^1, \mathbb{R}^d)$ itself.

We denote the Euclidean inner product on $\mathbb{R}^d$ by $\langle \cdot, \cdot \rangle$. Differentiation with respect to the curve parameter $\theta \in S^1$ is written as $c_\theta = \partial_\theta c = c'$. For any fixed curve c, we denote differentiation and integration with respect to arc length by $D_s = \frac{1}{|c_\theta|} \partial_\theta$ and $\mathrm{d}s = |c_\theta| \, \mathrm{d}\theta$, respectively. A path of curves is a smooth map $c : [0, 1] \rightarrow \mathrm{Imm}(S^1, \mathbb{R}^d)$ and we denote the space of all paths by $\mathcal{P} = C^\infty([0, 1], \mathrm{Imm}(S^1, \mathbb{R}^d))$. The velocity of a path c is denoted by $c_t = \partial_t c = \dot{c}$.

Definition 1. *A second order Sobolev metric with constant coefficients is a Riemannian metric on the space* $\mathrm{Imm}(S^1, \mathbb{R}^d)$ *of parametrized curves of the form*

$$G_c(h, k) = \int_{S^1} a_0 \langle h, k \rangle + a_1 \langle D_s h, D_s k \rangle + a_2 \langle D_s^2 h, D_s^2 k \rangle \, \mathrm{d}s \,, \tag{2}$$

where $h, k \in T_c \mathrm{Imm}(S^1, \mathbb{R}^d)$ *are tangent vectors,* $a_j \in \mathbb{R}_{\geq 0}$ *are constants and* $a_0, a_2 > 0$. *If* $a_2 = 0$ *and* $a_1 > 0$, *then* G *is a first order metric and if* $a_1 = a_2 = 0$ *it is a zero order or* L^2-*metric.*

Note that the symbols D_s and ds hide the nonlinear dependency of G_c in the base point c. We use arc length operations in the definition of G to ensure that the resulting metric is invariant under the action of the diffeomorphism group of S^1. The invariance property in turn allows us to define, using G, a Riemannian metric on the shape space of unparametrized curves.

The Riemannian length of a path $c \colon [0,1] \to \mathrm{Imm}(S^1, \mathbb{R}^d)$ is defined via

$$L(c) = \int_0^1 \sqrt{G_{c(t)}(c_t(t), c_t(t))} \, dt. \tag{3}$$

The induced geodesic distance between two given curves c_0, c_1 of the Riemannian metric G is then the infimum of the lengths of all paths connecting these two curves, i.e.,

$$\mathrm{dist}(c_0, c_1) = \inf \left\{ L(c) : c \in \mathcal{P}, \, c(0) = c_0, \, c(1) = c_1 \right\}.$$

We can find critical points of the length functional by looking for critical points of the energy

$$E(c) = \int_0^1 G_{c(t)}(c_t(t), c_t(t)) \, dt. \tag{4}$$

The geodesic equation which corresponds to the first order condition for critical points, $DE(c) = 0$, is in the case of Sobolev metrics a partial differential equation for the function $c = c(t, \theta)$. Solutions of this equation are called geodesics, and are locally distance-minimizing paths. Local and global existence results for geodesics of Sobolev metrics were proven recently in [3, 4, 12] and they serve as the theoretical foundation of the proposed numerical framework: they tell us that the geodesic distance between two curves can always be realized by a path between them, i.e. we can compute the geodesic distance by finding the energy-minimizing path.

Unparametrized Curves. Two curves that differ only by their parametrization represent the same geometric object. In the context of shape analysis it is therefore natural to consider them equal, i.e., we identify the curves c and $c \circ \varphi$, where φ is a reparametrization. We use as the reparametrization group the group,

$$\mathrm{Diff}(S^1) = \left\{ \varphi \in C^\infty(S^1, S^1) : \varphi' > 0 \right\},$$

of smooth diffeomorphisms of the circle. This is an infinite-dimensional regular Fréchet Lie group [10]. Reparametrizations act on curves by composition from the right, i.e., $c \circ \varphi$ is a reparametrization of c.

To define the quotient space of unparametrized curves we need to restrict ourselves to *free immersions*, i.e. those upon which the diffeomorphism group acts freely. In other words

$$c \in \mathrm{Imm}_f(S^1, \mathbb{R}^d) \quad \Leftrightarrow \quad \left(c \circ \varphi = c \Rightarrow \varphi = \mathrm{Id}_{S^1} \right).$$

This restriction is necessary for technical reasons; in applications almost all curves are freely immersed. The space

$$B_{i,f}(S^1, \mathbb{R}^d) = \mathrm{Imm}_f(S^1, \mathbb{R}^d)/\mathrm{Diff}(S^1), \tag{5}$$

of unparametrized curves is the orbit space of the group action restricted to free immersions. This space is again a Fréchet manifold although constructing charts is nontrivial in this case [5].

A Riemannian metric G on $\mathrm{Imm}(S^1, \mathbb{R}^d)$ is said to be *invariant* with respect to reparametrizations if is satisfies

$$G_{c \circ \varphi}(h \circ \varphi, k \circ \varphi) = G_c(h, k),$$

for all $\varphi \in \mathrm{Diff}(S^1)$. Sobolev metrics with constant coefficients are invariant with respect to reparametrizations and we have the following result concerning induced metrics on the quotient space.

Theorem 2. *An Sobolev metric with constant coefficients on* $\mathrm{Imm}(S^1, \mathbb{R}^d)$ *induces a metric on* $B_{i,f}(S^1, \mathbb{R}^d)$ *such that the projection* $\pi : \mathrm{Imm}_f(S^1, \mathbb{R}^d) \to B_{i,f}(S^1, \mathbb{R}^d)$ *is a Riemannian submersion.*

The geodesic distance of the induced Riemannian metric on $B_{i,f}(S^1, \mathbb{R}^d)$ can be calculated using paths in $\mathrm{Imm}(S^1, \mathbb{R}^d)$ connecting c_0 to the orbit $c_1 \circ \mathrm{Diff}(S^1)$, i.e., for $\pi(c_0), \pi(c_1) \in B_{i,f}(S^1, \mathbb{R}^d)$ we have,

$$\mathrm{dist}\big(\pi(c_0), \pi(c_1)\big) = \inf \big\{ L(c) : c \in \mathcal{P}, \, c(0) = c_0, \, c(1) \in c_1 \circ \mathrm{Diff}(S^1) \big\} .$$

In the same way, the action of other groups can be factored out if the metric has a corresponding invariance property. We will consider later the action of the group of orientation-preserving Euclidean motions $SE(d) = SO(d) \ltimes \mathbb{R}^d$,

$$(A, b).c = A.c + b, \quad (A, b) \in SO(d) \ltimes \mathbb{R}^d .$$

The corresponding geodesic distance on the space $B_i(S^1, \mathbb{R}^d)/SE(d)$ is then

$$\mathrm{dist}\big(\pi(c_0), \pi(c_1)\big) = \inf \big\{ L(c) : c \in \mathcal{P}, \, c(0) = c_0, \, c(1) \in c_1 \circ SE(d) \times \mathrm{Diff}(S^1) \big\} .$$

2.2 Varifold Distance on the Space of Curves

A second construction of a distance on the space of curves arises from the framework of geometric measure theory by interpreting curves as currents or varifolds. These concepts go back to the works of Federer but have been recently revisited within the field of shape analysis as practical fidelity terms for diffeomorphic registration methods [6,8]. Instead of relying on a quotient space representation, the core idea is to embed curves in a space of distributions. While the most general approach is explained in [9], the following gives a condensed overview adapted to the case of interest to this paper.

Let $C_0(\mathbb{R}^d \times S^1)$ be the space of continuous functions vanishing at infinity.

Definition 3. *A varifold is an element of the distribution space* $C_0(\mathbb{R}^d \times S^1)^*$. *The varifold application* $\mu : c \mapsto \mu_c$ *associates to any curve* $c \in \mathrm{Imm}(S^1, \mathbb{R}^d)$ *the varifold* μ_c *defined, for any* $\omega \in C_0(\mathbb{R}^d \times S^1)$, *by*

$$\mu_c(\omega) = \int_{S^1} \omega\left(c(\theta), \frac{c'(\theta)}{|c'(\theta)|}\right) ds. \tag{6}$$

The essential property is that μ_c is actually independent of the parametrization in the sense that for any reparametrization $\varphi \in \mathrm{Diff}(S^1)$, one has $\mu_{c\circ\varphi} = \mu_c$. Thus the map $c \mapsto \mu_c$ projects to a well-defined map from $B_{i,f}(S^1, \mathbb{R}^d)$ into the space of varifolds. Note however that the space of varifolds contains many other objects as well.

Distances between curves can be defined by restricting a distance or pseudo-distance defined on the space of varifolds. A simple approach leading to closed form expressions is to introduce a *reproducing kernel Hilbert space* (RKHS) of test functions and to use the corresponding kernel metric. Specifically, we consider kernels on $\mathbb{R}^d \times S^1$ of the form $k(x, u, y, v) \doteq \rho(|x-y|^2).\gamma(u \cdot v)$, i.e., k is the product of a positive, continuous radial basis function ρ on $\mathbb{R}^d$ and a positive, continuous zonal function γ on S^1. To any such k corresponds a RKHS $\mathcal{H}$ of functions, embedded in $C_0(\mathbb{R}^d \times S^1)$ with a dual metric $\langle \cdot, \cdot \rangle_{\mathrm{Var}}$ on the corresponding dual space $\mathcal{H}^*$ of varifolds. The reproducing kernel property implies—cf. [9] for details—that for any curves c_1, c_2 we have

$$\langle \mu_{c_1}, \mu_{c_2} \rangle_{\mathrm{Var}} = \iint_{S^1 \times S^1} \rho(|c_1(\theta_1) - c_2(\theta_2)|^2) \gamma\left(\frac{c_1'(\theta_1)}{|c_1'(\theta_1)|} \cdot \frac{c_2'(\theta_2)}{|c_2'(\theta_2)|}\right) ds_1 \, ds_2. \tag{7}$$

Now, taking $d^{\mathrm{Var}}(c_1, c_2) = \|\mu_{c_1} - \mu_{c_2}\|_{\mathrm{Var}} = \langle \mu_{c_1} - \mu_{c_2}, \mu_{c_1} - \mu_{c_2} \rangle_{\mathrm{Var}}^{1/2}$, the results of [9] imply the following theorem.

Theorem 4. *If* ρ *and* γ *are* C^1 *functions,* ρ *is* c_0-*universal and* $\gamma(1) > 0$, *then* d^{Var} *defines a distance between any two closed, unparametrized, oriented and embedded curves. In addition, the distance is invariant with respect to the action of rigid transformations.*

Note that we require the stronger condition that the curves under consideration have to be embedded. On the bigger space of immersions, as considered in the previous section, the induced distance can degenerate.

Invariance to rigid transformations means that for any $(A, b) \in SE(d)$, $d^{\mathrm{Var}}(A.c_1 + b, A.c_2 + b) = d^{\mathrm{Var}}(c_1, c_2)$. It is also possible to construct distances that are invariant with respect to changes of orientation: to achieve this one simply selects kernels satisfying $\gamma(-t) = \gamma(t)$.

Broadly speaking, the varifold distance (7) results in a localized comparison between the relative positions of points and tangent lines of the the two curves, quantified by the choice of kernel functions ρ and γ. As such, they do not derive from a Riemannian structre and there is no notion of geodesics in a shape space of curves. However, they provide a very efficient framework for defining and computing fidelity terms in relaxed matching problems as explained below.

2.3 Inexact Matching on the Shape Space of Curves

In this section we combine Sobolev metrics and varifold distances to compute geodesics on shape space via a relaxed optimization problem. Because reparametrizations lie in the kernel of the varifold distance,

$$d^{\mathrm{Var}}(c_0, c_1 \circ \varphi) = \|\mu_{c_0} - \mu_{c_1 \circ \varphi}\|_{\mathrm{Var}} = \|\mu_{c_0} - \mu_{c_1}\|_{\mathrm{Var}} = d^{\mathrm{Var}}(c_0, c_1),$$

we can reformulate the problem of finding geodesics as a constrained minimization problem,

$$\mathrm{dist}(\pi(c_0), \pi(c_1))^2 = \inf \left\{ E(c) : c \in \mathcal{P}, \, c(0) = c_0, \, d^{\mathrm{Var}}(c(1), c_1) = 0 \right\}. \quad (8)$$

where $d^{\mathrm{Var}}(c(1), c_1)$ is the varifold distance between the endpoint of the path $c(1)$ and the target curve c_1.

Because it is difficult to numerically encode the constraint $d^{\mathrm{Var}}(c(1), c_1) = 0$, we instead minimize the relaxed functional given by

$$\mathrm{dist}(\pi(c_0), \pi(c_1))^2 \approx \inf \left\{ E(c) + \lambda d^{\mathrm{Var}}(c(1), c_1)^2 : c \in \mathcal{P}, \, c(0) = c_0 \right\}. \quad (9)$$

If we minimize the relaxed functionals with an increasing sequence $\lambda \to \infty$, we would expect the minimizers to converge to the solution of the constrained minimization problem. For now we solve the problem with a fixed, large value of λ. This does not yield a geodesic with the correct endpoint, but for sufficiently large λ we can expect a good matching, see the beginning of Sect. 4. In the future we plan to analyze the problem using an augmented Lagrangian approach to automatically choose a suitable value for λ.

Considering additionally the action of the Euclidean motion group $SE(d)$ and using the invariance of the varifold distance under this group action we obtain the minimization problem

$$\inf \left\{ E(c) + \lambda d^{\mathrm{Var}}(c(1), A.c_1 + b)^2 : c \in \mathcal{P}, \, c(0) = c_0, \, (A, b) \in SE(d) \right\}. \quad (10)$$

to find geodesics on the space $B_{i.f}(S^1, \mathbb{R}^d)/SE(d)$.

3 Implementation

The H^2-metric on spline-curves. In order to discretize the Riemannian energy term in the optimization problem (9), we discretize paths of curves using tensor product B-splines with $N_t \times N_\theta$ knots of orders $n_t = 2$ and $n_\theta = 3$,

$$c(t, \theta) = \sum_{i=1}^{N_t} \sum_{j=1}^{N_\theta} c_{i,j} B_i(t) C_j(\theta). \quad (11)$$

Here $B_i(t)$ are B-splines defined by an equidistant simple knot sequence on $[0, 1]$ with full multiplicity at the boundary points, and $C_j(\theta)$ are defined by an equidistant simple knot sequence on $[0, 2\pi]$ with periodic boundary conditions; for details see [1]. Note that the full multiplicity of boundary knots in t implies

$$c(0, \theta) = \sum_{j=1}^{N_\theta} c_{1,j} C_j(\theta) \,, \qquad c(1, \theta) = \sum_{j=1}^{N_\theta} c_{N_t,j} C_j(\theta) \,.$$

Thus the end curve $c(1)$ is given by the control points $c_{N_t,j}$. We approximate the integrals in the energy functional (4) using Gaussian quadrature with quadrature sites placed between knots.

Some notes on previous work: to solve the geodesic boundary value problem on shape space, we have proposed in [1] a method that involves discretizing the reparametrization group $\mathrm{Diff}(S^1)$ using B-splines. However, the action of the reparametrization group is by composition, which does not preserve the B-spline space. To overcome this we added a projection step, where we project the composition $c \circ \varphi$ back into the spline space. This has the disadvantage that the projection smoothes out details of the original curve, depending on how many control points are used and which parts of the curve are reparametrized. Furthermore, this methods requires a good choice of an initial path, which turned out to be a nontrivial obstacle in examples where the shapes under consideration are sufficiently different from each other. These considerations are our motivation to consider inexact matching with a varifold distance.

The Varifold Distance on Spline Curves. Our discretization of the varifold distance on spline curves builds on existing code for polygonal curves. Given two spline curves $c_1 = \sum_{j=1}^{N_\theta} c_{1,j} C_j$ and $c_2 = \sum_{j=1}^{N_\theta} c_{2,j} C_j$, a simple way of discretizing the varifold distance (7) is to approximate the splines by polygonal curves, i.e., choose sample vertices $v_{1,k} = c_1(\theta_k)$ and $v_{2,k} = c_2(\theta_k)$ with $\theta_k \in S^1$ for $1 \leq k \leq P$ and $\theta_{P+1} = \theta_1$. In future work we plan to calculate the varifold distance directly for spline curves, without the approximating step used here.

Denoting the edge vectors $e_{1,k} = v_{1,k+1} - v_{1,k}$ and $e_{2,k} = v_{2,k+1} - v_{2,k}$, the inner product (7) for the two polygonal curves $\tilde{c}_1$ and $\tilde{c}_2$ becomes

$$\langle \mu_{\tilde{c}_1}, \mu_{\tilde{c}_2} \rangle_{\mathrm{Var}} =$$

$$\sum_{k,l=1}^{P} |e_{1,k}| \cdot |e_{2,l}| \cdot \gamma \left(\frac{e_{1,k}}{|e_{1,k}|} \cdot \frac{e_{2,l}}{|e_{2,l}|} \right) \iint_{[0,1]^2} \rho(|v_{1,k} + t_1 e_{1,k} - v_{2,l} - t_2 e_{2,l}|^2) \, dt_1 \, dt_2 \,.$$

In general, there are no closed form expressions for such integrals and hence we use a numerical approximation: we evaluate the integrand at the central point $(t_1, t_2) = (\frac{1}{2}, \frac{1}{2})$, leading to the discrete approximation

$$\langle \mu_{c_1}, \mu_{c_2} \rangle_{\mathrm{Var}} \approx$$

$$\sum_{k,l=1}^{P} |e_{1,k}| \cdot |e_{2,l}| \cdot \gamma \left(\frac{e_{1,k}}{|e_{1,k}|} \cdot \frac{e_{2,l}}{|e_{2,l}|} \right) \cdot \rho \left(\left| \frac{v_{1,k} + v_{1,k+1}}{2} - \frac{v_{2,l} + v_{2,l+1}}{2} \right|^2 \right)$$

and the corresponding expression for the distance d^{Var}. The total error resulting from both the polygonal approximation and the integral approximation can be shown to be of the order of $O(\max\{|\theta_{k+1} - \theta_k|\})$.

Additionally, we can compute the gradient of the discrete inner product with respect to, say, the spline coefficients $c_{1,j}$, using the chain rule. Indeed, denoting A the approximation of $\langle \mu_{c_1}, \mu_{c_2} \rangle_{\mathrm{Var}}$,

$$\partial_{v_1} A = \partial_{x_1} A . \partial_{v_1} x_1 + \partial_{e_1} A . \partial_{v_1} e_1$$

where $x_{1,k} = (v_{1,k} + v_{1,k+1})/2$ is the edge midpoint. The gradients $\partial_{x_1} A$ and $\partial_{e_1} A$ are easily computed from the expression for A, while $\partial_{v_{1,l}} x_{1,k} = (\delta_{k-1}(l) + \delta_k(l))/2$ and $\partial_{v_{1,l}} e_{1,k} = \delta_{k-1}(l) - \delta_k(l)$. Finally, to obtain the gradient with respect the $c_{1,j}$ we apply the chain rule a second time, noting that $\partial_{c_{1,j}} v_{1,k} = C_j(\theta_k)$.

Our implementation includes many different choices of admissible kernel functions ρ and γ, including the ones presented in [9].

The Inexact Matching Functional. With the discretization described above, the optimization problem (10) becomes an unconstrained optimization problem for the control points $c_{i,j}$ the rotation matrix A and the translation vector b. We choose a Limited-memory BFGS (L-BFGS) method to solve this problem, as implemented in the HANSO library [11] for Matlab, where we supply the formula for the gradient of the target function, see [1,9] for the specific formulas.

We initialize the optimization problem with the constant path $c(t, \theta) = c_0(\theta)$. Note that this overcomes one of the major drawbacks of the framework developed in [1], which requires an initial path without singularities connecting the given curves c_0 and c_1. To speed up the optimization we implemented a multigrid method, i.e., we first solve the geodesic problem with a coarser spline discretization and use the resulting optimal path to initialize the minimization of the original problem. A comparison of the resulting computation times can be seen in Table 1. The obtained computation times are of the same order of magnitude as those of the SRV framework [15][1].

Table 1. Average computation time (3.5 Ghz Core i7U) of the geodesic distance between mosquito wings (first line) and between shapes from the Surrey fish database (second line). The used methods are: L-BFGS without multigrid, with multigrid and with gradient calculation done via automatic differentiation (without multigrid).

Computation times	L-BFGS	Multigrid	Aut. Diff
Mosquito wings	1.9 s	1.0 s	3.0 s
Surrey fish	3.1 s	1.7 s	4.7 s

---

[1] We used the publicly available Matlab implementation, which can be downloaded at http://ssamg.stat.fsu.edu/software.

We also experimented with an implementation using automatic differentiation for the gradient calculation. While our implementation of the gradient is approximatively three times faster then the gradient computated with automatic differentiation, the resulting computation time for the optimization differed in average only by 51%, see Table 1. Automatic differentiation will allow us to implement, with little additional effort, a much wider class of Riemannian metrics, including curvature- and length-weighted metrics. See [2, 12] for an overview of several Riemannian metrics on the space of curves.

For our previous method [1] we achieved a great speed-up of the optimization using a second order trust-region method—requiring us to compute the Hessian of the Riemannian energy. We tried this as well for this problem, but achieved no improvement in convergence. We speculate that this is due to the fact that the Hessian of the varifold distance is degenerate due to its kernel containing reparametrizations.

4   Experiments

Influence of the weight λ. The weight λ for the fidelity term has a big influence on the quality of the matching. The solution of the optimization problem for different values of λ is depicted in Fig. 1, and one can see that a good final matching requires a choice of a large enough λ. Choosing λ too large, on the other hand, will make the functional too rigid, and the resulting deformation will be far from a geodesic. In the presence of noice, a large λ might also result in overfitting. In future work we plan to investigate how to choose this parameter.

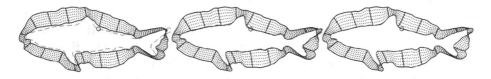

Fig. 1. Influence of the weight λ on the quality of the matching: Minimizers of (10) for $\lambda = 0.3, 1$ and 5. The target curve is depicted in blue. (Color figure online)

Towards a Comparison with LDDMM Curve Matching. Curve matching frameworks based on the LDDMM model such as [8, 9] are also formulated as relaxed optimizations involving the same varifold fidelity terms like (9) with the difference that curve evolution is governed by an extrinsic and dense deformation of the plane and the metric on the shape space is now induced from a metric on the diffeomorphism group. Yet the parallels between the two formulations and algorithms should allow one to draw some insightful comparisons of the two models. Although this topic will need to be treated more extensively in future work, we show in Fig. 2 a simple example illustrating the difficulty, in the LDDMM setting, to generate a deformation that is able to stretch a thin structure in contrast with the intrinsic metric approach of this paper.

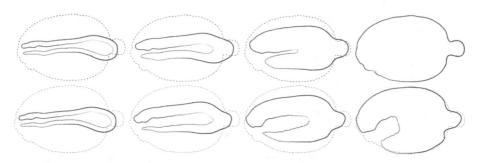

Fig. 2. Geodesics at time steps $0, 0.3, 0.6, 1$. First row: Inexact H^2-metric. Second row: LDDMM matching obtained using the algorithm of [9]. Note that in the latter case, increasing the weight of the fidelity term or varying deformation scales do not in fact lead to significanty better matching results than shown here.

Shape Clustering. We next illustrate the discriminative power of our method for the problem of finding different clusters within a population of shapes. We focus on a small subset of $n = 54$ shapes from the Surrey fish dataset and compute all the pairwise matchings between them. We then obtain a distance matrix given by the geodesic distance of the H^2-metric. Due to the asymmetry of inexact matching, we symmetrize the distance matrix a posteriori. In order to extract meaningful clusters, we use the spectral clustering framework presented in [16]: the p-nearest neighbour graph is constructed based on the distance matrix (we use $p = 12$ here) and the eigenvectors of the Jordan & Weiss normalized graph Laplacian are computed. Then each shape i is mapped as the i-th row vector of the $n \times k$ matrix of the first k eigenvectors and a k-means algorithm is used to separate those points into k clusters.

The results of this approach for $k = 7$ clusters is shown in Fig. 3. Overall, up to a few exceptions, the method is able to discriminate well between the different classes of this particular population with an accuracy comparable to using the LDDMM framework for measuring shape distances but with significantly faster computation of the distance matrix.

Mosquito Wings. Finally we want to demonstrate our numerical framework by providing a simple analysis of a set of mosquito wings. The data consists of the boundary curves $c_1, \ldots, c_{126}$ of 126 mosquito wings. The acquisition of the data is described in the article [13], where the authors analyzed the data using a polar coordinate system to describe each wing via the distance function from its centroid. Using inexact geodesic matching we use as a template the Karcher mean $\bar{c}$ of the data, with respect to the Sobolev metric. In the tangent space of the mean we represent each curve c_j by the initial velocity $v_j = \text{Log}_{\bar{c}(c_j)}$ to the geodesic connecting $\bar{c}$ and c_j. We then do a PCA with respect to the inner product $G_{\bar{c}}$ of the data in the linear tangent space. Figure 4 depicts the data set after projecting onto the subspace spanned by the first two principal components, and the geodesic in the direction of these to directions. It seems to

162   M. Bauer et al.

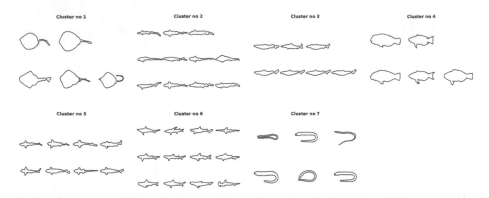

Fig. 3. The results of the cluster analysis for 54 shapes from the Surrey fish dataset obtained from the spectral clustering method.

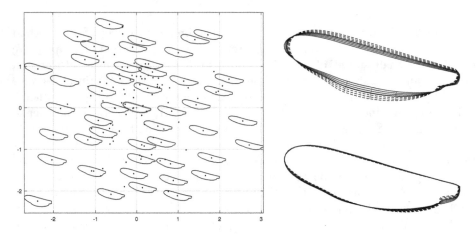

Fig. 4. Left: Wings projected to the plane in the tangent space of the mean, spanned by the first two principal directions. Right: Geodesics from the mean in the two first principal directions.

suggest that the two principal directions control the thickness of the wings, and the depth of the fold at the end, respectively.

5   Conclusions

In this article we present a new numerical method to compute geodesics for second order Sobolev metrics. The proposed algorithm is based on previous work on Sobolev metrics [1] and the varifold distance [9]. Since reparametrizations are in the kernel of the varifold distance we avoid having to discretize the reparametrization group $\mathrm{Diff}(S^1)$ to solve the geodesic boundary value problem on shape space. This allows us to overcome certain problems of the framework presented in [1]. Furthermore this new approach is better suited for generalization to shape spaces of unparametrized surfaces. Additionally, since we are now using an L-BFGS method—this only requires the computation of the gradient but not of the Hessian—it will be possible to generalize this framework with little additional effort to a much wider class of metrics. We plan to follow these lines of research in future work and use it to investigate methods for a data-driven choice of a Riemannian metric for applications in shape analysis.

References

1. Bauer, M., Bruveris, M., Harms, P., Møller-Andersen, J.: A numerical framework for Sobolev metrics on the space of curves. SIAM J. Imaging Sci. **10**(1), 47–73 (2017)
2. Bauer, M., Bruveris, M., Michor, P.W.: Overview of the geometries of shape spaces and diffeomorphism groups. J. Math. Imaging Vis. **50**, 60–97 (2014)
3. Bruveris, M.: Completeness properties of Sobolev metrics on the space of curves. J. Geom. Mech. **7**(2), 125–150 (2015)
4. Bruveris, M., Michor, P.W., Mumford, D.: Geodesic completeness for Sobolev metrics on the space of immersed plane curves. Forum Math. Sigma **2**, e19 (2014)
5. Cervera, V., Mascaró, F., Michor, P.W.: The action of the diffeomorphism group on the space of immersions. Differ. Geom. Appl. **1**(4), 391–401 (1991)
6. Charon, N.: Analysis of geometric and functional shapes with extensions of currents. Application to registration and atlas estimation. Ph.D. thesis, ENS Cachan (2013)
7. Mokhtarian, F., Abbasi, S., Kittler, J.: Efficient and robust shape retrieval by shape content through curvature scale space. In: Proceedings of First International Conference on Image Database and Multi-Search, pp. 35–42 (1996)
8. Glaunès, J., Qiu, A., Miller, M., Younes, L.: Large deformation diffeomorphic metric curve mapping. Int. J. Comput. Vis. **80**(3), 317–336 (2008)
9. Kaltenmark, I., Charlier, B., Charon, N.: A general framework for curve and surface comparison and registration with oriented varifolds. In: Computer Vision and Pattern Recognition (CVPR) (2017)
10. Kriegl, A., Michor, P.W.: The Convenient Setting of Global Analysis. Mathematical Surveys and Monographs, vol. 53. American Mathematical Society, Amsterdam (1997)
11. Lewis, A.S., Overton, M.L.: Nonsmooth optimization via quasi-Newton methods. Math. Program. **141**, 1–29 (2013)
12. Michor, P.W., Mumford, D.: An overview of the Riemannian metrics on spaces of curves using the Hamiltonian approach. Appl. Comput. Harmon. Anal. **23**(1), 74–113 (2007)
13. Rohlf, F.J., Archie, J.W.: A comparison of Fourier methods for the description of wing shape in mosquitoes (Diptera: Culicidae). Syst. Biol. **33**(3), 302–317 (1984)
14. Srivastava, A., Klassen, E.: Functional and Shape Data Analysis. Springer Series in Statistics. Springer, New York (2016)
15. Srivastava, A., Klassen, E., Joshi, S.H., Jermyn, I.H.: Shape analysis of elastic curves in Euclidean spaces. IEEE Trans. Pattern Anal. **33**(7), 1415–1428 (2011)
16. Von Luxburg, U.: A tutorial on spectral clustering. Stat. Comput. **17**(4), 395–416 (2007)

Computational Anatomy in Theano

Line Kühnel[(⊠)] and Stefan Sommer

Department of Computer Science, University of Copenhagen,
Copenhagen, Denmark
{kuhnel,sommer}@di.ku.dk

Abstract. To model deformation of anatomical shapes, non-linear statistics are required to take into account the non-linear structure of
the data space. Computer implementations of non-linear statistics and
differential geometry algorithms often lead to long and complex code
sequences. The aim of the paper is to show how the Theano framework
can be used for simple and concise implementation of complex differential geometry algorithms while being able to handle complex and high-
dimensional data structures. We show how the Theano framework meets
both of these requirements. The framework provides a symbolic language
that allows mathematical equations to be directly translated into Theano
code, and it is able to perform both fast CPU and GPU computations on
high-dimensional data. We show how different concepts from non-linear
statistics and differential geometry can be implemented in Theano, and
give examples of the implemented theory visualized on landmark representations of Corpus Callosum shapes.

Keywords: Computational anatomy · Differential geometry · Non-
linear statistics · Theano

1 Introduction

Euclidean statistical methods can generally not be used to analyse anatomical
shapes because of the non-linearity of shape data spaces. Taking into account
non-linearity and curvature of the data space in statistical analysis often requires
implementation of concepts from differential geometry.

Numerical implementation of even simple concepts in differential geometry
is often a complex task requiring manual implementation of long and complicated expressions involving high-order derivatives. We propose to use the Theano
framework in Python to make implementation of differential geometry and non-
linear statistics algorithms a simpler task. One of the main advantages of Theano
is that it can perform symbolic calculations and take symbolic derivatives of even
complex constructs such as symbolic integrators. As a consequence, mathematical equations can almost directly be translated into Theano code. For more
information on the Theano framework, see [8].

Even though Theano make use of symbolic calculations, it is still able to
perform fast computations on high-dimensional data. A main reason why Theano

© Springer International Publishing AG 2017
M.J. Cardoso et al. (Eds.): GRAIL/MFCA/MICGen 2017, LNCS 10551, pp. 164–176, 2017.
DOI: 10.1007/978-3-319-67675-3_15

can handle complicated data is the opportunity to use both CPU and GPU for calculations. As an example, Fig. 1 shows matching of 20000 landmarks on two different ellipsoids performed on a 40000-dimensional landmark manifold. The matching code was implemented symbolically using no explicit GPU code.

The paper will discuss multiple concepts in differential geometry and non-linear statistics relevant to computational anatomy and provide corresponding examples of Theano implementations. We start by considering simple theoretical concepts and then move to more complex constructions from sub-Riemannian geometry on fiber bundles. Examples of the implemented theory will be shown for landmark representations of Corpus Callosum shapes using the Riemannian manifold structure on the landmark space defined in the Large Deformation Diffeomorphic Metric Mapping (LDDMM) framework.

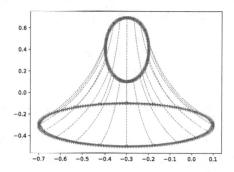

Fig. 1. Matching of 20000 landmarks on two ellipsoids. Only the matching curve for 20 landmarks have been plotted to make the plot interpretable. The GPU computation is automatic in Theano and no explicit GPU code is used for the implementation.

The presented Theano code is available in the Theano Geometry repository http://bitbucket.org/stefansommer/theanogeometry that includes Theano implementations of additional differential geometry, Lie group, and non-linear statistics algorithms. The described implementations are not specific to the LDDMM landmark manifold used for examples here. The code is completely general and can be directly applied to analysis of data modelled in spaces with different non-linear structures. For more examples of Theano implementation of algorithms directly targeting landmark dynamics, see [1,2].

The paper is structured as follows. Section 1.1 gives a short introduction to the LDDMM manifold. Section 2 concerns Theano implementation of geodesics as solution to Hamilton's equations. In Sect. 3, we use Christoffel symbols to define and implement parallel transport of tangent vectors. In Sect. 4, the Fréchet mean algorithm is considered, while stochastics, Brownian motions, and normal distributions are described in Sect. 5. Section 6 gives an example of calculating sample mean and covariance by estimating the Fréchet mean on the frame bundle. The paper ends with concluding remarks.

1.1 Background

The implemented theory is applied to data on a landmark manifold defined in the LDDMM framework [9]. More specifically, we will exemplify the theoretical concepts with landmark representations of Corpus Callosum (CC) shapes.

Consider a landmark manifold, $\mathcal{M}$, with elements $q = (x_1^1, x_1^2, \ldots, x_n^1, x_n^2)$ as illustrated in Fig. 2. In the LDDMM framework, deformation of shapes are modelled as a flow of diffeomorphisms. Let V denote a Reproducing Kernel Hilbert Space (RKHS) of vector fields and let $K \colon V \times V \to \mathbb{R}$ be the reproducing kernel, i.e. a vector field $v \in V$ satisfies $v(q) = \langle K_q, v \rangle_V$ for all $q \in \mathcal{M}$ with $K_q = K(., q)$. Deformation of shapes in $\mathcal{M}$ are then modelled by flows φ_t of diffeomorphisms acting on the landmarks. The flow solves the ordinary differential equation $\partial_t \varphi_t = v(t) \circ \varphi_t$, for $v \in V$. With suitable conditions on K, the norm on V defines a right-invariant metric on the diffeomorphism group that descends to a Riemannian structure on $\mathcal{M}$. The induced cometric $g_q^* \colon T_q^* \mathcal{M} \times T_q^* \mathcal{M} \to \mathbb{R}$ takes the form

$$g_q^*(\nu, \xi) = \sum_{i,j=1}^{n} \nu_i K(\boldsymbol{x}_i, \boldsymbol{x}_j) \xi_j, \tag{1}$$

where $\boldsymbol{x}^i = (x_i^1, x_i^2)$ for $i \in \{1, \ldots, n\}$. The coordinate matrix of the cometric is $g^{ij} = K(\boldsymbol{x}_i, \boldsymbol{x}_j)$ which results in the metric g having coordinates $g_{ij} = K^{-1}(\boldsymbol{x}_i, \boldsymbol{x}_j)$.

In the examples, we use 39 landmarks representing the CC shape outlines, and the kernel used is a Gaussian kernel defined by $K(\boldsymbol{x}_i, \boldsymbol{x}_j) = \mathrm{Exp}\left(-\frac{\|\boldsymbol{x}_i - \boldsymbol{x}_j\|^2}{2\sigma^2}\right)$ with variance parameter σ set to the average distance between landmarks in the CC data. Samples of CC outlines are shown in the right plot of Fig. 2.

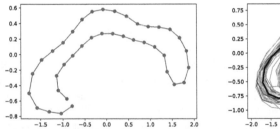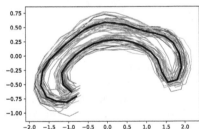

Fig. 2. (left) An example of a point in $\mathcal{M}$. (right) A subset of the data considered in the examples of this paper. The black curve represents the mean CC of the data.

2 Geodesics

Geodesics on $\mathcal{M}$ can be obtained as the solution to Hamilton's equations used in Hamiltonian mechanics to describe the change in position and momentum of a particle in a physical system. Let (U, φ) be a chart on $\mathcal{M}$ and assume $(\mathcal{M}, g)$ is a Riemannian manifold. The Hamiltonian H describes the total amount of energy in the physical system. From the cometric g^*, the Hamiltonian can be defined as $H(q,p) = \frac{1}{2}p^T g_q^* p$, where $g_q^* = (g^{ij})$ is the component matrix of g^* at q. Hamilton's equations are given as the system of ordinary differential equations

$$dq_t = \nabla_p H(q,p), \quad dp_t = -\nabla_q H(q,p).$$

Using the symbolic derivative feature of Theano, the system of ODE's can be represented and discretely integrated with the following code snippet:

```
"""
Hamiltonian function and equations
"""
# Hamiltonian function:
H = lambda q,p: 0.5*T.dot(p,T.dot(gMsharp(q),p))
# Hamiltonian equations:
dq = lambda q,p: T.grad(H(q,p),p)
dp = lambda q,p: -T.grad(H(q,p),q)

def ode_Ham(t,x):
    dqt = dq(x[0],x[1])
    dpt = dp(x[0],x[1])
    return T.stack((dqt,dpt))
# Geodesic:
Exp = lambda q,v: integrate(ode_Ham,T.stack((q,gMflat(v))))
```

where gMflat is the $\flat$ map turning tangent vectors in $T\mathcal{M}$ to elements in $T^*\mathcal{M}$. integrate denotes a function that integrates the ODE by finite time discretization. For the examples considered here, we use a simple Euler integration method. Higher-order integrators are available in the implemented repository mentioned in Sect. 1. A great advantage of Theano is that such integrators can be implemented symbolically as done below using a symbolic for -loop specified with theano.scan. The actual numerical scheme is only available after asking Theano to compile the function.

```
"""
Numerical Integration Method
"""
def integrator(ode_f):
    def euler(*y):
        t = y[-2]
        x = y[-1]
        return (t+dt,x+dt*ode_f(*y))
    return euler

def integrate(ode,x):
    (cout, updates) = theano.scan(fn=integrator(ode),
            outputs_info=[x],sequences=[*y], n_steps=n_steps)
    return cout
```

In the above, `integrator` specifies the chosen integration method, in this example the Euler method. Since the `integrate` function is a symbolic Theano function, symbolic derivatives can be obtained for the integrator, allowing e.g. gradient based optimization for the initial conditions of the ODE. As the derivatives of the integration schemes are symbolic, the schemes remain compatible.

An example of a geodesic found as the solution to Hamilton's equations is visualized in the right plot of Fig. 3. The initial point $q_0 \in \mathcal{M}$ was set to the average CC for the data shown in Fig. 2 and the initial tangent vector $v_0 \in T_{q_0}\mathcal{M}$ was given as the tangent vector plotted in Fig. 3.

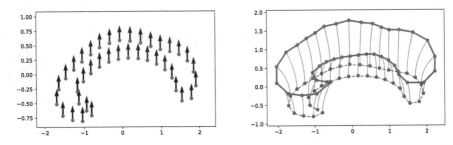

Fig. 3. (left) The initial point and tangent vector for the geodesic. (right) A geodesic obtained as solution to Hamilton's equations.

The exponential map, $\mathrm{Exp}_x : T_x\mathcal{M} \to \mathcal{M}$, $x \in \mathcal{M}$ is defined as $\mathrm{Exp}_x(v) = \gamma_1^v$, where γ_t^v, $t \in [0,1]$ is a geodesic with $\dot{\gamma}_0^v = v$. The inverse of the exponential map is called the logarithm map, denoted Log. Given two points $q_1, q_2 \in \mathcal{M}$, the logarithm map retuns the tangent vector $v \in T_{q_1}\mathcal{M}$ that results in the minimal geodesic from q_1 to q_2, i.e. v satisfies $\mathrm{Exp}_{q_1}(v) = q_2$. The logarithm map can be implemented using derivative based optimization by taking a symbolic derivative of the exponential map, `Exp`, implemented above:

```
"""
Logarithm map
"""
# Loss function for landmarks:
loss = lambda v,q1,q2: 1./d*T.sum(T.sqr(Exp(q1,v)-q2))
dloss = lambda v,q1,q2: T.grad(loss(v,q1,q2),v)
# Logarithm map: (v0 initial guess)
Log = minimize(loss, v0, jac=dloss, args=(q1,q2))
```

The use of the derivative features provided in Theano to take symbolic derivatives of a discrete integrator makes the implementation of the logarithm map extremely simple. The actual compiled code internally in Theano corresponds to a discrete backwards integration of the adjoint of the Hamiltonian system. An example of matching shapes by the logarithm map was shown in Fig. 1. Here two ellipsoids of 20000 landmarks were matched by applying the above `Log` function.

3   Christoffel Symbols

We here describe how Christoffel symbols can be computed and used in the Theano framework. A connection ∇ defines links between tangent spaces on $\mathcal{M}$ and describes how tangent vectors for different tangent spaces relate. Let (U, φ) denote a coordinate chart on $\mathcal{M}$ with basis coordinates ∂_i, $i = 1, \ldots, d$. The connection ∇ is uniquely described by its Christoffel symbols, Γ_{ij}^k, defined as $\nabla_{\partial_i} \partial_j = \Gamma_{ij}^k \partial_k$.

An example of a frequently used connection is the Levi-Civita connection for Riemannian manifolds. Based on the metric g on $\mathcal{M}$, the Levi-Civita Christoffel symbols are found by

$$\Gamma_{ij}^k = \frac{1}{2} g^{kl} (\partial_i g_{jl} + \partial_j g_{il} - \partial_l g_{ij}). \tag{2}$$

The Theano implementation below of the Christoffel symbols directly translates (2) into code:

```
"""
Christoffel Symbols
"""
## Cometric:
gsharp = lambda q: T.nlinalg.matrix_inverse(g(q))
## Derivative of metric:
Dg = lambda q: T.jacobian(g(q).flatten(),q).reshape((d,d,d))
## Christoffel symbols:
Gamma_g = lambda q: 0.5*(T.tensordot(gsharp(q),Dg(q),axes = [1,0])\
    + T.tensordot(gsharp(q),Dg(q),axes = [1,0]).dimshuffle(0,2,1)\
    - T.tensordot(gsharp(q),Dg(q),axes = [1,2]))
```

The connection, ∇, and Christoffel symbols, Γ_{ij}^k, can be used to define parallel transport of tangent vectors on $\mathcal{M}$. Let $\gamma \colon I \to \mathcal{M}$ be a curve and let $t_0 \in I$. A vector field V is said to be parallel along γ if the covariant derivative of V along γ is zero, i.e. $\nabla_{\dot{\gamma}_t} V = 0$. For a tangent vector $v_0 = v_0^i \partial_i \in T_{\gamma_{t_0}} \mathcal{M}$, there exists a unique parallel vector field V along γ s.t. $V_{t_0} = v_0$. Assume $V_t = v^i(t) \partial_i$, then the vector field V is parallel along γ if the coordinates follows the differential equation,

$$\dot{v}^k(t) + \Gamma_{ij}^k(\gamma_t) \dot{\gamma}_t^i v^j(t) = 0, \tag{3}$$

with initial values $v^i(0) = v_0^i$. In Theano code the ODE can be written as,

```
"""
Parallel transport
"""
def ode_partrans(gamma,dgamma,t,x):
    dpt = - T.tensordot(T.tensordot(dgamma, Gamma_gM(gamma),
                                     axes = [0,1]),x, axes = [1,0])
    return dpt


pt = lambda v,gamma,dgamma: integrate(ode_partrans,v,gamma,dgamma)
```

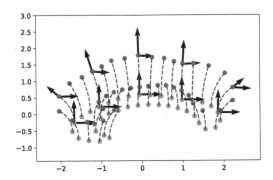

Fig. 4. Example of parallel transport of basis vectors v_1, v_2 along the geodesic with initial values q_0, v_2. The parallel transported vectors are only plotted for 5 landmarks.

Let q_0 be the mean CC plotted in Fig. 3 and consider $v_1, v_2 \in T_{q_0}\mathcal{M}$ s.t. v_1 is the vector consisting of 39 copies (one for each landmark) of $e_1 = (1,0)$ and v_2, the vector of 39 copies of $e_2 = (0,1)$. The tangent vector v_2 is shown in Fig. 3. Define γ as the geodesic calculated in Sect. 2 with initial values (q_0, v_2). The parallel transport of v_1, v_2 along γ is visualized in Fig. 4. To make the plot easier to interpret, the parallel transported vectors are only shown for five landmarks.

4   Fréchet Mean

The Fréchet mean [4] is a generalization of the Euclidean mean value to manifolds. Let d be a distance map on $\mathcal{M}$. The Fréchet mean set is defined as $F(x) = \arg\min_{y \in \mathcal{M}} \mathbb{E}d(y, x)^2$. For a sample of data points $x_1, \ldots, x_n \in \mathcal{M}$, the empirical Fréchet mean is

$$F_{\bar{x}} = \arg\min_{y \in \mathcal{M}} \frac{1}{n} \sum_{i=1}^{n} d(y, x_i)^2. \tag{4}$$

Letting d be the Riemannian distance function determined by the metric g, the distance can be formulated in terms of the logarithm map, defined in Sect. 2, as $d(x, y) = \|\mathrm{Log}(x, y)\|^2$. In Theano, the Fréchet mean can be obtained by optimizing the function implemented below, again using symbolic derivatives.

```
"""
Frechet Mean
"""
def Frechet_mean(q,y):
    (cout,updates) = theano.scan(fn=loss, non_sequences=[v0,q],
                    sequences=[y], n_steps=n_samples)
    return 1./n_samples*T.sum(cout)
dFrechet_mean = lambda q,y: T.grad(Frechet_mean(q,y),q)
```

The variable v0 denotes the optimal tangent vector found with the Log function in each iteration of the optimization procedure.

Consider a sample of 20 observations of the CC data shown in the right plot of Fig. 5. To calculate the empirical Fréchet mean on $\mathcal{M}$, the initial point $q_0 \in \mathcal{M}$ was set to one of the CC observations plotted in the left plot of Fig. 5. The result of the optimization is shown in Fig. 5 (bold outline).

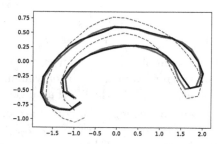 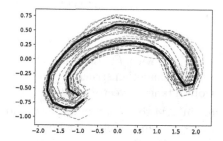

Fig. 5. (left) The estimated empirical Fréchet mean (black), the initial value (blue) and the Euclidean mean of the 20 samples (red). (right) Plot of the 20 samples of CC, with the Fréchet mean shown as the black curve. (Color figure online)

So far we have shown how Theano can be used to implement simple and frequently used concepts in differential geometry. In the following sections, we will exemplify how Theano can be used for stochastic dynamics and for implementation of more complex concepts from sub-Riemannian geometry on the frame bundle of $\mathcal{M}$.

5 Normal Distributions and Stochastic Development

We here consider Brownian motion and normal distributions on manifolds. Brownian motion on Riemannian manifolds can be constructed in several ways. Here, we consider two definitions based on stochastic development and coordinate representation of Brownian motion as an Itô SDE. The first approach [3] allows anisotropic generalizations of the Brownian motion [5,7] as we will use later.

Stochastic processes on $\mathcal{M}$ can be defined by transport of processes from $\mathbb{R}^m$, $m \leq d$ to $\mathcal{M}$ by the stochastic development map. In order to describe stochastic development of processes onto $\mathcal{M}$, the frame bundle has to be considered.

The frame bundle, $F\mathcal{M}$, is the space of points $u = (q, \nu)$ s.t. $q \in \mathcal{M}$ and ν is a frame for the tangent space $T_q\mathcal{M}$. The tangent space of $F\mathcal{M}$, $TF\mathcal{M}$, can be split into a vertical subspace, $VF\mathcal{M}$, and a horizontal subspace, $HF\mathcal{M}$, i.e. $TF\mathcal{M} = VF\mathcal{M} \oplus HF\mathcal{M}$. The vertical space, $VF\mathcal{M}$, describes changes in the frame ν, while $HF\mathcal{M}$ defines changes in the point $x \in \mathcal{M}$ when the frame ν is fixed in the sense of having zero acceleration measured by the connection. The frame bundle can be equipped with a sub-Riemannian structure by considering the distribution $HF\mathcal{M}$ and a corresponding degenerate cometric $g^*_{F\mathcal{M}} : TF\mathcal{M}^* \to HF\mathcal{M}$. Let (U, φ) denote a chart on $\mathcal{M}$ with coordinates $(x^i)_{i=1,\dots,d}$ and coordinate frame

$\partial_i = \frac{\partial}{\partial x^i}$ for $i = 1, \ldots, d$. Let ν_α $\alpha = 1, \ldots, d$ denote the basis vectors of the frame ν. Then (q, ν) have coordinates (q^i, ν_α^i) where $\nu_\alpha = \nu_\alpha^i \partial_i$ and ν_i^α defines the inverse coordinates of ν_α. The coordinate representation of the sub-Riemannian cometric is then given as

$$(g_{F\mathcal{M}})^{ij} = \begin{pmatrix} W^{-1} & -W^{-1}\Gamma^T \\ -\Gamma W^{-1} & \Gamma W^{-1}\Gamma^T \end{pmatrix}, \tag{5}$$

where W is the matrix with components $W_{ij} = \delta_{\alpha\beta}\nu_i^\alpha\nu_j^\beta$ and $\Gamma = (\Gamma_j^{h\gamma})$ for $\Gamma_j^{h\gamma} = \Gamma_{ji}^h \nu_\gamma^i$ with Γ_{ji}^h denoting the Christoffel symbols for the connection, ∇. The sub-Riemannian structure restricts infinitesimal movements to be only along horizontal tangent vectors. Let $\pi_{(q,\nu)}^*: T_q\mathcal{M} \to H_{(q,\nu)}F\mathcal{M}$ be the lift of a tangent vector in $T\mathcal{M}$ to its horizontal part and let $e \in \mathbb{R}^d$ be given. A horizontal vector at $u = (q, \nu)$ can be defined as the horizontal lift of the tangent vector $\nu e \in T_q\mathcal{M}$, i.e. $H_e(u) = (\nu e)^*$. A basis for the horizontal subspace at $u \in F\mathcal{M}$ is then defined as $H_i = H_{e_i}(u)$, where $e_1, \ldots, e_d$ denote the canonical basis of $\mathbb{R}^d$.

Let W_t denote a stochastic process on $\mathbb{R}^m$, $m \leq d$. A stochastic process U_t on $F\mathcal{M}$ can be obtained by the solution to the stratonovich stochastic differential equation, $dU_t = \sum_{i=1}^m H_i(U_t) \circ dW_t^i$, with initial point $u_0 \in F\mathcal{M}$. A stochastic process on $\mathcal{M}$ can then be defined as the natural projection of U_t to $\mathcal{M}$. In Theano, the stochastic development map is implemented as

```
"""
Stochastic Development
"""
def sde_SD(dWt,t,q,nu):
    return T.tensordot(Hori(q,nu), dWt, axes = [1,0])
stoc_dev = lambda q,u,dWt: integrate_sde(sde_SD,
                          integrator_stratonovich,q,u,dWt)[1]
```

Here, `integrate_sde` is a function performing stochastic integration of the SDE. The `integrate_sde` is defined in a similar manner as `integrate` described in Sect. 2. In Fig. 6 is given an example of stochastic development of a stochastic process W_t in $\mathbb{R}^2$ to the landmark manifold. Notice that for $m < d$, only the first m basis vectors of the basis H_i is used in the stochastic development.

Given the stochastic development map, Brownian motions on $\mathcal{M}$ can be defined as the projection of the stochastic development of Brownian motions in $\mathbb{R}^d$. Defining Brownian motions by stochastic development makes it possible to consider Brownian motions with anisotropic covariance by choosing the initial frame as not being orthonormal.

However, if one is only interested in isotropic Brownian motions, a different definition can be applied. In [6], the coordinates of a Brownian motion is defined as solution to the Itô integral,

$$dq_t^i = g_q^{kl}\Gamma_{kl}^i dt + \sqrt{g_q^*}^i dW_t. \tag{6}$$

This stochastic differential equation is implemented in Theano by the following code.

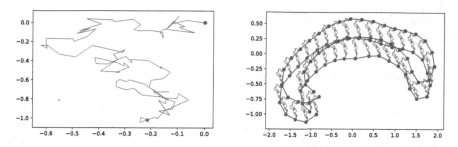

Fig. 6. (left) Stochastic process W_t on $\mathbb{R}^2$. (right) The stochastic development of W_t on $\mathcal{M}$. The blue points represents the initial point chosen as the mean CC. The red points visualize the endpoint of the stochastic development. (Color figure online)

```
"""
Brownian Motion in Coordinates
"""
def sde_Brownian_coords(dW,t,q):
    gMsharpq = gMsharp(q)
    X = theano.tensor.slinalg.Cholesky()(gMsharpq)
    det = T.tensordot(gMsharpq,Gamma_gM(q),((0,1),(0,1)))
    sto = T.tensordot(X,dW,(1,0))
    return (det,sto,X)
Brownian_coords = lambda x,dWt: integrate_sde(sde_Brownian_coords,
                                              integrator_ito,x,dWt)
```

An example of an isotropic Brownian motion found by the solution of (6) is shown in Fig. 7.

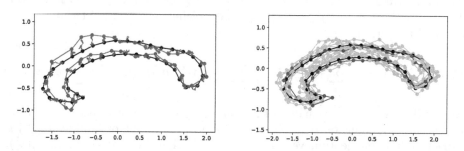

Fig. 7. (left) Brownian motion on $\mathcal{M}$. (right) Samples drawn from an isotropic normal distribution defined as the transition distribution of a Brownian motion obtained as a solution to (6).

In Euclidean statistical theory, a normal distribution can be considered as the transition distribution of a Brownian motion. A similar definition was described in [7]. Here a normal distribution on $\mathcal{M}$ is defined as the transition distribution of a Brownian motion on $\mathcal{M}$. In Fig. 7 is shown samples drawn from a normal distribution on $\mathcal{M}$ with mean set to the average CC shown in Fig. 2 and isotropic covariance. The Brownian motions are in this example defined in terms of (6).

6   Fréchet Mean on Frame Bundle

A common task in statistical analysis is to estimate the distribution of data samples. If the observations are assumed to be normally distributed, the goal is to estimate the mean vector and covariance matrix. In [7], it was proposed to estimate the mean and covariance of a normal distribution on $\mathcal{M}$ by the Fréchet mean on the frame bundle.

Consider Brownian motions on $\mathcal{M}$ defined as the projected stochastic development of Brownian motions on $\mathbb{R}^d$. A normal distribution on $\mathcal{M}$ is given as the transition distribution of a Brownian motion on $\mathcal{M}$. The initial point for the stochastic development, $u_0 = (q_0, \nu_0) \in F\mathcal{M}$, corresponds to the mean and covariance, i.e. $q_0 \in \mathcal{M}$ denotes the mean shape and ν_0 the covariance of the normal distribution. As a consequence, normal distributions with anisotropic covariance can be obtained by letting ν_0 be a non-orthonormal frame.

In Sect. 4, the Fréchet mean on $\mathcal{M}$ was defined as the point $y \in \mathcal{M}$, minimizing the average geodesic distance to the observations. However, as only a sub-Riemannian structure is defined on $F\mathcal{M}$, the logarithm map does not exist and hence the geodesic distance cannot be used to define the Fréchet mean on $F\mathcal{M}$. Instead, the distance function will be defined based on the most probable paths (MPP) defined in [5]. In this section, a slightly different algorithm for estimating the mean and covariance for a normal distribution is proposed compared to the one defined in [7].

Let $u = (q, \nu) \in F\mathcal{M}$ be given such that q, ν is the mean and covariance of a normal distribution on $\mathcal{M}$. Assume that observations $y_1, \ldots, y_n \in \mathcal{M}$ have been observed and let $p_1, \ldots, p_n \in H^* F\mathcal{M}$. The Fréchet mean on $F\mathcal{M}$ can then be obtained by optimizing,

$$F_{F\mathcal{M}} = \underset{(u, p_1, \ldots, p_n)}{\arg\min} \frac{1}{n} \sum_{i=1}^{n} \|p_i\|_{g_{F\mathcal{M}}^*}^2 + \frac{\lambda}{n} \sum_{i=1}^{n} d_{\mathcal{M}}(\pi(\mathrm{Exp}_u(p_i^\sharp)), y_i)^2 - \frac{1}{2}\mathrm{Log}(\det \nu),$$

where $\sharp$ denotes the sharp map on $F\mathcal{M}$ changing a momentum vector in $T^* F\mathcal{M}$ to the corresponding tangent vector in $T F\mathcal{M}$. The point of minimizing with respect to the momentum vector $p_1, \ldots, p_n$ is that the geodesics, $\mathrm{Exp}_u(p_i^\sharp)$, becomes MPPs on $F\mathcal{M}$, i.e. the first term penalizes the momentum vector. The second term decreases the distance of the mean to each data point as in the empirical Fréchet mean on $\mathcal{M}$, while the last term ensures that the covariance frame does not tend to 0.

The Fréchet mean on FM is implemented in Theano and numpy as,

```
"""
Frechet Mean on FM
"""
detg = lambda q,nu: T.nlinalg.Det()(T.tensordot(nu.T,
                  T.tensordot(gM(q),nu,axes=(1,0)),axes=(1,0)))

lossf = lambda q1,q2: 1./d.eval()*np.sum((q1-q2)**2)

def Frechet_meanFM(u,p,y0):
    q = u[0:d.eval()]
    nu = u[d.eval():].reshape((d.eval(),rank.eval()))
for i in range(n_samples):
    distv[i,:] = lossf(Expfmf(u,p[i,:])[0:d.eval()],y0)
    normp[i,:] = 2*Hfm(u,p[i,:]) # Hamiltonian on FM
return 1./n_samples*np.sum(normp)
   +lambda0/n_samples*np.sum(distv**2)-1./2*np.log(detgf(x,u))
```

7   Conclusion

In the paper, it has been shown how different concepts in differential geometry and non-linear statistics can be implemented using the Theano framework. Integration of geodesics, computation of Christoffel symbols and parallel transport, stochastic development and Fréchet mean estimation were considered and demonstrated on landmark shape manifolds. In addition, we showed how the Fréchet mean on the frame bundle FM can be computed for estimating the mean and covariance of an anisotropic normal distribution on $\mathcal{M}$.

Theano has, for the cases shown in this paper, been a very efficient framework for implementation of differential geometry concepts and for non-linear statistics in a simple and concise way yet allowing efficient and fast computations. We emphasize that Theano is able to perform calculations on high-dimensional manifolds using either CPU or GPU computations. In the future, we plan to extend the presented ideas to derive Theano implementations of differential geometry concepts in more general fiber bundle and Lie group geometries.

Acknowledgments. This work was supported by Centre for Stochastic Geometry and Advanced Bioimaging (CSGB) funded by a grant from the Villum foundation.

References

1. Arnaudon, A., Holm, D., Pai, A., Sommer, S.: A Stochastic Large Deformation Model for Computational Anatomy, December 2016. arXiv:1612.05323 [cs, math]
2. Arnaudon, A., Holm, D., Sommer, S.: A Geometric Framework for Stochastic Shape Analysis, March 2017. arXiv:1703.09971 [cs, math]

3. Elworthy, D.: Geometric aspects of diffusions on manifolds. In: Hennequin, P.-L. (ed.) École d'Été de Probabilités de Saint-Flour XV–XVII, 1985–87. LNM, vol. 1362, pp. 277–425. Springer, Heidelberg (1988). doi:10.1007/BFb0086183

4. Fréchet, M.: L'intégrale abstraite d'une fonction abstraite d'une variable abstraite et son application a la moyenne d'un élément aléatoire de nature quelconque. La Revue Scientifique (1944)

5. Sommer, S.: Anisotropic distributions on manifolds: template estimation and most probable paths. In: Ourselin, S., Alexander, D.C., Westin, C.-F., Cardoso, M.J. (eds.) IPMI 2015. LNCS, vol. 9123, pp. 193–204. Springer, Cham (2015). doi:10.1007/978-3-319-19992-4_15

6. Sommer, S., Arnaudon, A., Kühnel, L., Joshi, S.: Bridge Simulation and Metric Estimation on Landmark Manifolds, May 2017. arXiv:1705.10943 [cs]

7. Sommer, S., Svane, A.M.: Modelling Anisotropic Covariance using Stochastic Development and Sub-Riemannian Frame Bundle Geometry, December 2015. arXiv:1512.08544

8. Theano Development Team. Theano: A Python framework for fast computation of mathematical expressions. arXiv e-prints, abs/1605.02688

9. Younes, L.: Shapes and Diffeomorphisms. Springer, Heidelberg (2010)

Rank Constrained Diffeomorphic Density Motion Estimation for Respiratory Correlated Computed Tomography

Markus Foote[1]([✉]), Pouya Sabouri[2], Amit Sawant[2], and Sarang Joshi[1]

[1] Department of Bioengineering, Scientific Computing and Imaging Institute,
University of Utah, Salt Lake City, UT, USA
foote@sci.utah.edu
[2] University of Maryland School of Medicine, Baltimore, MD, USA

Abstract. Motion estimation of organs in a sequence of images is important in numerous medical imaging applications. The focus of this paper is the analysis of 4D Respiratory Correlated Computed Tomography (RCCT) Imaging. It is hypothesized that the quasi-periodic breathing induced motion of organs in the thorax can be represented by deformations spanning a very low dimension subspace of the full infinite dimensional space of diffeomorphic transformations. This paper presents a novel motion estimation algorithm that includes the constraint for low-rank motion between the different phases of the RCCT images. Low-rank deformation solutions are necessary for the efficient statistical analysis and improved treatment planning and delivery. Although the application focus of this paper is RCCT the algorithm is quite general and applicable to various motion estimation problems in medical imaging.

Keywords: Diffeomorphisms · Image registration

1 Introduction

In this paper we consider the image registration problem for a set of images acquired over the breathing cycle by Respiratory Correlated Computed Tomography (RCCT). This problem has widespread medical applications, in particular 4D radiation therapy for lung cancer patients which considers lung deformations during treatment planning and delivery. Fundamental to the application of 4D motion modeling to improve radiation treatment planning and delivery is the statistical analysis of organ motion which can vary significantly from one breathing cycle to another [6]. Shown in Fig. 1 is a sample breathing trace captured by an abdominal belt in lung cancer radiation treatment patient. This cycle-to-cycle variability has recently been accounted for by live surface tracking methods in conjunction with Principal Component Analysis (PCA) of the

S. Joshi—This work was partially supported through research funding from the National Institute of Health (R01CA169102).

© Springer International Publishing AG 2017
M.J. Cardoso et al. (Eds.): GRAIL/MFCA/MICGen 2017, LNCS 10551, pp. 177–185, 2017.
DOI: 10.1007/978-3-319-67675-3_16

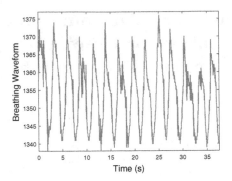

Fig. 1. Breathing waveform of a RCCT subject. Variation in breathing intensity, rate, and pattern is apparent between respiratory cycles.

deformation fields to develop a low dimensional representation of the motion (usually two). The use of Principal Component Analysis (PCA) to draw statistical relations between surface tracking data and RCCT is inherently lossy due to truncation of deformation fields to the few largest principal components [6,12].

We extend pairwise weighted density matching first developed by Rottman et al. [10] for application to statistical analysis of the breathing cycle by incorporating a direct constraint on the rank of the estimated deformations and by considering an entire image series in single optimization problem. This method allows for the preservation of more descriptive deformations in downstream statistical processing that is dependent upon the rank of the deformation fields. Physiologically, the basis of density matching provides for tissue expansion and compression to occur within the lung while the low-rank optimization relates motion between all images in the series to describe the basic inhale-exhale breathing process very well, along with respiratory hysteresis.

Although the rank constraint introduced in this paper is applicable to any image registration algorithm, we focus on the Diffeomorphic Density Matching framework. Density matching has previously been shown to be very effective in pairwise RCCT image registration [10]. Considering the image volumes as densities provides the mathematical foundation to consider conservation of mass between images. Density action of the deformation on the image provides a mechanism through which compression of tissue results in an increased reported density by the deformed CT image, or vice-versa with tissue expansion [1]. This mathematical foundation also provides an efficient method for diffeomorphic registration, as integration of geodesic equations is avoided (contrary to methods like LDDMM [3]).

2   Low Rank Motion Estimation

Our problem extends the diffeomorphic density matching problem [11] to find a set of diffeomorphic transformations between one base image and a set of related images which exist in a low-rank subspace of the space of diffeomorphisms, Diff(Ω).

Measuring the rank of the set of deformations is accomplished by the surrogate nuclear norm of the deformation matrix [9]. Formal rank of the matrix, the number of non-zero eigenvalues, is avoided due to the non-smooth nature of the rank function. Instead, the nuclear norm serves as a convex surrogate function. The nuclear norm for a matrix X is defined as

$$\|X\|_* = \text{trace}\left(\sqrt{X^*X}\right) = \sum_{i}^{\min\{m,n\}} \sigma_i(X) \tag{1}$$

σ_i is the i-th singular value of the $m \times n$ matrix X. Note that the singular values σ_i are positive. We interpret each vectorized deformation field as a row of this matrix,

$$X = \begin{bmatrix} \varphi_1^{-1}(x) - x \\ \varphi_2^{-1}(x) - x \\ \vdots \\ \varphi_{N-1}^{-1}(x) - x \end{bmatrix} = \{\varphi_i^{-1}(x) - x\} \tag{2}$$

where φ_i^{-1} is the inverse of the deformation from the i-th image in the image series to a selected reference image. We can thus define the nuclear norm for deformations between N images as

$$\|X\|_* = \sum_{i}^{N-1} \sigma_i(X) \tag{3}$$

as there are $N-1$ deformations between N images, giving only $N-1$ singular values. The nuclear norm measure on this grouped deformation matrix effectively constrains the rank of the deformation set because of the summation of the singular values.

The rank minimization builds upon the density matching framework, summarized here for completeness [1,10]. A density or volume form $I\,dx$ is acted upon by a diffeomorphism φ to compensate for changes of the density by the deformation:

$$(\varphi, I\,dx) \mapsto \varphi_*(I\,dx) = \left(\varphi^{-1}\right)^*(I\,dx) = \left(|D\varphi^{-1}|I \circ \varphi^{-1}\right)dx \tag{4}$$

where $|D\varphi^{-1}|$ denotes the Jacobian determinant of φ^{-1}. The Riemannian geometry of the group of diffeomorphisms with a suitable Sobolev H^1 metric is linked to the Riemannian geometry of densities with the Fisher-Rao metric [1,5,7]. The Fisher-Rao metric is used due to the property that it is invariant to the action of diffeomorphisms:

$$d_F^2(I_0\,dx, I_1\,dx) = \int_\Omega \left(\sqrt{I_0} - \sqrt{I_1}\right)^2 dx. \tag{5}$$

The linkage between a suitable Sobolev H^1 metric and the Fisher-Rao metric allows for evaluation of the distance in the space of diffeomorphisms in closed form. The Fisher-Rao metric and an incompressibility measure can then be used to match an image pair by minimizing the energy functional:

$$E\left(\varphi\right) = \int_{\Omega} \left(\sqrt{|D\varphi^{-1}|\, I_1 \circ \varphi^{-1}} - \sqrt{I_0}\right)^2 dx + \int_{\Omega} \left(\sqrt{|D\varphi^{-1}|} - 1\right)^2 f\, dx. \quad (6)$$

The first term here penalizes dissimilarity between the two densities. The second term penalizes deviations from a volume-preserving deformation. The penalty function f acts as weighting of the volume-preserving measure. A change of volume is penalized more (or less) where f is large (or small).

This problem has been solved by taking the Sobolev gradient of this energy functional and performing Euler integration of the gradient flow [10]:

$$\delta E = -\Delta^{-1}(-\nabla(f \circ \varphi^{-1}(\sqrt{|D\varphi^{-1}|}))$$
$$- \sqrt{|D\varphi^{-1}|\, I_1 \circ \varphi^{-1}} \nabla(\sqrt{I_0}) + \nabla(\sqrt{|D\varphi^{-1}|\, I_1 \circ \varphi^{-1}})\sqrt{I_0}) \quad (7)$$

$$\varphi_{j+1}^{-1}(x) = \varphi_j^{-1}(x + \epsilon\delta E) \quad (8)$$

We approach the rank constrained density matching problem by including the nuclear norm measure of the deformation fields matrix in the minimization problem and extending pairwise matching to the collective matching of a group of images to the reference image. We therefore seek to solve the following:

$$\min_{\{\varphi_i^{-1}\}} \sum_{i}^{N-1} \int_{\Omega} \left(\sqrt{|D\varphi_i^{-1}|\, I_i \circ \varphi_i^{-1}} - \sqrt{I_0}\right)^2 dx + \int_{\Omega} \left(\sqrt{|D\varphi_i^{-1}|} - 1\right)^2 f\, dx$$
$$s.t. \quad \left\|\{\varphi_i^{-1}(x) - x\}\right\|_* < k \quad (9)$$

where I_0 is a chosen base or reference image and I_i are the other $N-1$ images in the series. We re-frame the rank constraint as a Lagrange multiplier to include the nuclear norm rank measure as a penalty function. This formulation allows us to directly apply the rank minimization strategies such as the iterative shrinkage-thresholding algorithm (ISTA) outlined by Cai et al. [4]. Our problem can thus be written as the minimization of the following energy functional:

$$E(\{\varphi_i\}) = \sum_{i}^{N-1} \left[\int_{\Omega} \left(\sqrt{|D\varphi_i^{-1}|\, I_i \circ \varphi_i^{-1}} - \sqrt{I_0}\right)^2 dx\right.$$
$$\left. + \int_{\Omega} \left(\sqrt{|D\varphi_i^{-1}|} - 1\right)^2 f\, dx\right] + \alpha \sum_{i}^{N-1} \sigma_i\left(\{\varphi_i^{-1}(x) - x\}\right). \quad (10)$$

3   Singular Value Thresholding and Implementation

In this section we describe in detail our implementation of the solution to (9) by the ISTA algorithm, with special consideration for efficient acceleration by GPGPU programming through the PyCA software package [8].

This problem seeks to minimize the singular values of the deformations, so we perform ISTA [4] on the singular value decomposition of the ideal H^1 gradient of the diffeomorphisms. The shrinkage-thresholding algorithm is employed by the shrinkage operator [4]:

$$\mathcal{D}_\tau\left(\Sigma\right) = \text{diag}\left(\{\sigma_i - \tau\}_+\right) \tag{11}$$

where the singular value decomposition is noted as $X = U\Sigma V^*$, thus the shrinkage acts only on the singular values, and $t_+ = \max(0, t)$.

The solution to (9) can therefore be found through an ISTA approach by first finding an optimal update for the density matching problem of each image pair, then performing the shrinkage operation on singular values of the updated fields, and finally replacing the deformations with reconstructions by SVD of the shrunken singular values. In our implementation, we choose to perform SVD on the deformation gram matrix XX^*, as our GPU image processing library lacks an SVD algorithm. This allows for accelerated computation of the gram matrix instead of an accelerated SVD, and only a small penalty for performing SVD on a small 9×9 matrix on the host CPU. Combining the solution to a single density matching problem with our singular value thresholding algorithm gives the algorithm:

Algorithm 1. GPU Accelerated Algorithm

Choose step size $\epsilon > 0$
Choose rank weighting parameter $\alpha > 0$
Set $\varphi_i^{-1} = \text{id}$
Set $\left|D\varphi_i^{-1}\right| = 1$
for $iter = 1 ..$ NumIter **do**
    for i $= 1 .. N - 1$ **do**
        Compute $\varphi_{*i} I_i = I_i \circ \varphi_i$
        Compute $u = -\nabla\left(f \circ \varphi_i^{-1}(1 - \sqrt{|D\varphi_i^{-1}|})\right) - \sqrt{\varphi_{*i} I_i}\nabla\sqrt{I_0} + \nabla(\sqrt{\varphi_{*i} I_i})\sqrt{I_0}$
        Compute $v = -\Delta^{-1}(u)$
        Update $\varphi_i^{-1} \rightarrow \varphi_i^{-1}(x + \epsilon v)$
    end for
    Compute $\boldsymbol{K} = XX^*$
    Compute $\boldsymbol{U\Sigma V^*} = \boldsymbol{K}$ on host CPU
    Compute $\boldsymbol{W} = \boldsymbol{U}\mathcal{D}_{\epsilon\alpha}(\boldsymbol{\Sigma})$ on host CPU
    Update $\{\varphi_i^{-1}\} \rightarrow \boldsymbol{W}X + x$
    Compute $\left|D\varphi_i^{-1}\right|$
end for

We further accelerate the above algorithm by implementing a multi-scale approach. Rather than use the full resolution data from initialization, the algorithm is instead initialized at a lower resolution with down-sampled data. After convergence at the lower resolution, a lower down-sampling factor is selected, resulting in a resolution closer to full resolution. At each scale level change the current deformation field estimates are up-sampled to the new scale and the data is again down-sampled from the original, full resolution images. The final scale level is at the same resolution of the original data.

This multi-scale approach requires two special considerations for tracking the energy being minimized. First, as the volume of a voxel is not constant, the penalties from a voxel must be scaled by the current voxel volume. In other words, the energy must be considered volumetrically, not simply as a data grid. Second, the gram matrix K must be divided by the number of voxels, as a scale change results in the summation over millions more voxels of the deformation fields which would otherwise greatly increase the singular values. Inclusion of these two scale-dependent factors allows the total energy of (10) to be tracked over the multiple scale levels without massive increases when the scale level is changed.

4 Application to Respiratory 4DCT Phase Registration

A RCCT of a radiotherapy patient was acquired at University of Maryland and provided as 10 respiratory phase-binned images. The full exhale image was chosen as the reference image for the registration problem. Image intensities were modified with an exponential function as in [11] to transform the intensity such that the volume exhibits conservation of mass. The final deformations were computed at the resolution of the original 3D volume ($320 \times 256 \times 144$); all the figures show the same middle sagittal, coronal, and axial slices of the volume.

For the compressibility penalty f, we used a soft thresholding of the intensity values of the base image using the logistic function. High intensity regions were penalized with 5σ as dense, incompressible tissue, and vice-versa for low intensity regions (0.2σ). The incompressibility parameter, σ, was set at 0.01 for all runs. The algorithm was implemented on a single Nvidia GTX Titan X GPU, which runs 1000 iterations of the full-resolution volume in approximately 17 min for all 10 images. Lower scales of the multi-scale optimization run significantly faster, mainly due to the $O(n^2)$ complexity of calculating the gram matrix.

Deformations were calculated from each of the 9 other images with rank weighting parameter α of 0, 0.01, 0.02, and 0.05. Figure 2 shows the result of registration for one of the nine pairings, full inhale to full exhale. These deformations have geometric accuracy similar to that attained by the density matching without a rank constraint, as measured by the DICE coefficient between reference and deformed volumes (Fig. 3).

Deformations resulting from the rank constrained algorithm are physiologically relevant, as with previous density matched results, because compression occurs predominantly within the lung tissue. Additionally, the confinement to a low-rank subspace of deformations requires relation to develop between the deformation fields, resulting in linkage of the generally reverse relation between inhalation and exhalation. This added rank constraint results in even better geometric accuracy of some motion estimates as measured by the DICE coefficients.

Increased weighting of the rank term in the minimization problem produces sets of deformations that can be explained by fewer principal components

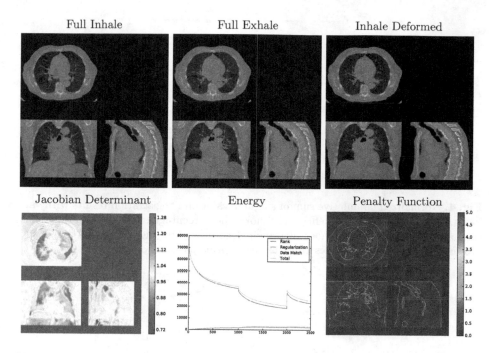

Fig. 2. Registration results for $\alpha = 0.01$. Top row: Full inhale image, full exhale image, and registered inhale image to exhale. Bottom row: Jacobian determinant of the deformation to full exhale, energy plot, and penalty function for density matching algorithm. Note the energy plot shows three scale levels of a multi-scale run; the increase at 2000 is due to the first two scale levels having a blurring applied in the down-sampling procedure which removes noise in the data.

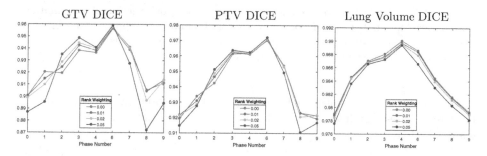

Fig. 3. DICE coefficients for registration results with various rank weightings, α. GTV - Gross Tumor Volume, PTV - Planned Treatment Volume

(Fig. 4). The resulting deformations preserve geometric accuracy better when using PCA to truncate the deformation fields to the largest principal components. The average GTV DICE coefficient across all phases is shown for each number of principal components included in the reconstructed deformation field for a motion estimate performed with and without rank constraint in Fig. 5.

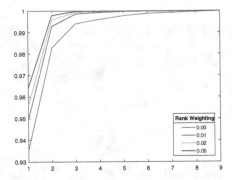

Fig. 4. Normalized cumulative sum of singular values for registration results with various rank weightings, α. This effectively shows the percentage of the deformation fields that are explained by a number of principal components. Increased rank weighting produces deformations well-described by fewer principal components.

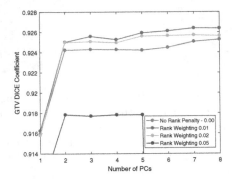

Fig. 5. DICE Coefficients averaged across phases after reconstruction of deformations using a variable number of principal components. Including an appropriate rank constraint in the minimization results in more accurate deformation fields after a statistical truncation of the lower principal components.

Further increase of the rank weighting (such as 0.05), while effective at minimizing rank, causes significant loss in the anatomical accuracy of the deformation estimates (Fig. 3).

5   Discussion

In this paper, we have shown that including rank minimization in the motion estimation problem improves deformation accuracy in later statistical analysis while improving anatomic accuracy. We implemented ISTA to minimize the rank of the deformations between a set of CT images throughout a breathing cycle. In particular, a rank weighting of 0.01 produces better overall geometric accuracy with a significant shift in the rank of the deformations which preserves the deformation accuracy through PCA treatment planning procedures. The geometric accuracy improvement may arise from increased physiologic relevance of the low-rank deformations matching well with the general reversal process of an inhale-exhale cycle, along with hysteresis in other components. Substantial improvement in speed of our algorithm could be achieved by implementing a FISTA technique [2]. Additional parallelization from upcoming multi-GPU systems would provide a speedup with low complexity increase, as the density matching portion of the algorithm is completely independent between phases.

References

1. Bauer, M., Joshi, S., Modin, K.: Diffeomorphic density matching by optimal information transport. SIAM J. Imaging Sci. **8**(3), 1718–1751 (2015)
2. Beck, A., Teboulle, M.: A fast iterative shrinkage-thresholding algorithm. Soc. Ind. Appl. Math. J. Imaging Sci. **2**(1), 183–202 (2009)
3. Beg, M.F., Miller, M.I., Trouvé, A., Younes, L.: Computing large deformation metric mappings via geodesic flows of diffeomorphisms. Int. J. Comput. Vis. **61**(2), 139–157 (2005)
4. Cai, J.F., Candès, E.J., Shen, Z.: A singular value thresholding algorithm for matrix completion. SIAM J. Optim. **20**(4), 1956–1982 (2010)
5. Khesin, B., Lenells, J., Misiołek, G., Preston, S.C.: Geometry of diffeomorphism groups, complete integrability and geometric statistics. Geom. Funct. Anal. **23**(1), 334–366 (2013)
6. Li, R., Lewis, J.H., Jia, X., Zhao, T., Liu, W., Wuenschel, S., Lamb, J., Yang, D., Low, D.A., Jiang, S.B.: On a PCA-based lung motion model. Phys. Med. Biol. **56**(18), 6009–6030 (2011)
7. Modin, K.: Generalized hunter-saxton equations, optimal information transport, and factorization of diffeomorphisms. J. Geom. Anal. **25**(2), 1306–1334 (2015)
8. Preston, J., Hinkle, J., Singh, N., Rottman, C., Joshi, S.: PyCA: Python for Computational Anatomy. https://bitbucket.org/scicompanat/pyca
9. Recht, B., Fazel, M., Parrilo, P.A.: Guaranteed minimum-rank solutions of linear matrix equations via nuclear norm minimization. SIAM Rev. **52**(3), 471–501 (2010)
10. Rottman, C., Bauer, M., Modin, K., Joshi, S.C.: Weighted diffeomorphic density matching with applications to thoracic image registration. In: 5th MICCAI Workshop on Mathematical Foundations of Computational Anatomy (MFCA 2015), pp. 1–12 (2015)
11. Rottman, C., Larson, B., Sabouri, P., Sawant, A., Joshi, S.: Diffeomorphic density registration in thoracic computed tomography. In: Ourselin, S., Joskowicz, L., Sabuncu, M.R., Unal, G., Wells, W. (eds.) MICCAI 2016. LNCS, vol. 9902, pp. 46–53. Springer, Cham (2016). doi:10.1007/978-3-319-46726-9_6
12. Sabouri, P., Foote, M., Ranjbar, M., Tajdini, M., Mossahebi, S., Joshi, S., Sawant, A.: A novel method using surface monitoring to capture breathing-induced cycle-to-cycle variations with 4DCT. In: 59th Annual Meeting of The American Association of Physicists in Medicine. Denver, CO (2017)

Efficient Parallel Transport in the Group of Diffeomorphisms via Reduction to the Lie Algebra

Kristen M. Campbell$^{(\boxtimes)}$ and P. Thomas Fletcher

Scientific Computing and Imaging Institute, University of Utah,
Salt Lake City, UT, USA
kris@sci.utah.edu

Abstract. This paper presents an efficient, numerically stable algorithm for parallel transport of tangent vectors in the group of diffeomorphisms. Previous approaches to parallel transport in large deformation diffeomorphic metric mapping (LDDMM) of images represent a momenta field, the dual of a tangent vector to the diffeomorphism group, as a scalar field times the image gradient. This "scalar momenta" constraint couples tangent vectors with the images being deformed and leads to computationally costly horizontal lifts in parallel transport. This paper uses the vector momenta formulation of LDDMM, which decouples the diffeomorphisms from the structures being transformed, e.g., images, point sets, etc. This decoupling leads to parallel transport expressed as a linear ODE in the Lie algebra. Solving this ODE directly is numerically stable and significantly faster than other LDDMM parallel transport methods. Results on 2D synthetic data and 3D brain MRI demonstrate that our algorithm is fast and conserves the inner products of the transported tangent vectors.

1 Introduction

Analysis of anatomical shape changes from longitudinal medical imaging requires comparing the changes over time of subjects in disparate groups. For instance, imaging studies have shown that the hippocampi of subjects with Alzheimer's disease atrophy significantly more over time than those of healthy aging subjects. Trajectories of anatomical shape change can be estimated from sequences of images using regression methods in the space of diffeomorphisms. When trajectories are modeled as geodesics, they can be represented by their initial velocity. However, these velocities are defined with respect to different coordinate systems associated with the baseline image of each subject. As such, they are not directly comparable. In order to perform statistical analysis of these trajectories, multiple researchers have proposed using parallel transport to bring these subject-specific trajectories into a common coordinate system for comparison.

One of the preferred techniques for analyzing images in this context is large deformation diffeomorphic metric mapping (LDDMM) [2], which is a mathematical framework for finding smooth diffeomorphic transformations between

© Springer International Publishing AG 2017
M.J. Cardoso et al. (Eds.): GRAIL/MFCA/MICGen 2017, LNCS 10551, pp. 186–198, 2017.
DOI: 10.1007/978-3-319-67675-3_17

images. The main benefits of LDDMM are that the deformations between images are smooth and invertible and that a metric allows distances between diffeomorphisms to be computed in a meaningful way. Existing methods for parallel translation within the LDDMM setting work well in practice and have been used for longitudinal shape analysis [11,12]. However, these approaches require computing horizontal lifts at each time step, an expensive computation involving solving a linear system for the scalar momenta using an iterative conjugate gradient method [16]. Additionally, these methods approximate each time step of parallel transport with a short time step evolution of Jacobi fields. Instead of that approximation, this paper works directly with the parallel translation equation.

Another method [4,5] uses a sparse parameterization of the diffeomorphism by using control points. Other approaches involve using stationary velocity fields (SVFs) to generate the diffeomorphisms. These methods use Schild's ladder to approximate parallel transport along a curve by taking small steps in the associated tangent space at each time [6]. However, as each rung of Schild's ladder requires two imperfect, computationally-intensive image registrations, the Schild's ladder steps are then further approximated using the Baker-Campbell-Hausdorff (BCH) formula. This results in fast parallel transport, however, much like the Jacobi field approximation for LDDMM [16], each time step is an approximation to the direct parallel transport equation. Also, the SVF formulation is different from LDDMM in that it does not result in a distance metric on the space of diffeomorphisms.

This paper uses the vector momenta [13] formulation of LDDMM to decouple the diffeomorphisms from the image data. This decoupling allows us to work in the full Lie algebra of the space of diffeomorphisms, and we can then directly implement the parallel translation equations in terms of right-invariant tangent vectors to this space of diffeomorphisms. This results in a linear ordinary differential equation (ODE) that can be solved with a standard, numerically stable scheme that avoids the need to perform computationally-expensive horizontal lifts to the constraint of scalar momenta, as is done in [16]. Additionally, we use the Fourier approximations of vector fields from [17] to gain more numeric stability as well as a more efficient algorithm.

We perform experiments with 2D synthetic data and 3D brain MRIs in order to show the effectiveness of our approach and demonstrate that we can transport realistic vector fields even for quite large deformations. Our results show that our approach is quite fast, indeed it is two orders of magnitude faster than the LDDMM image matching that is also performed using the efficient Fourier-approximated vector fields. Additionally, we demonstrate conservation of the inner product of the tangent vectors being transported. This approaches nearly exact conservation as we increase the number of time steps in the numerical integration scheme.

2   Background on Diffeomorphisms and LDDMM

We provide a brief review of diffeomorphisms, associated Lie group operators and the LDDMM formulation, highlighting the math relevant to parallel transport of diffeomorphisms and the links to diffeomorphic image registration.

2.1   Diffeomorphisms

Let $\Omega = \mathbb{R}^d/\mathbb{Z}^d$ be a d-dimensional toroidal image domain. A toroidal domain is the natural setting for defining the Fourier transform and assuming cyclical boundary conditions. A diffeomorphism of Ω is a bijective, C^∞ mapping $\phi : \Omega \to \Omega$ whose inverse, ϕ^{-1}, is also C^∞. We will denote the space of all such diffeomorphisms as $\mathrm{Diff}(\Omega)$. We are particularly interested in time-varying diffeomorphisms, $\phi(t,x) : [0,1] \times \Omega \to \Omega$, which can be generated as flows of time-varying velocity fields $v(t,x) : [0,1] \times \Omega \to \mathbb{R}^d$. These will be referred to in this paper as $\phi_t(x)$ and $v_t(x)$, where $t \in [0,1]$ and $x \in \Omega$. Note that $\phi_t(x)$ is generated by the flow $t \mapsto \phi_t \in \mathrm{Diff}(\Omega)$ by integrating the ODE

$$\frac{d\phi_t}{dt} = v_t \circ \phi_t. \tag{1}$$

We know that $\mathrm{Diff}(\Omega)$ is an infinite-dimensional Lie group, whose associated Lie algebra, $V = \mathfrak{X}(\Omega)$, consists of all C^∞ vector fields on Ω. For two vector fields $v, w \in V$, the Lie bracket is defined as $[v, w] = Dv \cdot w - Dw \cdot v$. Here D is the first derivative operator and $\cdot$ is element-wise matrix-vector multiplication.

In order to define distances on the manifold $\mathrm{Diff}(\Omega)$, we need an appropriate Riemannian metric. Here we use a weak metric

$$\langle v, w \rangle_V = \int_\Omega \langle Lv(x), w(x) \rangle \, dx, \tag{2}$$

where $L : V \to V$ is a positive-definite, self-adjoint differential operator. In this paper, L is chosen to be a Laplacian operator of the form $L = (-\alpha\Delta + I)^c$ where $\alpha > 0$, $c > 0$ and I is the $d \times d$ identity matrix. In order to compute the inner product of vector fields v and w that belong to the tangent space of any other element $\phi \in \mathrm{Diff}(\Omega)$, we need to pull back the velocities to the tangent space at identity by using a right-invariant metric such as

$$\langle v, w \rangle_{T_\phi \mathrm{Diff}(\Omega)} = \langle v \circ \phi^{-1}, w \circ \phi^{-1} \rangle_V. \tag{3}$$

Then the distance between ϕ and id becomes

$$\mathrm{dist}(\mathrm{id}, \phi) = \int_0^1 \|v_t\|_V \, dt. \tag{4}$$

2.2   LDDMM Image Registration

For the image registration application, we will be looking at how to find an optimal diffeomorphism that takes us from image I_0 to image I_1, where optimal will mean that the diffeomorphism is as small as possible and that $I_0 \circ \phi_1^{-1}$ is as close to I_1 as possible. The LDDMM formulation will formulate this problem as an energy-minimization problem. Before we get to the more specific notion of diffeomorphisms acting on images, we look at the geodesic equations in the general Lie group setting.

First, we will need to define some fundamental operators from Lie group theory. We define the adjoint action of $\mathrm{Diff}(\Omega)$ on $\mathfrak{X}(\Omega)$, $\mathrm{Ad}_\psi : V \to V$, as

$$\mathrm{Ad}_\psi(v) = \frac{d}{dt} \left(\psi \circ \phi_t \circ \psi^{-1} \right) \big|_{t=0}, \tag{5}$$

where $\phi_0 = \mathrm{id}$ and $\frac{d\phi}{dt}\big|_{t=0} = v$. Note that if ϕ_t and ψ commuted, we would simply end up with ϕ_t, thus Ad_ψ is evaluating how well all infinitesimal deformations commute with ψ. Now we let ψ be time-varying and we define the adjoint action, ad, of $\mathfrak{X}(\Omega)$ on itself by

$$\mathrm{ad}_u v = \frac{d}{ds} \left(\mathrm{Ad}_{\psi_s} v \right) \big|_{s=0}, \tag{6}$$

where $\psi_0 = \mathrm{id}$ and $\frac{d\psi}{ds}\big|_{s=0} = u$. In the case of the Lie group $\mathrm{Diff}(\Omega)$, the adjoint action is given by the formula

$$\mathrm{ad}_u v = [u, v] = Du \cdot v - Dv \cdot u. \tag{7}$$

For the energy optimization, we will use results from Arnold [1] and Miller et al. [9] that show that geodesics are extremal curves that satisfy the Euler-Poincaré equations for diffeomorphisms (EPDiff):

$$\frac{dv_t}{dt} = -\mathrm{ad}_{v_t}^\dagger w_t, \tag{8}$$

where $\mathrm{ad}^\dagger$, the adjoint of the ad operator, is

$$\mathrm{ad}_{v_t}^\dagger w_t = K \left[(Dv_t)^T L w_t + D(L w_t) v_t + L w_t \, \mathrm{div} \, v_t \right]. \tag{9}$$

Here div denotes the divergence operator. The process of finding the unique geodesic path, ϕ_t by integrating an initial velocity, $v_0 \in V$ at $t = 0$ forward in time according to (8) is known as geodesic shooting.

Now let's look more specifically at diffeomorphisms acting on images $I \in L^2(\Omega, \mathbb{R})$, meaning that images are square-integrable functions defined on Ω. Diffeomorphic image registration is looking for a v_t that minimizes an energy function, $E(v_t)$, that measures how well $I_0 \circ \phi_1^{-1}$ matches I_1 while preferring small diffeomorphisms by adding a regularization term.

$$E(v_t) = \frac{1}{2\sigma^2} \| I_0 \circ \phi_1^{-1} - I_1 \|_{L^2}^2 + \int_0^1 \| v_t \|_V^2 \, dt, \tag{10}$$

where σ^2 represents image noise variance.

Vialard et al. [14] and Younes et al. [15] showed that it is only necessary to estimate the initial velocity, v_0. Therefore, we can rewrite (10) as

$$E(v_0) = \frac{1}{2\sigma^2}\|I_0 \circ \phi_1^{-1} - I_1\|_{L^2}^2 + \|v_0\|_V^2, \qquad \text{s.t. EPDiff (8) holds.} \qquad (11)$$

2.3 Decoupling Diffeomorphisms from Images

In the original LDDMM formulation, Beg et al. [2] showed that the initial vector fields that are minimizers of the diffeomorphic image registration energy (11) are of the form $\hat{v}_0 = K(s\nabla I_0)$, where $s : \Omega \to \mathbb{R}$ is a scalar field. In other words, the initial momenta $m_0 = Lv_0 = s\nabla I_0$ is constrained to be a scalar field times the image gradient. The scalar momenta constraint was also used in the derivation of geodesic shooting by Vialard [14]. This constraint has the practical benefit that it reduces the size needed to represent the initial conditions, i.e., we can discretize the scalar field s, rather than the vector field v_0. However, Singh et al. [13] showed that removing the scalar momenta constraint, that is, optimizing over initial momenta m_0 that are vector fields, was more numerically stable and converged to better local optima of the target energy.

Removing the scalar momenta constraint also has the effect of *decoupling* the diffeomorphisms from the images that they are acting on. This decoupling has advantages in Bayesian formulations of diffeomorphic image registration and atlas building, as developed by Zhang et al. [19]. In this approach, the decoupling enables formulation of diffeomorphisms as latent random variable with a prior that does not depend on the images (data) in any way. Furthermore, elements of the Lie algebra V are spatially smooth vector fields, and as such, are easier to deal with numerically than non-smooth momenta fields. Zhang and Fletcher [17] used this fact to show that initial velocities could be efficiently represented in the Fourier domain by low-frequency approximations, resulting in much faster image registration and even better optimization of the LDDMM energy. Similarly, we show in the next section that parallel translation benefits from this same decoupling of the diffeomorphisms from images. By working in the full Lie algebra of the space of diffeomorphisms, we can directly implement the equations for parallel translation in terms of right-invariant tangent vectors to $\text{Diff}(\Omega)$. As such, we avoid the need to perform computationally-expensive horizontal lifts to the constraint of scalar momenta, as used in [16]. We are also able to use the Fourier approximations of vector fields from [17]. The end result is an efficient and numerically stable algorithm for directly computing parallel transport in the space of diffeomorphisms.

3   Parallel Transport

In order to do comparisons of trajectories defined by geodesic segments in the space of diffeomorphisms, we need a way to bring the initial velocities of these geodesics to the same reference point. One mechanism to do so is called parallel transport, a generalization of the Euclidean notion of parallel translation of one vector to the origin of another. When this happens in Euclidean space, the angle between the vectors is preserved and the magnitude of the vector is preserved. We will see below that parallel transport along a geodesic on a Riemannian manifold similarly preserves the inner product of the transported vector to the tangent vector of the geodesic and also preserves the norms of the transported vector and the tangent vector.

In this section, we will start from the definition of parallel transport on general Lie groups and then look more specifically at parallel transport on the manifold of diffeomorphisms, Diff(Ω). Then we will do a computational complexity analysis of parallel transport. We'll also talk about details related to implementing parallel transport of diffeomorphisms on a computer, including numerical integration details and using a Fourier-approximated Lie algebra to speed up the discrete computation.

3.1   Parallel Transport Equation

Let's start by looking generally at right-invariant vector fields v and w on a Lie group. We can look at how w varies in the direction v by looking at the covariant derivative $\nabla_v w$. Parallel transport of a tangent vector along a curve is defined by this covariant derivative of the transported vector being zero in the direction of the velocity of the curve. The covariant derivative for right-invariant vector fields (c.f. [3]) is given by the equation

$$\nabla_v w = -\frac{1}{2}\left(\mathrm{ad}_v^\dagger w + \mathrm{ad}_w^\dagger v - \mathrm{ad}_v w\right).\tag{12}$$

For our application, we want to transport along a curve ϕ_t in the space of diffeomorphisms. Remember that (1) says the change in ϕ_t over time is equal to a time-varying velocity field v_t composed with ϕ_t. Let's plug these time-varying right-invariant vector fields into (12) to get the following:

$$\nabla_{v_t} w_t = \frac{dw_t}{dt} - \frac{1}{2}\left(\mathrm{ad}_{v_t}^\dagger w_t + \mathrm{ad}_{w_t}^\dagger v_t - \mathrm{ad}_{v_t} w_t\right),\tag{13}$$

where the dw_t/dt comes from needing to take the total derivative since w_t varies with time. Let's set this covariant derivative to 0 and substitute the definitions for $\mathrm{ad}_{v_t} w_t$ and $\mathrm{ad}_{v_t}^\dagger w_t$ from (7) and (9) to get:

$$\begin{aligned}
\frac{dw_t}{dt} = -\frac{1}{2}(&K\left[(Dv_t)^T L w_t + D(Lw_t)v_t + Lw_t \operatorname{div} v_t\right]\\
+ &K\left[(Dw_t)^T L v_t + D(Lv_t)w_t + Lv_t \operatorname{div} w_t\right]\\
- &Dv_t w_t + Dw_t v_t).
\end{aligned}\tag{14}$$

Notice that this becomes the geodesic equation when $w_t = v_t$.

3.2   Computational Complexity Analysis

The computational complexity of solving (14) is $O(NM \log M)$ where M is the number of voxels in the image and N is the number of time steps taken. If we instead solve (14) in the Fourier-approximated space, the complexity improves to $O(Nm \log m)$, where m is number of frequencies used in the reduced space. We use $m = 16^3$ in the real data experiments below. Note that computing Jacobi fields in the Lie algebra would be the same complexity. But our method avoids computing the horizontal lifts needed in order to enforce the scalar momenta constraint used by other LDDMM parallel transport methods. These horizontal lifts involve solving an M-dimensional system of linear equations using an iterative conjugate gradient method.

3.3   Implementation Details

In order to gain the performance benefits from performing operations in the Fourier-approximated Lie algebra (FLASH) [17], we implemented parallel translation in the Flash C++ environment [18], which is built on top of PyCA [10]. Additionally, we implemented a more accurate numerical integration scheme for both forward integrating v_0 at each time step $t = 1/N, 2/N..., 1$ and for solving the parallel translation ODE (13) numerically using N time steps. We provide both an Euler first-order scheme and a Runge-Kutta fourth-order (RK4) scheme to perform these integrations, with the RK4 integration happening independently for w_t and v_t. Ideally, since w_t and v_t are coupled, the integration would be even more accurate by doing a coupled symplectic integration scheme. Below we run experiments in order to find a reasonably small N that gives good enough stability.

4   Experiments

We ran experiments with both synthetic images and real 3D MR images of human brains to explore the accuracy, stability and speed of our parallel translation approach. In all of our experiments, we follow the same general setup. First we use Flash C++ to do image matching between two time points of the first subject, I_0 and I_n, to find a diffeomorphism between the two images represented by an initial velocity w_{0_n}. Then we do image matching between the first subject, I_0 and the template image, T_0 to find a diffeomorphism between the subject and the template represented by the initial velocity v_0. At this point, we parallel translate w_{0_n} in the direction of v_0 to get the translated diffeomorphism represented by the initial velocity $\pi(w_{0_n})$ as shown in Fig. 1. The values $\langle Lv, v \rangle$, $\langle Lv, w \rangle$, and $\langle Lw, w \rangle$, while different from each other, should each remain constant throughout integration. We measure the percent change of these inner products at each time step of the integration in order to quantify the stability.

4.1   Synthetic Data

We modeled our synthetic data experiments to follow the approach of Lorenzi and Pennec [7] that was also used by [8]. These experiments consist of 2D images of size 256×256 pixels. The subject's initial image, I_0, at time 0 is composed of centered black and white semi-circles with a 21 pixel radius surrounded by a centered grey circle with a 42 pixel radius. Brain atrophy over 3 time steps is modeled by decreasing the volume of the outer grey circle by 5% of the initial time point at each time increment, while simultaneously increasing the volume of the inner semi-circles by 5%. A second image, T_0, which can represent either a template image, atlas image, or second subject, is composed of the same black and white semi-circles found in I_0, while the outer grey circle has been deformed into an ellipse by stretching the top and bottom edges an amount equal to 10% of the diameter of the grey circle in I_0 and then rotating the ellipse by 45°.

The initial velocities $v_0, w_{0_1}, w_{0_2}, w_{0_3}$ of the deformations are found with 100 iterations of Flash C++'s image matching using a truncation dimension of 16 and the parameters $\alpha = 3.0, s = 3.0, \sigma = 0.03, \gamma = 0.2$. The results of transporting these velocities between I_0 and each time point $I_n, n \in \{1, 2, 3\}$ can be seen in Fig. 1.

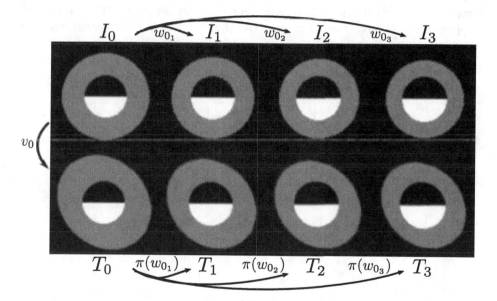

Fig. 1. Results of parallel translating w_{0_n} for each $I_0 \cdots I_3$ to the template space T_0 to produce the transformed images T_1, T_2, T_3.

Numerical Stability. We expect to see that the stability of parallel translation improves as the number of time steps of numerical integration increase for a particular integration scheme, or improves for higher order numerical schemes. Additionally, we want to characterize the stability of translation as the deformations grow larger. Therefore, we compare the percent change relative to the value at $t = 0$ of the norms, $\langle Lv, v \rangle = \|v\|^2, \langle Lw, w \rangle = \|w\|^2$, and the relative percent change of the inner product, $\langle Lv, w \rangle$, all of which should be 0 since these inner products remain constant throughout parallel translation. We look at how the stability changes as we do either 10, 20 or 100 time steps of both an Euler first-order numerical integration scheme and a Runge-Kutta 4 (RK4) fourth-order integration scheme. We then do this same comparison for the 5%, 10%, and 15% volume change to see how the implementation behaves as deformations grow larger. As you can see in Fig. 2, the relative change approaches 0 as expected as the number of integration steps increases and as the numerical scheme changes from Euler to RK4 where it becomes effectively 0 for 100 steps of RK4. While it is more expensive to compute this many steps of RK4, it provides excellent preservation of the relationship between v and w throughout the parallel transport. From these results, we see that 20 iterations of RK4 gives reasonable performance without being too computationally intensive. Therefore, we chose to do 20 iterations of RK4 for the real data experiments below. Note also that the percent relative change for the angle between v and w, $\langle Lv, w \rangle$, increases somewhat as the amount of deformation increases from 5% simulated atrophy in the top row to 10% atrophy in the center row to the 15% simulated atrophy in the bottom row. It is expected that the larger deformation leads to somewhat larger errors.

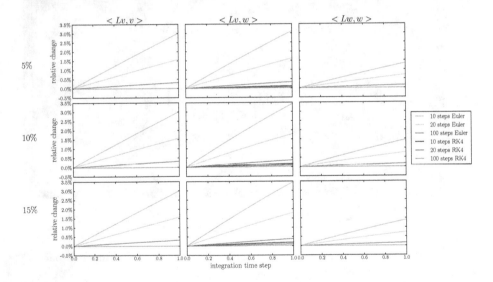

Fig. 2. Percent relative change of the inner product over the integration time from 0 to 1. Where relative percent change of $x = \langle \cdot, \cdot \rangle$ is computed by $100 * (x_t - x_0)/x_0$ for each time step t. The rows correspond to results for 5%, 10% and 15% simulated atrophy respectively.

4.2   Real Data

We looked at performance of our parallel translation in the context of 3D brain MRIs from the OASIS database in order to see how well it captures known atrophy associated with the progression of Alzheimer's disease. We did pairwise comparison of every combination of 11 healthy subjects and 10 subjects with Alzheimers. We start with images of size $128 \times 128 \times 128$ that have had the skulls stripped out, intensities normalized, and are then rigidly co-registered. For each pair, the subject with Alzheimer's is I_0, and I_1 is the same subject's scan at a later time, between 2 and 5 years later. The healthy subject's initial scan is T_0. I_0 is deformably registered to each of I_1 and T_0 using 200 iterations of image matching from Flash C++ with truncated dimension of 16 and parameters $\alpha = 3.0, s = 3.0, \sigma = 0.03, \gamma = 1.0$. The results for a typical pair are shown in Fig. 3.

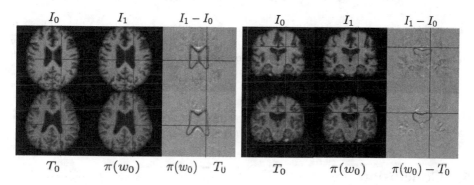

Fig. 3. Axial and coronal views of the results of parallel translating w_0 along v_0 to the template space T_0 to produce the transformed image $\pi(w_0)$. The top row in each group consists of the original images from a subject with Alzheimer's, I_0 and I_1 as well as the difference image $I_1 - I_0$. The bottom row in each group consists of the original template image from a control subject T_0, the parallel translated image $\pi(w_0)$, and the difference image $\pi(w_0) - T_0$.

One of the benefits of this parallel transport is that it is significantly faster than the image matching registrations used to produce the diffeomorphisms to be transported. For our experiments with real data, the image registration of one pair of 3D images took on the order of 800 s while the parallel transport of 3D vector fields from one subject to another took on the order of 8 s. Since parallel transport is consistently 2 orders of magnitude faster than the image matching, it becomes an essentially free operation for an image analysis pipeline.

Numerical Stability. In order to evaluate the numerical stability, we look at the maximum percent change of the inner products $\langle Lv, v \rangle, \langle Lv, w \rangle, \langle Lw, w \rangle$ as w is transported along v. A plot of the maximum percent change across all 106 pairs of subjects can be found in Fig. 4. The largest maximum relative change across all subjects in $\langle Lv, w \rangle$ is 8.6%. The associated $\langle Lv, v \rangle$ is 0.0009% and the $\langle Lw, w \rangle$ is 0.0000% for this same pair of subjects. In order to understand why this pair had such a large value compared to other pairs, we ran the same pair

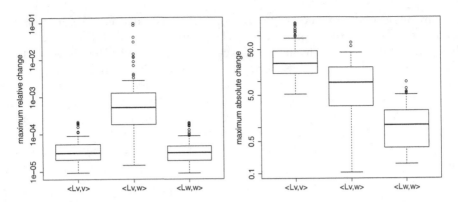

Fig. 4. Maximum amount of change in inner products for each subject. The left plot shows the maximum relative change of each subject $x = \langle \cdot, \cdot \rangle$ is computed by $\max_{0 \le t \le 1} \left((x_t - x_0)/x_0 \right)$. The right plot shows the maximum absolute change of each subject, computed as $\max_{0 \le t \le 1} (x_t - x_0)$.

for 100 steps of RK4. That experiment resulted in much smaller percent change of $\langle Lv, w \rangle = 1.51\%, \langle Lv, v \rangle = 0.00086\%, \langle Lw, w \rangle = 0.0000\%$.

5   Conclusion

We presented a method to perform parallel translation in the space of diffeomorphisms, allowing us to work with the parallel translation equations directly instead of approximating them. Further, we were able to use FLASH to speed up computations further by performing them in a smaller Fourier-approximated space. We demonstrated that our method is numerically stable and that preservation of the inner products throughout parallel translation can be improved in a predictable manner by increasing the number of integration steps and/or using the RK4 scheme with a modest associated computational cost.

We look forward to applying this method to studying trajectories of anatomical shape change in a variety of medical image analysis contexts. Also, this method is one example of how formulating problems directly in the space of diffeomorphisms and working with that Lie algebra combined with efficiencies gained from FLASH techniques allows us to perform computations efficiently and stably. We expect that this same approach could work well for other analysis such as working with Sasaki metrics.

Acknowledgments. This work was supported by NIH grant R01EB022876. The OASIS data was provided by the following grants: P50 AG05681, P01 AG03991, R01 AG021910, P20 MH071616, U24 RR021382.

References

1. Arnold, V.: Sur la géométrie différentielle des groupes de lie de dimension infinie et ses applications à l'hydrodynamique des fluides parfaits. Annales de l'institut Fourier **16**, 319–361 (1966)
2. Beg, M.F., Miller, M.I., Trouvé, A., Younes, L.: Computing large deformation metric mappings via geodesic flows of diffeomorphisms. Int. J. Comput. Vision **61**(2), 139–157 (2005)
3. Cheeger, J., Ebin, D.G., Ebin, D.G.: Comparison Theorems in Riemannian geometry, vol. 9. North-Holland Publishing Company, Amsterdam (1975)
4. Durrleman, S., Prastawa, M., Gerig, G., Joshi, S.: Optimal data-driven sparse parameterization of diffeomorphisms for population analysis. In: Székely, G., Hahn, H.K. (eds.) IPMI 2011. LNCS, vol. 6801, pp. 123–134. Springer, Heidelberg (2011). doi:10.1007/978-3-642-22092-0_11
5. Durrleman, S., Prastawa, M., Charon, N., Korenberg, J.R., Joshi, S., Gerig, G., Trouvé, A.: Morphometry of anatomical shape complexes with dense deformations and sparse parameters. NeuroImage **101**, 35–49 (2014)
6. Lorenzi, M., Ayache, N., Pennec, X.: Schild's ladder for the parallel transport of deformations in time series of images. In: Székely, G., Hahn, H.K. (eds.) IPMI 2011. LNCS, vol. 6801, pp. 463–474. Springer, Heidelberg (2011). doi:10.1007/978-3-642-22092-0_38
7. Lorenzi, M., Pennec, X.: Geodesics, parallel transport & one-parameter subgroups for diffeomorphic image registration. Int. J. Comput. Vision **105**(2), 111–127 (2013)
8. Matsui, J.T.: Development of image processing tools and procedures for analyzing multi-site longitudinal diffusion-weighted imaging studies (2014)
9. Miller, M.I., Trouvé, A., Younes, L.: Geodesic shooting for computational anatomy. J. Mathe. Imaging Vision **24**(2), 209–228 (2006)
10. Preston, J.S.: Python for computational anatomy (2016). Commit e649151. https://bitbucket.org/scicompanat/pyca
11. Qiu, A., Albert, M., Younes, L., Miller, M.I.: Time sequence diffeomorphic metric mapping and parallel transport track time-dependent shape changes. NeuroImage **45**(1), S51–S60 (2009)
12. Qiu, A., Younes, L., Miller, M.I., Csernansky, J.G.: Parallel transport in diffeomorphisms distinguishes the time-dependent pattern of hippocampal surface deformation due to healthy aging and the dementia of the alzheimer's type. NeuroImage **40**(1), 68–76 (2008)
13. Singh, N., Hinkle, J., Joshi, S., Fletcher, P.T.: A vector momenta formulation of diffeomorphisms for improved geodesic regression and atlas construction. In: 2013 IEEE 10th International Symposium on Biomedical Imaging (ISBI), pp. 1219–1222. IEEE (2013)
14. Vialard, F.X., Risser, L., Rueckert, D., Cotter, C.J.: Diffeomorphic 3D image registration via geodesic shooting using an efficient adjoint calculation. Int. J. Comput. Vision **97**(2), 229–241 (2012)
15. Younes, L., Arrate, F., Miller, M.I.: Evolutions equations in computational anatomy. NeuroImage **45**(1), S40–S50 (2009)
16. Younes, L., Qiu, A., Winslow, R.L., Miller, M.I.: Transport of relational structures in groups of diffeomorphisms. J. Mathe. Imaging Vision **32**(1), 41–56 (2008)

17. Zhang, M., Fletcher, P.T.: Finite-dimensional lie algebras for fast diffeomorphic image registration. In: Ourselin, S., Alexander, D.C., Westin, C.-F., Cardoso, M.J. (eds.) IPMI 2015. LNCS, vol. 9123, pp. 249–260. Springer, Cham (2015). doi:10. 1007/978-3-319-19992-4_19
18. Zhang, M., Fletcher, P.T.: Flashc++ (2016). Commit 33cfd0e. https://bitbucket. org/FlashC/flashc
19. Zhang, M., Singh, N., Fletcher, P.T.: Bayesian estimation of regularization and atlas building in diffeomorphic image registration. IPMI **23**, 37–48 (2013)

Third International Workshop on Imaging Genetics, MICGen 2017

Multi-modal Image Classification Using Low-Dimensional Texture Features for Genomic Brain Tumor Recognition

Esther Alberts[1,2,3(✉)], Giles Tetteh[2], Stefano Trebeschi[2], Marie Bieth[2], Alexander Valentinitsch[1,2], Benedikt Wiestler[1], Claus Zimmer[1], and Bjoern H. Menze[2,3]

[1] Neuroradiology, Klinikum Rechts der Isar, TU München, Munich, Germany
esther.alberts@tum.de
[2] Department of Computer Science, TU München, Munich, Germany
[3] Institute for Advanced Study, TU München, Munich, Germany

Abstract. In this paper, we present a multi-modal medical image classification framework classifying brain tumor glioblastomas in genetic classes based on DNA methylation status. The framework makes use of computationally efficient 3D implementations of short local image descriptors, such as LBP, BRIEF and HOG, which are processed by a Bag-of-Patterns model to represent image regions, as well as deep-learned features acquired by denoising auto-encoders and hand-crafted shape features calculated on segmentation masks. The framework is validated against a cohort of 116 brain tumor patients from the TCIA database and is shown to obtain high accuracies even though the same image-based classification task is hardly possible for medical experts.

1 Introduction

Currently the most aggressive brain tumors are categorized in World Health Organisation (WHO) Grade III (anaplastic gliomas) and Grade IV (glioblastomas). [1] proposes to group brain tumors in three genomic classes based on DNA methylation patterns: CIMP-Codel, CIMP-Non-Codel and CIMP-Neg. The authors showed that these genomic classes have clear links with underlying biology and a significant association with clinical outcome. In this study, we aim to detect these genomic groups using image-based biomarkers such as tumor texture and shape features in standard MR modalities: T1, T1gd, T2 and FLAIR. Examples of the image data for each of the genomic classes are depicted in Fig. 1.

Predicting labels from image evidence is a hot topic in medical image analysis, studied with the purpose of disease detection [2–4], genetic labelling [5] or outcome prediction [6]. Medical image classification methods majorly differ in feature generation and classification algorithms. Features reflecting image evidence are often implemented as texture and shape representations. *Classical texture descriptors* based on filter banks, Haar wavelets, Haralick features of

© Springer International Publishing AG 2017
M.J. Cardoso et al. (Eds.): GRAIL/MFCA/MICGen 2017, LNCS 10551, pp. 201–209, 2017.
DOI: 10.1007/978-3-319-67675-3_18

gray-level co-occurence matrices (GLCM) and histogram of gradients (HOG) are still popular [2], but are known to suffer from normalisation problems, lack of (local) rotation invariance, poor local organization of image directions and non-trivial 3D extensions. Wavelet and space-frequency representations, such as the ones generated by Riesz wavelets [3] and polar S-transforms [5] have been forwarded as an attempt to deal with these caveats. However, when working with multi-modal 3D medical images for which one needs to calculate, store and match a large number of descriptors, adopting *short descriptors* has prominent advantages in terms of memory-efficiency and computation time. Short descriptors can be generated from full descriptors (such as wavelet representations or traditional descriptors such as SIFT [7] and SURF [8]), by means of dimensionality reduction, quantization into integers or binarization. A computationally efficient alternative is to directly extract short descriptors as binary strings calculated over image patches, as proposed for local binary patterns (LBP) [9] and BRIEF features [10]. Next to classical texture descriptors, we want to consider another strong category of texture descriptors generated by *deep learning*. Neural nets have been shown to learn meaningfull texture representations, either in supervised contexts (using convolutional neural networks (CNN)) or unsupervised contexts (using auto-encoders (AE), deep belief networks (DBN) or restricted Boltzmann machines (RBM)) [4].

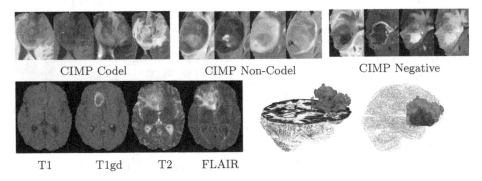

Fig. 1. *Top*: Close-up of tumor texture in T1, T1gd, T2 and FLAIR resp. for three samples with different genetic labels. *Bottom*: Image data of one sample i with four image modalities $\{I_i^m\}_{m=1}^4$ (left) and two ROIs (active tumor in red and edema in blue) $\{S_i^k\}_{k=1}^2$ (right). (Color figure online)

For medical image classification, traditional classifiers typically obtain good accuracies, as shown in [3] using softmax classifiers, [5] using l1-regularized neural nets and [2] using random forests (RF). The high-dimensional nature of the feature space p and the sparse availability of data samples N, denoted as $p \gg N$, makes the classification task particularly challenging, leading to overfitting. Therefore, most studies include feature dimensionality reduction or specialized task-dependant feature selection models [2,6,11] in order to facilitate the classification task.

In this paper, we aim to build a multi-modal image classifier making use of traditional hand-crafted features, modern local image texture features and features learned through a deep neural network. More in particular, we adopt a mathematically sound extension of LBPs towards 3D based on spherical harmonics [12], as well as a 3D version of the BRIEF [13] and HOG [14] features. In parallel, inspired by the success of deep learning in texture analysis [4], we also include features learned by unsupervised auto-encoders (AEs). We validate the framework on a brain tumor dataset with different genetic classes, using several state-of-the-art classifiers in conjunction with feature dimensionality reduction by means of principal component analysis (PCA).

2   Methods

An overview of the framework is depicted in Fig. 2. In this section, we discuss the feature extraction based on local image features (I.) and deep learned features (II.). Hand-crafted shape and texture features (III.) are directly calculated on segmented regions of interest (ROIs) using criteria such as volume, surface, flatness, roundness and elongation and on the image intensities within the ROIs using the first four statistical moments (mean, variance, skewness and kurtosis) for each of the image modalities.

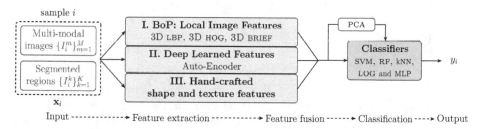

Fig. 2. Overview of the proposed framework. Each sample consist of several image modalities and segmented regions. Features are generated by a Bag-of-Patterns (BoP) model performed on local image features, a deep learned auto-encoder and traditional shape and texture features. Feature dimension reduction through principal component analysis (PCA) is investigated before the features are being fed to the classifiers.

Notation. Given a training set of N samples $\{(\boldsymbol{x}_i, y_i)\}_{i=1}^{N}$, with $\boldsymbol{x}_i = \{I_i^m|_{m=1}^{M}, S_i^k|_{k=1}^{K}\}$ the image data consisting of M image modalities and K segmentation ROIs, and $y_i \in \{1, \ldots, C\}$ the labels associated with each sample (cfr. Fig. 1).

2.1   Bag-of-Patterns: From Local Image Features to Image Region Descriptors

We investigate three types of *local image features*: LBP, BRIEF and HOG. To compute the LBP features, 42 offsets are taken on an icosahedron of radius r

centered around the center voxel (Fig. 3, left), each offset denoted by its spherical coordinates (θ, ϕ). Next, binary intensity comparisons $f(\theta, \phi) \in \{0, 1\}$ are made between the discrete offsets (θ, ϕ) and the center voxel, and a continuous approximation $\tilde{f}(\theta, \phi)$ is made by a linear combination of spherical harmonics Y_l^m of degree l and order m: $\tilde{f}(\theta, \phi) = \sum_{l=1}^{n} \sum_{m=-l}^{l} c_l^m Y_l^m(\theta, \phi)$. The 3D rotationally invariant LBP features are then set to $(\|f_0\|, \ldots, \|f_n\|, k)$ with $\|f_l\| = (\sum_\theta \sum_\phi (\sum_{m=-l}^{l} c_l^m Y_l^m(\theta, \phi))^2)^{1/2}$ and k the kurtosis over the intensities. We use spherical harmonics up to degree $n = 3$. To compute the BRIEF features, images where smoothed with a Gaussian kernel and 64 binary intensity comparisons are made around the center voxel, including comparisons between pairs of offset locations (Fig. 3, middle). A binary string is constructed from the results of the binary comparisons and is stored as a 64-bit float. Next to the binary descriptors, we explore histogram of gradient (HOG) features as presented in [14]. We quantized gradient orientations on an icosahedron, categorizing opposite directions in one bin, which leaves us with 10 gradient orientations as visualised in the rightmost plot in Fig. 3. Gradients are first calculated along the three dimensions using point derivative discrete masks and are then projected on the 10 aforementioned gradient orientations to get the local image descriptor.

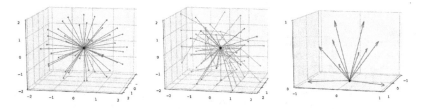

Fig. 3. Sampled offset locations in the voxel grid for the LBP (left) and BRIEF (middle) features ($r = 2\,\text{mm}$) and HOG gradient orientation quantization (right). Binary intensity comparisons are made between offset locations and the center (blue lines) and among pairs of offset locations (orange lines). (Color figure online)

Local image features are calculated over image patches centered at voxel locations. We use a Bag-of-Patterns (BoP) model to generate *image region descriptors*, describing texture over image regions of arbitrary size. Analogous to the Bag-of-Words (BoW) model in computer vision [15], the BoP model consists of two steps: first, a *codebook of patterns* is learned and secondly, a *bag of visual patterns* is calculated over an image region, as visualised in Fig. 4. The patterns in the codebook are learned, for example by means of dictionary learning, on a (large) set of local image features acquired over several images. Each of the codebook patterns represent a subspace of the local image feature space. The bag of visual patterns can be obtained by collecting the closest pattern for each of the local image features within an image region. The image region descriptor is then set as the occurrence count of each of the patterns in the bag of visual patterns and is fed to the classifier.

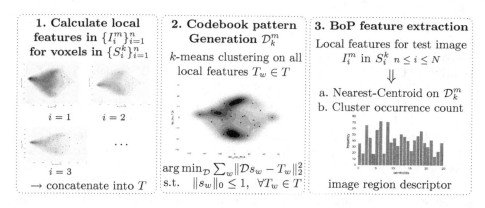

Fig. 4. Generation of image region descriptors based on the BoP model. Local image features are calculated on n images of modality m for all voxels j in a ROI $S_i^k(j) > 0$. A codebook pattern is then generated by means of k-means clustering. The image region descriptor for an (unseen) image i is set as the codebook pattern occurrence count predicted over its local image features.

2.2 Unsupervised Feature Learning Based on Deep Auto-Encoders

An auto-encoder (AE) is an unsupervised deep neural network used for non-linear dimensionality reduction, image reconstruction or image denoising. By means of stacked convolutional, activation and pooling layers, the input image in space $\mathcal{X}$ is reduced to a feature vector in space $\mathcal{F}$. This part of the AE is denoted as the encoder: $\phi : \mathcal{X} \rightarrow \mathcal{F}$, whereas the decoder maps the feature vector back to the input image space: $\psi : \mathcal{F} \rightarrow \mathcal{X}$. The filters in the convolutional layers of the AE architecture are learned trough backpropagation of the reconstruction error $\mathcal{L}(I_i^m, \tilde{I}_i^m)$, defined between the original image I_i^m and the reconstructed image $\tilde{I}_i^m = (\psi \circ \phi)(I_i^m)$.

Network Architecture. Let $\mathsf{C_k}$ denote a $(3 \times 3 \times 3)$ convolutional layer with k filter banks, S a sigmoid activation layer, R a ReLu activation layer and $\mathsf{P_{s_1 s_2 s_3}}$ a pooling layer with $(\mathsf{s}_1 \times \mathsf{s}_2 \times \mathsf{s}_2)$ filters. We implemented an AE of five layers, which we can then write as: $\mathsf{C_4 S P_{444}} - \mathsf{C_8 R P_{333}} - \mathsf{C_{16} R P_{355}} - \mathsf{C_{32} R P_{222}} - \mathsf{C_{64} S P_{333}}$. Taking a 3D volume with fixed dimensions as an input, the AE generates a feature vector of length 512.

Implementation Details. The AE is trained with tied weights and input images are corrupted with noise in order to force the AE to generate features that are robustly representing the input distribution, similar to denoising AE [16]. Moreover, during training, the reconstruction error is only calculated within the segmentation masks, as we are only interested in reconstructing features representing texture within the segmentation masks.

3 Experiments

We conduct experiments on a brain tumor dataset from "The Cancer Imaging Archive" (TCIA). For each patient genetic labels, CIMP Codel, CIMP Non-Codel or CIMP Negative, are available. These genetic classes are originally acquired by biopsies. Medical experts are not able to differentiate between these classes solely based on image evidence, making the classification task particularly challenging. We constructed a training set of 92 patients and a test set of 24 patients by means of stratified sampling. The genetic classes are rather unbalanced with 19, 25 and 48 respective label occurrences in the training dataset and 5, 7 and 12 in the test set. T1, T1gd, T2 and FLAIR are skull stripped, co-registered and resampled to the same resolution and image dimensions. Brain tumor segmentations for whole tumor and active tumor are calculated using a brain tumor Expectation-Maximisation algorithm [17] for which the code is online available[1].

LBP and BRIEF features are generated for radii of 2, 3, 4 and 5 mm. Figure 5 visualizes LBP and BRIEF features calculated over the entire brain region. Using 50 patients randomly sampled from the training set, pattern codebooks are learned for each modality for LBP, BRIEF and HOG. Only whole tumor masks were used, because active tumor regions do not contain much texture information. Image patches representing the codebook patterns learned for LBP, BRIEF and HOG in FLAIR images are visualized in Fig. 6. Each codebook consists of 50 patterns, resulting in image region descriptors of length $4 \times 50 = 200$ of for each local image feature type. Average runtimes[2] for LBP, BRIEF and HOG feature calculation for one sample x_i (including all four modalities masked over the whole tumor region) are about 81, 5 and 9 s.

We train AEs on FLAIR and on T1c images separately, each time using the whole tumor masks when calculating the reconstruction error. We denote the concatenation of the features generated by these two AEs as AE_{texture}. A third AE, generating features denoted as AE_{shape}, is trained on ternary tumor mask images (background, edema and active tumor encoded as 0, 1 and 2 resp.) to learn tumor shape features. Training was done on 50 patients randomly sampled from the training set. Each AE was randomly initialized and ran during 200 iterations. The reconstruction error is set to the mean squared error and 30% of the voxels in each input volume were corrupted (setting voxel intensities to zero). An example of the input and reconstruction of an AE trained on FLAIR images is shown in Fig. 7. Average runtime[3] for the AE feature calculation (including AE_{texture} and AE_{shape}) for one sample x_i is < 1 s.

Table 1 shows the results of all classifiers using different feature sets. For each classifier and feature set, classifier-specific parameters were learned by cross-validation on the training set using grid search. Best accuracies on the test set are obtained by using all features together with random forests (0.83). LBP,

---

[1] https://bitbucket.org/s0216660/brain_tumor_segmentation_em.
[2] Intel® Xeon® Processor E3-1225 v3.
[3] GeForce GTX Titan X (VRAM 12 GB).

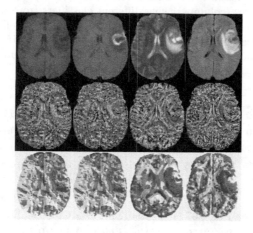

Fig. 5. Local image features ($r = 5\,\mathrm{mm}$) calculated in the full brain mask for modalities T1, T1gd, T2 and FLAIR (top). LBP features are visualised as RGB channels over the first three LBP features corresponding to the order of the spherical harmonics: $[\|f_0\|, \|f_1\|, \|f_2\|]$ (middle row). BRIEF features are visualised as their 64-bit float representation.

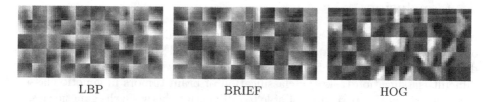

| LBP | BRIEF | HOG |

Fig. 6. Pattern codebooks learned over 50 FLAIR images within the whole tumor regions for the three local image features. Patterns are visualised by averaging patches ($\varnothing 7\,\mathrm{mm}$) collected in the normalized FLAIR images for which the local image features of the center voxel are nearest to the pattern centroids (2D cross-sections are shown).

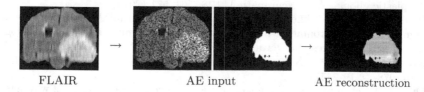

FLAIR   AE input   AE reconstruction

Fig. 7. Auto-encoder reconstruction results learned on FLAIR and whole tumor masks. Inputs are corrupted by a noise level of 30%.

Table 1. Three-class classification accuracies (training score/test score) acquired with different sets of features (columns) using different classifiers (rows). For comparison, a majority-vote classifier would obtain a test score of 0.50. Classifiers include nearest neighbour (NN), logistic regression (LOG), multi-layer perceptron (MLP), random forests (RF) and support vector machines (SVM), optionally in combination with PCA.

Train/test	LBP	BRIEF	HOG	Shape	$AE_{texture}$	AE_{shape}	All
k-NN	0.66/0.50	0.66/0.50	0.66/0.50	0.70/0.42	0.74/**0.75**	0.74/**0.75**	0.66/0.46
- w/ PCA	0.72/0.50	0.72/0.50	0.72/0.50	0.72/0.38	0.73/**0.75**	0.73/**0.71**	0.66/0.42
LOG	1.00/0.67	1.00/0.67	1.00/0.67	0.65/0.50	0.64/0.63	0.55/0.54	1.00/0.71
- w/ PCA	0.99/**0.75**	0.99/**0.75**	1.00/**0.75**	0.70/0.38	0.64/0.63	0.55/0.54	0.89/0.63
MLP	1.00/0.67	0.92/0.54	1.00/0.63	0.74/0.33	0.69/0.63	0.52/0.50	0.63/0.42
- w/ PCA	1.00/0.63	1.00/0.67	1.00/0.63	0.46/0.42	0.64/0.54	0.94/0.67	0.73/0.42
RF	1.00/0.58	1.00/0.67	1.00/0.63	1.00/0.42	0.97/0.63	1.00/0.67	1.00/**0.83**
- w/ PCA	1.00/0.54	0.99/0.50	1.00/0.54	1.00/0.50	1.00/**0.79**	1.00/0.58	1.00/0.54
SVM	1.00/0.67	1.00/0.67	1.00/0.67	0.54/0.33	0.52/0.50	0.52/0.50	1.00/0.67

BRIEF or HOG features do remarkably well in combination with PCA and logistic regression (0.75), while the AE features perform well in combination with k-NN (0.71, 0.75) or with random forests in combination with PCA (0.75).

4   Conclusion

In this study, we present a multi-modal medical image classifier making use of modern 3D implementations of LBP, BRIEF and HOG features, as well as deep learned auto-encoder features. The framework is validated against a highly difficult classification task: the classification of brain tumors in genetic classes. Although medical experts are not able to differentiate between the genetic classes using only image evidence, the presented framework obtained an accuracy of 0.83 when using all features combined with PCA and RF classification.

References

1. Wiestler, B., Capper, D., Sill, M., et al.: Integrated DNA methylation and copy-number profiling identify three clinically and biologically relevant groups of anaplastic glioma. Acta Neuropathol. **128**, 561–571 (2014)
2. Paul, A., Dey, A., Mukherjee, D.P., Sivaswamy, J., Tourani, V.: Regenerative random forest with automatic feature selection to detect mitosis in histopathological breast cancer images. In: Navab, N., Hornegger, J., Wells, W.M., Frangi, A.F. (eds.) MICCAI 2015. LNCS, vol. 9350, pp. 94–102. Springer, Cham (2015). doi:10.1007/978-3-319-24571-3_12
3. Otálora, S., et al.: Combining unsupervised feature learning and riesz wavelets for histopathology image representation: application to identifying anaplastic medulloblastoma. In: Navab, N., Hornegger, J., Wells, W.M., Frangi, A.F. (eds.) MICCAI 2015. LNCS, vol. 9349, pp. 581–588. Springer, Cham (2015). doi:10.1007/978-3-319-24553-9_71

4. Chen, X., Xu, Y., Yan, S., Wong, D.W.K., Wong, T.Y., Liu, J.: Automatic feature learning for glaucoma detection based on deep learning. In: Navab, N., Hornegger, J., Wells, W.M., Frangi, A.F. (eds.) MICCAI 2015. LNCS, vol. 9351, pp. 669–677. Springer, Cham (2015). doi:10.1007/978-3-319-24574-4_80

5. Levner, I., Drabycz, S., Roldan, G., Robles, P., Cairncross, J.G., Mitchell, R.: Predicting MGMT methylation status of glioblastomas from MRI texture. In: Yang, G.-Z., Hawkes, D., Rueckert, D., Noble, A., Taylor, C. (eds.) MICCAI 2009. LNCS, vol. 5762, pp. 522–530. Springer, Heidelberg (2009). doi:10.1007/978-3-642-04271-3_64

6. Lian, C., Ruan, S., Denœux, T., Li, H., Vera, P.: Dempster-shafer theory based feature selection with sparse constraint for outcome prediction in cancer therapy. In: Navab, N., Hornegger, J., Wells, W.M., Frangi, A.F. (eds.) MICCAI 2015. LNCS, vol. 9351, pp. 695–702. Springer, Cham (2015). doi:10.1007/978-3-319-24574-4_83

7. Lowe, D.: Distinctive image features from scale-invariant keypoints. Int. J. Comput. Vis. **20**(2), 91–110 (2004)

8. Bay, H., Tuytelaars, T., Gool, L.: SURF: speeded up robust features. In: Leonardis, A., Bischof, H., Pinz, A. (eds.) ECCV 2006. LNCS, vol. 3951, pp. 404–417. Springer, Heidelberg (2006). doi:10.1007/11744023_32

9. Ojala, T., Pietikäinen, M., Mäenpää, T.: Multiresolution gray-scale and rotation-invariant texture classification with local binary patterns. IEEE Trans. Pattern. Anal. Mach. Intell. **24**, 971–987 (2002)

10. Calonder, M., Lepetit, V., Ozuysal, M., et al.: BRIEF: computing a local binary descriptor very fast. IEEE Trans. Pattern Anal. Mach. Intell. **34**(7), 1281–1298 (2012)

11. Chen, X., Xu, Y., Yan, S., Chua, T.-S., Wong, D.W.K., Wong, T.Y., Liu, J.: Discriminative feature selection for multiple ocular diseases classification by sparse induced graph regularized group lasso. In: Navab, N., Hornegger, J., Wells, W.M., Frangi, A.F. (eds.) MICCAI 2015. LNCS, vol. 9350, pp. 11–19. Springer, Cham (2015). doi:10.1007/978-3-319-24571-3_2

12. Banerjee, J., Moelker, A., Niessen, W.J., Walsum, T.: 3D LBP-based rotationally invariant region description. In: Park, J.-I., Kim, J. (eds.) ACCV 2012. LNCS, vol. 7728, pp. 26–37. Springer, Heidelberg (2013). doi:10.1007/978-3-642-37410-4_3

13. Heinrich, M.P., Blendowski, M.: Multi-organ segmentation using vantage point forests and binary context features. In: Ourselin, S., Joskowicz, L., Sabuncu, M.R., Unal, G., Wells, W. (eds.) MICCAI 2016. LNCS, vol. 9901, pp. 598–606. Springer, Cham (2016). doi:10.1007/978-3-319-46723-8_69

14. Kläser, A., Marszalek, M., Schmid, C.: A Spatio-Temporal Descriptor based on 3d-Gradients. In: BMVC (2008)

15. Csurka, G., Bray, C., Dance, C., et al.: Visual Categorization with Bags of Keypoints. In: ECCV Workshop on Statistical Learning in Computer Vision, pp. 1–22 (2004)

16. Vincent, P., Larochelle, H., Lajoie, I., et al.: Stacked denoising autoencoders: learning useful representations in a deep network with a local denoising criterion. J. Mach. Learn. Res. **11**, 3371–3408 (2010)

17. Menze, B.H., et al.: A generative probabilistic model and discriminative extensions for brain lesion segmentation - with application to tumor and stroke. IEEE Trans. Med. Imaging **35**(4), 933–946 (2016)

A Fast SCCA Algorithm for Big Data Analysis in Brain Imaging Genetics

Yuming Huang[1], Lei Du[1(✉)], Kefei Liu[2], Xiaohui Yao[2], Shannon L. Risacher[2], Lei Guo[1], Andrew J. Saykin[2], and Li Shen[2], and the Alzheimer's Disease Neuroimaging Initiative

[1] School of Automation, Northwestern Polytechnical University, Xi'an, China
dulei@nwpu.edu.cn
[2] Radiology and Imaging Sciences, Indiana University, School of Medicine, Indianapolis, IN, USA

Abstract. Mining big data in brain imaging genetics is an emerging topic in brain science. It can uncover meaningful associations between genetic variations and brain structures and functions. Sparse canonical correlation analysis (SCCA) is introduced to discover bi-multivariate correlations with feature selection. However, these SCCA methods cannot be directly applied to big brain imaging genetics data due to two limitations. First, they have cubic complexity in the size of the matrix involved and are computational and memory intensive when the matrix becomes large. Second, the parameters in an SCCA method need to be fine-tuned in advance. This further dramatically increases the computational time, and gets severe in high-dimensional scenarios. In this paper, we propose two fast and efficient algorithms to speed up the structure-aware SCCA (S2CCA) implementations without modification to the original SCCA models. The fast algorithms employ a divide-and-conquer strategy and are easy to implement. The experimental results, compared with conventional algorithms, show that our algorithms reduce the time usage significantly. Specifically, the fast algorithms improve the computational efficiency by tens to hundreds of times compared to conventional algorithms. Besides, our algorithms yield similar correlation coefficients and canonical loading profiles to the conventional implementations. Our fast algorithms can be easily parallelized to further reduce the computational

L. Du—This work was supported by NSFC (61602384), the Natural Science Basic Research Plan in Shaanxi Province of China (2017JQ6001), the China Postdoctoral Science Foundation (2017M613214), and the Fundamental Research Funds for the Central Universities (3102016OQD0065). This work was also supported by NIH R01 EB022574, R01 LM011360, U01 AG024904, P30 AG10133, R01 AG19771, UL1 TR001108, R01 AG 042437, R01 AG046171, and R01 AG040770, by DoD W81XWH-14-2-0151, W81XWH-13-1-0259, W81XWH-12-2-0012, and NCAA 14132004.

Data used in preparation of this article were obtained from the Alzheimer's Disease Neuroimaging Initiative (ADNI) database (adni.loni.usc.edu). As such, the investigators within the ADNI contributed to the design and implementation of ADNI and/or provided data but did not participate in analysis or writing of this report. A complete listing of ADNI investigators can be found at: http://adni.loni.usc.edu/wp-content/uploads/how_to_apply/ADNI_Acknowledgement_List.pdf.

M.J. Cardoso et al. (Eds.): GRAIL/MFCA/MICGen 2017, LNCS 10551, pp. 210–219, 2017.
DOI: 10.1007/978-3-319-67675-3_19

time. This indicates that the proposed fast scalable SCCA algorithms can be a powerful tool for big data analysis in brain imaging genetics.

1   Introduction

In brain science, mining big brain imaging genetics data is an emerging topic. The complex associations between genetic factors and brain structures or functions can help reveal interesting and meaningful biological mechanisms, including the genetic basis of brain disorders [11,12]. The genetic factors such as the single nucleotide polymorphisms (SNPs) are usually huge in size. The neuroimaging phenotypic data such as the quantitative traits (QTs) are also very large if we intend to analyze the brain imaging in fine resolution. Therefore, efficient identification of complex multi-SNP-multi-QT associations for large imaging genetics data becomes an urgent topic in brain science.

Sparse canonical correlation analysis (SCCA) [13] is a multi-view learning technique which discovers the relationship between two views of data with sparse output. It has been broadly applied to imaging genetics studies [1–5]. The imaging genetics data usually have a small number of observations with a huge size of features. This incurs severe computational burden to the SCCA analysis. To reduce the time complexity and memory usage, as well as the computational difficulty, most studies assume the covariance matrix of both SNPs and QTs data to be an identity matrix [1,2,9,13]. Du et al. [4] have proposed the structure-aware SCCA (S2CCA) to address this issue, but their S2CCA suffers from heavy computational cost and is memory expensive since it involves big matrix manipulation in high-dimensional settings. Furthermore, there are four parameters to be fine-tuned in the S2CCA model.

In this study, we propose a fast algorithm to address the ℓ_1-norm based and the combined ℓ_1-norm and ℓ_1/ℓ_2-norm based S2CCA problems, without assuming covariance structure being an identity matrix. To improve both time and memory efficiency, we take advantage of the group-like structure (e.g., voxels in an ROI or SNPs in an LD block), other than just incorporating it like S2CCA [3,4]. The proposed algorithms employ the divide-and-conquer strategy and block matrix decomposition, and are easy to implement. In the rest of this paper, we call the proposed algorithms fast ℓ_1-S2CCA and fast ℓ_1/ℓ_2-S2CCA, and use ℓ_1-S2CCA to denote the conventional implementation of ℓ_1-norm based S2CCA, and ℓ_1/ℓ_2-S2CCA to denote the conventional implementation of the combined ℓ_1-norm and ℓ_1/ℓ_2-norm based S2CCA. Experimental results on both synthetic and real imaging genetic data show that, compared with the ℓ_1-S2CCA and ℓ_1/ℓ_2-S2CCA, our fast algorithms gain substantial time efficiency enhancement, e.g. several hundred fold in some cases. More interestingly, the speedup grows as fast as the number of features increases. The performance in term of canonical correlation coefficients and canonical weight profiles shows no significant difference between the fast and conventional algorithms. These promising results demonstrate the potential and power of our fast algorithms in big brain imaging genetics analysis.

2   The Fast SCCA Algorithm

In this paper, a vector is denoted by a lowercase boldface letter, and a matrix is denoted by an uppercase one. Let $\mathbf{X} \in \mathcal{R}^{n \times p}$ denote the SNP data matrix with n observations and p SNPs, and $\mathbf{Y} \in \mathcal{R}^{n \times q}$ be the QT one with q QTs, the SCCA and S2CCA problems can be uniformly defined as

$$\min_{\mathbf{u}, \mathbf{v}} -\mathbf{u}^\top \mathbf{X}^\top \mathbf{Y} \mathbf{v} + \Omega(\mathbf{u}) + \Omega(\mathbf{v}) \tag{1}$$

$s.t.$ $||\mathbf{X}\mathbf{u}||_2^2 = 1, ||\mathbf{Y}\mathbf{v}||_2^2 = 1$, where $\Omega(\mathbf{u})$ and $\Omega(\mathbf{v})$ are two norm functions to pursuit sparsity [3, 4, 9, 13, 14]. Suppose $\Omega(\mathbf{u}) = \lambda_1 ||\mathbf{u}||_1 + \beta_1 ||\mathbf{u}||_G$, we have

$$\min_{\mathbf{u}, \mathbf{v}} -\mathbf{u}^\top \mathbf{X}^\top \mathbf{Y} \mathbf{v} + \lambda_1 ||\mathbf{u}||_1 + \beta_1 ||\mathbf{u}||_G + \gamma_1 ||\mathbf{X}\mathbf{u}||_2^2 + \lambda_2 ||\mathbf{v}||_1 + \beta_2 ||\mathbf{v}||_G + \gamma_2 ||\mathbf{Y}\mathbf{v}||_2^2 \tag{2}$$

based on the Lagrangian method, where $||\cdot||_G$ is the ℓ_1/ℓ_2-norm function. According to S2CCA algorithm [4], we have the closed-form updating expressions

$$\mathbf{u} = (\lambda_1 \mathbf{D}_1 + \beta_1 \tilde{\mathbf{D}}_1 + \gamma_1 \mathbf{X}^\top \mathbf{X})^{-1} \mathbf{X}^\top \mathbf{Y} \mathbf{v}, \tag{3}$$

$$\mathbf{v} = (\lambda_2 \mathbf{D}_2 + \beta_2 \tilde{\mathbf{D}}_2 + \gamma_2 \mathbf{Y}^\top \mathbf{Y})^{-1} \mathbf{Y}^\top \mathbf{X} \mathbf{u}, \tag{4}$$

where $\mathbf{D}_1$ is a diagonal matrix with each diagonal element being $\frac{1}{|u_i|}(i \in [1, p])$, and $\tilde{\mathbf{D}}_1$ is a diagonal matrix with each diagonal element being $\tilde{\mathbf{D}}_1(i, i) = \frac{1}{||\mathbf{u}_{k_1}||_2}$, if $u_i \in \mathbf{u}_{k_1}$ where k_1 is the index of the LD block. $\mathbf{D}_2$ and $\tilde{\mathbf{D}}_2$ have the same entries with respect to $\mathbf{v}$. $\mathbf{u}$ and $\mathbf{v}$ can be solved using the alternative iteration algorithm [6], which however is quite time intensive for high-dimensional data.

We propose the fast SCCA algorithm based on the following theorem.

Theorem 1. *Given both $\mathbf{X}^\top \mathbf{X}$ and $\mathbf{Y}^\top \mathbf{Y}$ are block diagonal matrices, the S2CCA can be equivalently solved via*

$$\mathbf{u} = \oplus_{k_1=1}^{|G_1|} \mathbf{u}_{k_1}, where \ \mathbf{u}_{k_1} = (\lambda_1 \mathbf{D}_{1,k_1} + \beta_1 \tilde{\mathbf{D}}_{1,k_1} + \gamma_1 \mathbf{X}_{k_1}^\top \mathbf{X}_{k_1})^{-1} \mathbf{X}_{k_1}^\top \mathbf{Y} \mathbf{v}, \tag{5}$$

$$\mathbf{v} = \oplus_{k_2=1}^{|G_2|} \mathbf{v}_{k_2}, where \ \mathbf{v}_{k_2} = (\lambda_2 \mathbf{D}_{2,k_2} + \beta_2 \tilde{\mathbf{D}}_{2,k_2} + \gamma_2 \mathbf{Y}_{k_2}^\top \mathbf{Y}_{k_2})^{-1} \mathbf{Y}_{k_2}^\top \mathbf{X} \mathbf{u}, \tag{6}$$

where $\oplus$ denotes the concatenate operator for vectors, $|G_1|$ is the number of LD block for SNPs, and $|G_2|$ is the number of ROI block for voxels.

Proof. We first prove the $\mathbf{u}$-update. Denoting $\mathbf{X} = (\mathbf{x}_1, \cdots, \mathbf{x}_{k_1}, \cdots, \mathbf{x}_{|G_1|})^\top$, letting k_1 be the index of the blocks, the block diagonal matrix $\mathbf{X}^\top \mathbf{X}$ can be represented as

$$\mathbf{X}^\top \mathbf{X} = \begin{bmatrix} \mathbf{x}_1^\top \mathbf{x}_1 & & \\ & \ddots & \\ & & \mathbf{x}_{|G_1|}^\top \mathbf{x}_{|G_1|} \end{bmatrix}.$$

Since both $\mathbf{D}_1$ and $\tilde{\mathbf{D}}_1$ are diagonal matrices, they are diagonal separable. Thus we have

$$\mathbf{u} = \left(\lambda_1 \begin{bmatrix} \mathbf{D}_{1,1} & & \\ & \ddots & \\ & & \mathbf{D}_{1,|G_1|} \end{bmatrix} + \beta_1 \begin{bmatrix} \tilde{\mathbf{D}}_{1,1} & & \\ & \ddots & \\ & & \tilde{\mathbf{D}}_{1,|G_1|} \end{bmatrix} + \gamma_1 \begin{bmatrix} \mathbf{x}_1^\top \mathbf{x}_1 & & \\ & \ddots & \\ & & \mathbf{x}_{|G_1|}^\top \mathbf{x}_{|G_1|} \end{bmatrix} \right)^{-1} \mathbf{X}^\top \mathbf{Y} \mathbf{v}$$

$$
= \left(\lambda_1 \begin{bmatrix} \mathbf{D}_{1,1} & & \\ & \ddots & \\ & & \mathbf{D}_{1,|G_1|} \end{bmatrix} + \beta_1 \begin{bmatrix} \tilde{\mathbf{D}}_{1,1} & & \\ & \ddots & \\ & & \tilde{\mathbf{D}}_{1,|G_1|} \end{bmatrix} + \gamma_1 \begin{bmatrix} \mathbf{x}_1^\top \mathbf{x}_1 & & \\ & \ddots & \\ & & \mathbf{x}_{|G_1|}^\top \mathbf{x}_{|G_1|} \end{bmatrix} \right)^{-1} \begin{bmatrix} \mathbf{X}_1^\top \\ \vdots \\ \mathbf{X}_{|G_1|}^\top \end{bmatrix} \mathbf{Yv}
$$

$$
= \begin{bmatrix} (\lambda_1 \mathbf{D}_{1,1} + \beta_1 \tilde{\mathbf{D}}_{1,1} + \gamma_1 \mathbf{x}_1^\top \mathbf{x}_1)^{-1} \mathbf{X}_1^\top \mathbf{Yv} \\ \vdots \\ (\lambda_1 \mathbf{D}_{1,|G_1|} + \beta_1 \tilde{\mathbf{D}}_{1,|G_1|} + \gamma_1 \mathbf{x}_{|G_1|}^\top \mathbf{x}_{|G_1|})^{-1} \mathbf{X}_{|G_1|}^\top \mathbf{Yv} \end{bmatrix} = \oplus_{k_1=1}^{|G_1|} \mathbf{u}_{k_1}.
$$

Equation (6) can be proved similarly. In this theorem, we divide the big matrix into a group of small ones with the dimensions equivalent to the LD (or ROI) block size, i.e. the number of SNPs (or the number of voxels). Then after the calculation, we concatenate $\mathbf{u}_{k_1}$'s ($\mathbf{v}_{k_2}$'s) to obtain the original solution. Thus the computational burden is greatly reduced. The procedure details are shown below.

Algorithm for fast SCCA

1. Initialize $\mathbf{u}$ and $\mathbf{v}$;
2. Repeat the following steps until convergence:
   (1) Calculate $\mathbf{u}_{k_1}$ according to Eq. (5), and then update $\mathbf{u} = \oplus_{k_1=1}^{|G_1|} \mathbf{u}_{k_1}$;
   (2) Calculate $\mathbf{v}_{k_2}$ according to Eq. (6), and then update $\mathbf{v} = \oplus_{k_2=1}^{|G_2|} \mathbf{v}_{k_2}$.

Time Complexity: In the S2CCA algorithm, the dominant computational burden of $\mathbf{u}$-update refers to calculating the inverse of matrix. This can be reduced to approximate quadratic complexity, i.e. $O(np^2)$, via solving a system of linear equations. In our fast algorithm, the main complexity is $O(np_{k_1}^2 |G_1|)$ where p_{k_1} denotes the dimension of the k_1-th block. In biomedical studies, both the sample size and the LD block size are usually much smaller than the total number of biomarkers, i.e. $\max(n, p_{k_1}) \ll p$ [10], thus the time complexity has been greatly reduced. In addition, the memory requirement can also be reduced since the algorithm only stores small matrices during the iteration. Moreover, each $\mathbf{u}_{k_1}$ can be independently solved, and thus our algorithm can be easily parallelized.

3   Experiments

Based on our motivation, we choose the S2CCA algorithm for comparison. Those $\mathbf{X}^\top \mathbf{X} = \mathbf{I}$ based methods are not included because they ignore the structure information of the covariance matrix. We implement ℓ_1-S2CCA ($\beta_1 = \beta_2 = 0$ in Eqs. (3–4)) and ℓ_1/ℓ_2-S2CCA algorithms as benchmarks. Since ℓ_1-S2CCA and ℓ_1/ℓ_2-S2CCA are time intensive, we cannot afford a grid search strategy in the experiments. We fine-tuned these parameters on a small data set for each method, and directly use them in the subsequent experiments. In this study, all methods use the same implementation except for the speedup design, run on the same platform and data partition, and employ the same stopping condition, i.e. $\max_i |u_i^{t+1} - u_i^t| \leq 10^{-5}$ and $\max_j |v_j^{t+1} - v_j^t| \leq 10^{-5}$.

3.1   Results on Synthetic Data

We simulated nine data sets with the number of features spanning from small to large for both $\mathbf{u}$ and $\mathbf{v}$. We also set the ground truth with sparse signals and the number of observations being small enough to simulate a *small-n-large-(p + q)* scenario. We first generated $\mathbf{u}$ and $\mathbf{v}$ with sparse entries, and then created a latent vector $\mathbf{z} \sim N(\mathbf{0}, \mathbf{I}_{n \times n})$. After that, the data matrices $\mathbf{X}$ and $\mathbf{Y}$ can be generated as $\mathbf{x}_i \sim N(z_i \mathbf{u}, \sum_x)$ and $\mathbf{y}_i \sim N(z_i \mathbf{v}, \sum_y)$. The true signal of every data set were shown in Fig. 1 (top row of $\mathbf{u}$-panel and $\mathbf{v}$-panel).

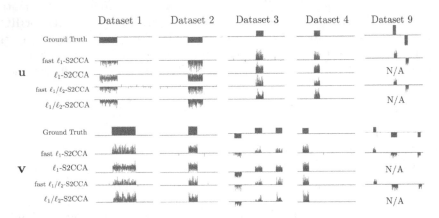

Fig. 1. Canonical weights estimated on synthetic data. The top half shows the estimated $\mathbf{u}$, and the bottom half shows $\mathbf{v}$. For each canonical weights, the first row shows the ground truth, and each remaining one shows a SCCA method. The 'N/A' means that a method is out of memory or no result is obtained after one hour run.

We first present canonical weights estimated from the training sets in Fig. 1. We observe that all S2CCA methods successfully find out the true signals from the first four data sets. From the fifth data set on, both ℓ_1-S2CCA and ℓ_1/ℓ_2-S2CCA fail since they either require too much time to yield the result or are out of memory. Our fast S2CCA algorithms run significantly fast and report the correct canonical weights which are consistent to the ground truth. Due to space limitation, we only show the estimated $\mathbf{u}$ and $\mathbf{v}$ for the ninth (largest) data set. The testing correlation coefficients are also contained in Table 1, where training ones are omitted for space constraint. The values again show that the fast methods hold higher scores than the conventional S2CCA methods.

Table 2 shows the runtime. The times of both fast algorithms drop significantly compared with their conventional opponents. They take much less time than conventional ones to obtain similar results. Further, the speedup, i.e. times/folds improved by the fast S2CCA against the conventional algorithms, reaches more than 700 folds for ℓ_1-S2CCA, and 400 folds for ℓ_1/ℓ_2-S2CCA on average. In Fig. 2, we clearly observe that the time efficiency of the fast

Table 1. Results on synthetic data. Testing results (training ones are omitted for space limitations) are shown. The '-' means that a method is out of memory or no result is given after one hour run.

Testing correlation coefficients ($mean \pm std$)				
Methods	fast ℓ_1-S2CCA	ℓ_1-S2CCA	fast ℓ_1/ℓ_2-S2CCA	ℓ_1/ℓ_2-S2CCA
Dataset1	0.91±0.03	0.88±0.01	0.95±0.01	0.93±0.03
Dataset2	0.90±0.04	0.91±0.02	0.97±0.01	0.96±0.01
Dataset3	0.87±0.05	0.83±0.03	0.97±0.01	0.95±0.01
Dataset4	0.85±0.04	0.83±0.03	0.97±0.00	0.95±0.01
Dataset5	0.95±0.01	-	1.00±0.00	-
Dataset6	0.97±0.02	-	1.00±0.00	-
Dataset7	0.94±0.02	-	1.00±0.00	-
Dataset8	0.93±0.01	-	1.00±0.00	-
Dataset9	0.92±0.02	-	1.00±0.00	-

Table 2. Runtime on synthetic data. The average value cross five folds are shown.

Runtime (sec.)				
Methods	fast ℓ_1-S2CCA	ℓ_1-S2CCA	fast ℓ_1/ℓ_2-S2CCA	ℓ_1/ℓ_2-S2CCA
Dataset1	0.05	3.14	0.11	1.03
Dataset2	0.11	22.94	0.22	8.09
Dataset3	0.39	116.87	0.51	66.94
Dataset4	1.14	829.1	1.2	489.46
Dataset5	3.49	-	3.67	-
Dataset6	7.33	-	7.08	-
Dataset7	11.24	-	9.73	-
Dataset8	22.73	-	20.22	-
Dataset9	53.28	-	57.62	-

methods shows significantly improvements. The folds keep ascending as the feature number increase. This is very promising, demonstrating that the proposed algorithms can not only enjoy promising time efficiency for big imaging genetics data analysis, but also outperform conventional S2CCA algorithms.

3.2 Results on Real Neuroimaging Genetics Data

The magnetic resonance imaging (MRI), amyloid imaging and SNP data were downloaded from the Alzheimer's Disease Neuroimaging Initiative (ADNI) database. One aim of ADNI has been to test whether serial MRI, positron emission tomography, other biological markers, and clinical and neuropsychological assess-

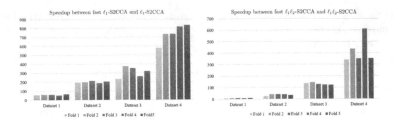

Fig. 2. Speedup comparison on synthetic data. The left panel shows the speedup between the ℓ_1-SCCA and fast ℓ_1-SCCA, and the right one shows the speedup between the ℓ_1/ℓ_2-SCCA and fast ℓ_1/ℓ_2-SCCA.

ment can be combined to measure the progression of mild cognitive impairment (MCI) and early AD. For up-to-date information, see www.adni-info.org.

In this study, we included 85 non-Hispanic Caucasian participants. Their amyloid imaging data from LONI (adni.loni.usc.edu) were preprocessed as described in [7]. After that, we used the regression to eliminate the effects of the baseline age, gender, education and handedness. Based on the MarsBaR AAL atlas, we extracted 191 ROI level mean amyloid measurements across the brain. The genotyping data were extracted from an imputed genetic data set including only SNPs in Illumina 610Q and/or OmniExpress arrays after basic quality control. We extracted 13,372 SNPs from the top 23 AD-risk genes, such as *APOE, CLU, INPP5D* etc., and the full list can be found in [8]. We intend to employ SCCA methods to evaluate the association between SNPs and brain ROIs, and identify the loci of those correlated SNPs and ROIs.

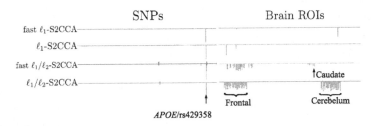

Fig. 3. Canonical loadings estimated on real imaging genetics data. Each row corresponds to an SCCA method. For each method, the estimated of **u** (genetic markers) is shown on the left panel, and **v** (brain ROIs) is shown on the right.

Figure 3 presents the estimated canonical weights, indicating which SNPs and amyloid measurements are selected and associated. All these four methods exhibit clear and sparse results for genetic markers, and the strongest signal comes from the rs429358 allele, located in the best-known AD-risk gene *APOE*. The top 5 SNPs except for rs429358 identified by both ℓ_1/ℓ_2-S2CCA are rs1081105 in *APOE*, rs12721051, rs56131196 and rs4420638 in *APOC1*, also from the region proximal to $APOE$. The results demonstrate that our fast algorithms do not limit the capability of the S2CCA model. On the brain side, both ℓ_1-S2CCA report a vary sparse signal, with only two markers coming from the frontal and cerebellum of the brain. While both ℓ_1/ℓ_2-S2CCA clearly show a group structure from the same brain regions. This assures the structure detection ability of the ℓ_1/ℓ_2-norm constraint. However, it seems strange that the fast ℓ_1/ℓ_2-S2CCA and ℓ_1/ℓ_2-S2CCA perform inconsistently. The reason could be that hyper-parameters for the conventional ℓ_1/ℓ_2-S2CCA are sub-optimal, which are tuned from a small data set as we stated in experimental setup. The training and testing correlation coefficients, as well as the runtime ($mean$) are all available in Table 3. These values show no significant difference between the fast and conventional algorithms, while their time consumptions vary distinctly. On this real data set, our fast algorithms only take around 10 s and 11 s, while two non-fast ones take around 690 s and 2300 s. This is a significant improvement in time efficiency. To sum up, results on this real data reveal that our fast algorithms reduce the time consumption dramatically, and they hold similar performances of correlation coefficients and canonical weights. This indicates that the fast algorithms could be a promising technique for genome-wide brain-wide imaging genetics.

Table 3. Results on real data. Training and testing correlation coefficients are shown. The $mean$ value are used for fast algorithms, and only an individual value for non-fast algorithms because they take too much time when using cross-validation.

	fast ℓ_1-S2CCA	ℓ_1-S2CCA	fast ℓ_1/ℓ_2-S2CCA	ℓ_1/ℓ_2-S2CCA
Training correlation coefficients	0.60	0.68	0.78	0.77
Testing correlation coefficients	0.54	0.54	0.68	0.65
Runtime (sec.)	10.35	687.22	11.22	2300.00

4   Conclusions

We have proposed two fast and efficient algorithms for the S2CCA models with ℓ_1-norm constraint, and combined ℓ_1-norm and ℓ_1/ℓ_2-norm constraint. Our algorithms make use of the structures of covariance matrices (without $\mathbf{X}^\top \mathbf{X} = \mathbf{I}$ assumption) [4]. They run significantly fast based on divide and conquer method. We compare our fast algorithms with two conventional S2CCA implementations using both synthetic data and real imaging genetic data. The results demonstrate that our methods run much more efficiently, and the speedup against S2CCA shows a growth trend with the increasing number of features. No significant differences are found between our fast algorithms and conventional S2CCA ones on both synthetic and real data. Actually, fast algorithms yield slightly better results regarding correlation coefficients in the simulation study. They find out a meaningful association between the SNP rs429358 ($APOE$) and frontal region in the AD cohort. This demonstrates that the proposed fast S2CCA algorithms can be a powerful method for massive brain imaging genetics analysis, making the genome-wide-brain-wide association studies possible. Future directions include (1) parallelizing our fast algorithm for further acceleration; (2) using massive imaging genetics data to evaluate our fast S2CCA algorithms in more realistic settings to verify their time and memory efficiency, as well as their capability to discovery meaningful association; and (3) studying fast methods for more general cases (e.g., non-overlapping blocks, data without block diagonal structure).

References

1. Chen, J., Bushman, F.D., et al.: Structure-constrained sparse canonical correlation analysis with an application to microbiome data analysis. Biostatistics **14**(2), 244–258 (2013)
2. Chen, X., Liu, H., Carbonell, J.G.: Structured sparse canonical correlation analysis. In: AISTATS (2012)
3. Du, L., Huang, H., Yan, J., Kim, S., Risacher, S.L., et al.: Structured sparse canonical correlation analysis for brain imaging genetics: an improved graphnet method. Bioinformatics **32**(10), 1544–1551 (2016)
4. Du, L., et al.: A novel structure-aware sparse learning algorithm for brain imaging genetics. In: Golland, P., Hata, N., Barillot, C., Hornegger, J., Howe, R. (eds.) MICCAI 2014. LNCS, vol. 8675, pp. 329–336. Springer, Cham (2014). doi:10.1007/978-3-319-10443-0_42
5. Du, L., et al.: Identifying associations between brain imaging phenotypes and genetic factors via a novel structured SCCA approach. In: Niethammer, M., Styner, M., Aylward, S., Zhu, H., Oguz, I., Yap, P.-T., Shen, D. (eds.) IPMI 2017. LNCS, vol. 10265, pp. 543–555. Springer, Cham (2017). doi:10.1007/978-3-319-59050-9_43
6. Gorski, J., Pfeuffer, F., Klamroth, K.: Biconvex sets and optimization with biconvex functions: a survey and extensions. Math. Methods Oper. Res. **66**(3), 373–407 (2007)
7. Jagust, W.J., Bandy, D., Chen, K., Foster, N.L., Landau, S.M., Mathis, C.A., Price, J.C., Reiman, E.M., Skovronsky, D., Koeppe, R.A., et al.: The Alzheimer's disease neuroimaging initiative positron emission tomography core. Alzheimer's Dement. **6**(3), 221–229 (2010)
8. Lambert, J.C., Ibrahim-Verbaas, C.A., Harold, D., Naj, A.C., Sims, R., Bellenguez, C., Jun, G., DeStefano, A.L., Bis, J.C., Beecham, G.W., et al.: Meta-analysis of 74,046 individuals identifies 11 new susceptibility loci for Alzheimer's disease. Nat. Genet. **45**(12), 1452–1458 (2013)
9. Parkhomenko, E., Tritchler, D., Beyene, J.: Sparse canonical correlation analysis with application to genomic data integration. Stat. Appl. Genet. Mol. Biol. **8**(1), 1–34 (2009)
10. Rosenfeld, J.A., Mason, C.E., Smith, T.M.: Limitations of the human reference genome for personalized genomics. PLoS ONE **7**(7), e40294 (2012)
11. Saykin, A.J., Shen, L., Yao, X., Kim, S., Nho, K., et al.: Genetic studies of quantitative MCI and ad phenotypes in ADNI: progress, opportunities, and plans. Alzheimer's Dement. **11**(7), 792–814 (2015)
12. Shen, L., Kim, S., Risacher, S.L., Nho, K., Swaminathan, S., West, J.D., Foroud, T., Pankratz, N., Moore, J.H., Sloan, C.D., et al.: Whole genome association study of brain-wide imaging phenotypes for identifying quantitative trait loci in MCI and AD: a study of the ADNI cohort. Neuroimage **53**(3), 1051–1063 (2010)

13. Witten, D.M., Tibshirani, R., Hastie, T.: A penalized matrix decomposition, with applications to sparse principal components and canonical correlation analysis. Biostatistics **10**(3), 515–534 (2009)
14. Yuan, M., Lin, Y.: Model selection and estimation in regression with grouped variables. J. R. Stat. Soc. Ser. B (Stat. Methodol.) **68**(1), 49–67 (2006)

Transcriptome-Guided Imaging Genetic Analysis via a Novel Sparse CCA Algorithm

Kefei Liu[1], Xiaohui Yao[1,2], Jingwen Yan[1,2], Danai Chasioti[1,2],
Shannon Risacher[1], Kwangsik Nho[1], Andrew Saykin[1], Li Shen[1,2(✉)],
and the Alzheimer's Disease Neuroimaging Initiative

[1] Department of Radiology and Imaging Sciences,
Indiana University School of Medicine, Indianapolis, IN 46202, USA
shenli@iu.edu
[2] School of Informatics and Computing, Indiana University,
Indianapolis, IN, USA

Abstract. Imaging genetics is an emerging field that studies the influence of genetic variation on brain structure and function. The major task is to examine the association between genetic markers such as single nucleotide polymorphisms (SNPs) and quantitative traits (QTs) extracted from neuroimaging data. Sparse canonical correlation analysis (SCCA) is a bi-multivariate technique used in imaging genetics to identify complex multi-SNP-multi-QT associations. In imaging genetics, genes associated with a phenotype should be at least expressed in the phenotypical region. We study the association between the genotype and amyloid imaging data and propose a transcriptome-guided SCCA framework that incorporates the gene expression information into the SCCA criterion. An alternating optimization method is used to solve the formulated problem. Although the problem is not biconcave, a closed-form solution has been found for each subproblem. The results on real data show that using the gene expression data to guide the feature selection facilities the detection of genetic markers that are not only associated with the identified QTs, but also highly expressed there.

1 Introduction

Brain imaging genetics is an emerging research field that studies the influence of genetic variation on brain structure and function. A fundamental problem in

This work was supported by NIH R01 EB022574, R01 LM011360, U01 AG024904, P30 AG10133, R01 AG19771, UL1 TR001108, R01 AG 042437, R01 AG046171, and R01 AG040770, by DoD W81XWH-14-2-0151, W81XWH-13-1-0259, W81XWH-12-2-0012, and NCAA 14132004.

Data used in preparation of this article were obtained from the Alzheimer's Disease Neuroimaging Initiative (ADNI) database (adni.loni.usc.edu). As such, the investigators within the ADNI contributed to the design and implementation of ADNI and/or provided data but did not participate in analysis or writing of this report. A complete listing of ADNI investigators can be found at: http://adni.loni.usc.edu/wp-content/uploads/how_to_apply/ADNI_Acknowledgement_List.pdf.

M.J. Cardoso et al. (Eds.): GRAIL/MFCA/MICGen 2017, LNCS 10551, pp. 220–229, 2017.
DOI: 10.1007/978-3-319-67675-3_20

brain imaging genetics is to investigate the association between genetic variations such as single nucleotide polymorphisms (SNPs) and phenotypes extracted
from multimodal neuroimaging data (e.g., anatomical, functional and molecular
imaging scans). Given the well-known importance of gene and imaging phenotype in brain function, bridging these two factors and exploring their connections
would lead to a better mechanistic understanding of normal or disordered brain
functions.

Sparse canonical correlation analysis (SCCA) has been widely adopted to
identify complex imaging genetic associations in both synthetic and real imaging
genetics data [2,3,6–8]. The prior graph or group structural knowledge among
variables (e.g., a number of genes form a group to participate in a particular
biological process to perform certain functionality in a cell) can be incorporated
into SCCA model to guide the association analysis [2,3,9], which can improve
the accuracy and stability in variable selection and facilitate the interpretability
of the identified associations.

In this work, we propose to take advantage of the brain wide gene expression
profile available in Allen human brain atlas (AHBA) and use it as a 2-D prior
to guide the brain imaging genetics association analysis. To account for such
2-D prior, we propose a transcriptome-guided SCCA (TG-SCCA) framework
that incorporates the gene expression information into traditional SCCA model.
A new regularization term is introduced to encourage the discovery of imaging
genomic associations so that the identified genes have relatively high expression level in their associated brain regions. To solve the formulated problem,
we employ an alternating optimization method and manage to find a closed-
form globally maximum solution for each of the two subproblems despite not
biconcave.

Notation: The superscript $^\mathrm{T}$ stands for the transpose of a matrix or vector.
The $\|u\|$ and $\|u\|_1$ denote the Euclidean norm and ℓ_1 norm of a vector u, respec-
tively. The operator $\odot$ represents the Hadamard product (entrywise product) of
two matrices of the same dimensions. The sign function of a real number x is
defined as follows: $\mathrm{sign}\{x\} = 1$ when $x \geq 0$ and $\mathrm{sign}\{x\} = -1$ when $x < 0$.

2 Problem Formulation

Let $X \in \mathbb{R}^{n \times p}$ be the genotype data (SNP) and $Y \in \mathbb{R}^{n \times q}$ be the imaging
quantitative traits (QT) data, where n, p and q are the numbers of participants,
SNPs and QTs, respectively. Sparse canonical correlation analysis (SCCA) aims
to find a linear combination of variables in X and Y to maximize the correlation:

$$\underset{u,v}{\text{maximize}}\; u^\mathrm{T} X^\mathrm{T} Y v \quad \text{subject to } \|u\|^2 \leq 1, \|v\|^2 \leq 1, \|u\|_1 \leq c_1, \|v\|_1 \leq c_2. \quad (1)$$

Suppose the p SNPs belong to G genes. Let $E = \{e_{gj}\} \in \mathbb{R}^{G \times q}$ be
the gene expression matrix with e_{gj} being the expression of gene g in brain
region j. Let the SNPs be ordered in terms of the genes they belong to.

Denote $\boldsymbol{u} = \begin{bmatrix} \boldsymbol{u}_1^{\mathrm{T}} \ \boldsymbol{u}_2^{\mathrm{T}} \ \cdots \ \boldsymbol{u}_G^{\mathrm{T}} \end{bmatrix}^{\mathrm{T}}$, where $\boldsymbol{u}_g = \begin{bmatrix} u_{g,1} \ u_{g,2} \ \cdots \ u_{g,p_g} \end{bmatrix}^{\mathrm{T}} \in \mathbb{R}^{p_g \times 1}$, $g = 1, 2, \ldots, G$, contains the canonical weights of the p_g SNPs in gene g, where p_g is the number of SNPs in gene g. We assume that each SNP belongs to only one gene such that $p_1 + p_2 + \cdots + p_G = p$. To exploit the gene expression information, we propose to extend the SCCA in (1) in the following way:

$$\underset{\boldsymbol{u},\boldsymbol{v}}{\text{maximize}} \quad (1 - \lambda)\boldsymbol{u}^{\mathrm{T}}\boldsymbol{X}^{\mathrm{T}}\boldsymbol{Y}\boldsymbol{v} + \lambda \sum_{g=1}^{G} \sum_{j=1}^{q} \max \left\{ |u_{g,1}|, |u_{g,2}|, \ldots, |u_{g,p_g}| \right\} e_{gj} |v_j| \quad (2)$$

$$\text{subject to} \quad \|\boldsymbol{u}\|^2 \le 1, \|\boldsymbol{v}\|^2 \le 1, \|\boldsymbol{u}\|_1 \le c_1, \|\boldsymbol{v}\|_1 \le c_2,$$

where $\boldsymbol{E} = \{e_{gj}\}$ is the gene expression matrix in which all the elements are equal to or greater than zero, and $\lambda \in [0, 1)$ is the weighting coefficient that reflects our confidence in imposing the correlation with the gene expression data. The regularization term encourages the selection of one SNP from each gene with relatively high expression in the relevant QTs. The intuition is that if a gene is related to a QT, it should be expressed in the corresponding brain tissue.

3   Methods

We employ an alternating optimization method to solve problem (2). Alternating optimization is an iterative procedure that proceeds in two alternating steps: update of $\boldsymbol{u}$ while holding $\boldsymbol{v}$ fixed and update of $\boldsymbol{v}$ while holding $\boldsymbol{u}$ fixed.

3.1   Update of $\boldsymbol{u}$ with $\boldsymbol{v}$ fixed

Denote

$$\boldsymbol{a} = (1 - \lambda)\boldsymbol{X}^{\mathrm{T}}\boldsymbol{Y}\boldsymbol{v} \in \mathbb{R}^{p \times 1}, \quad \boldsymbol{b} = \lambda\boldsymbol{E}|\boldsymbol{v}| \in \mathbb{R}^{G \times 1}.$$

The optimization of (2) with respect to $\boldsymbol{u}$ can be written as

$$\underset{\boldsymbol{u}}{\text{maximize}} \ \boldsymbol{a}^{\mathrm{T}}\boldsymbol{u} + \sum_{g=1}^{G} b_g \max \left\{ |u_{g,1}|, |u_{g,2}|, \ldots, |u_{g,p_g}| \right\} \quad \text{subject to} \ \|\boldsymbol{u}\|^2 \le 1, \|\boldsymbol{u}\|_1 \le c_1. \quad (3)$$

The problem in (3) is highly non-concave. Notice however, that if we know which is largest among the absolute values of the optimal $u_{g,1}, u_{g,2}, \ldots, u_{g,p_g}$, we can narrow down our search space for optimal solutions and move $|u_{g,1}|, |u_{g,2}|, \ldots, |u_{g,p_g}|$ outside the $\max\{\}$ operator in the objective function. Next we determine the largest absolute value among the optimal $u_{g,1}, u_{g,2}, \ldots, u_{g,p_g}$.
Define

$$h(\boldsymbol{u}_g) = \boldsymbol{a}_g^{\mathrm{T}}\boldsymbol{u}_g + b_g \max \left\{ |u_{g,1}|, |u_{g,2}|, \ldots, |u_{g,p_g}| \right\}, \quad (4)$$

where $\boldsymbol{a}_g \in \mathbb{R}^{p_g \times 1}$ is the subvector of $\boldsymbol{a}$ corresponding to the SNPs in gene g. The objective function in (3) can be written as $\sum\limits_{g=1}^{G} h(\boldsymbol{u}_g)$.

Consider the optimization problem:

$$\underset{\boldsymbol{u}_g}{\text{maximize}}\; h\left(\boldsymbol{u}_g\right) \quad \text{subject to } \|\boldsymbol{u}_g\|^2 \leq \mu^2, \|\boldsymbol{u}_g\|_1 \leq \nu, \tag{5}$$

where μ and ν are arbitrary positive constants.

Without loss of generality suppose

$$|a_{g,1}| = \max\left\{|a_{g,1}|, |a_{g,2}|, \ldots, |a_{g,p_g}|\right\}.$$

It can be shown that the optimal solutions of problem (5) satisfy

$$|u_{g,1}| = \max\left\{|u_{g,1}|, |u_{g,2}|, \ldots, |u_{g,p_g}|\right\}. \tag{6}$$

Equation (6) can be proved by contradiction. The idea is that if equation (6) does not hold, the objective value $h\left(\boldsymbol{u}_g\right)$ can be increased by swapping the absolute values of the first element and the element with the largest magnitude in $\boldsymbol{u}_g$. Moreover, $u_{g,1}$ has the same sign as $a_{g,1}$; otherwise, reversing the sign of $u_{g,1}$ increases the objective value, which contradicts $\boldsymbol{u}_g$ being the optimal solution.

Therefore, the objective function for problem (5) becomes

$$h\left(\boldsymbol{u}_g\right) = \left(a_{g,1} + b_g \operatorname{sign}\{a_{g,1}\}\right) u_{g,1} + a_{g,2}\, u_{g,2} + \cdots + a_{g,p_g}\, u_{g,p_g}.$$

For $g = 1, 2, \ldots, G$, let

$$\ell_g = \underset{k=1,2,\ldots,p_g}{\arg\max}\; |a_{g,k}| \tag{7}$$

and let $\boldsymbol{e}_{\ell_g}$ be a length-p_g column vector with 1 at location ℓ_g and 0 elsewhere. The problem (3) reduces to solving

$$\underset{\boldsymbol{u}}{\text{maximize}} \sum_{g=1}^{G} \left[\boldsymbol{a}_g + b_g \boldsymbol{e}_{\ell_g} \odot \operatorname{sign}\{\boldsymbol{a}_g\}\right]^{\mathrm{T}} \boldsymbol{u}_g \quad \text{subject to } \|\boldsymbol{u}\|^2 \leq 1, \|\boldsymbol{u}\|_1 \leq c_1. \tag{8}$$

Define

$$\boldsymbol{w} = \begin{pmatrix} \boldsymbol{a}_1 + b_1 \boldsymbol{e}_{\ell_1} \odot \operatorname{sign}\{\boldsymbol{a}_1\} \\ \boldsymbol{a}_2 + b_2 \boldsymbol{e}_{\ell_2} \odot \operatorname{sign}\{\boldsymbol{a}_2\} \\ \vdots \\ \boldsymbol{a}_G + b_G \boldsymbol{e}_{\ell_G} \odot \operatorname{sign}\{\boldsymbol{a}_G\} \end{pmatrix}. \tag{9}$$

The problem (8) is expressed in a more compact form as

$$\underset{\boldsymbol{u}}{\text{maximize}}\; \boldsymbol{w}^{\mathrm{T}} \boldsymbol{u} \quad \text{subject to } \|\boldsymbol{u}\|^2 \leq 1, \|\boldsymbol{u}\|_1 \leq c_1. \tag{10}$$

According to [7, Lemma 2.2], problem (10) has a closed-form solution which can be obtained by shrinking the elements in $\boldsymbol{w}$ toward zero by a non-negative constant and then normalizing the result to unit norm. Formally, the solution to (10) is

$$\boldsymbol{u}^* = \frac{S\left(\boldsymbol{w}, \Delta\right)}{\|S\left(\boldsymbol{w}, \Delta\right)\|} \tag{11}$$

with $\Delta = 0$ if this results in $\|u^*\|_1 \le c_1$; otherwise, Δ is a positive number that satisfies $\|u^*\|_1 = c_1$. In (11), $S(w, \Delta)$ is the soft-thresholding operator that is applied to each element of w, with

$$S(w_i, \Delta) = \begin{cases} w_i - \Delta, & w_i > \Delta \\ w_i + \Delta, & w_i < -\Delta \\ 0, & -\Delta \le w_i \le \Delta \end{cases}$$

3.2   Update of v with u fixed

Denote

$$\alpha = (1 - \lambda)Y^T X u \in \mathbb{R}^{q \times 1}.$$

The optimization of (2) with respect to v can be written as

$$\underset{v}{\text{maximize}} \sum_{j=1}^{q} \alpha_j v_j + \beta_j |v_j| \quad \text{subject to } \|v\|^2 \le 1, \|v\|_1 \le c_2. \tag{12}$$

where $\beta_j = \lambda \sum_{g=1}^{G} \max\left\{|u_{g,1}|, |u_{g,2}|, \ldots, |u_{g,p_g}|\right\} e_{gj}$, for $j = 1, 2, \ldots, q$.

Since $\beta_j \ge 0$ it can be shown that the optimal v_j has the same sign as α_j[1]. Define

$$\gamma = \begin{pmatrix} \alpha_1 + \beta_1 \operatorname{sign}\{\alpha_1\} \\ \alpha_2 + \beta_2 \operatorname{sign}\{\alpha_2\} \\ \vdots \\ \alpha_q + \beta_q \operatorname{sign}\{\alpha_q\} \end{pmatrix}. \tag{13}$$

The optimization problem in (12) boils down to solving the following problem:

$$\underset{v}{\text{maximize }} \gamma^T v \quad \text{subject to } \|v\|^2 \le 1, \|v\|_1 \le c_2. \tag{14}$$

According to [7, Lemma 2.2], the solution to (14) is

$$v^* = \frac{S(\gamma, \delta)}{\|S(\gamma, \delta)\|} \tag{15}$$

with $\delta = 0$ if this results in $\|v^*\|_1 \le c_2$; otherwise, δ is a positive number that satisfies $\|v^*\|_1 = c_2$.

Given an initial estimate for v, the TG-SCCA algorithm alternately update u and v in an iterative manner until convergence, as outlined in Algorithm 1.

Remark 1. Analysis shows that the optimization problem (2) is not biconcave in **u** and **v**: it is neither concave in **u** when **v** is fixed, nor concave in **v** when **u** is fixed[2]. Interestingly, the TG-SCCA algorithm finds the global maxima of the two subproblems in each iteration (i.e., Steps 5 and 6 of Algorithm 1).

---

[1] Otherwise, we can always increase the objective value by reversing the sign of v_j.

[2] The problem (2) is actually biconvex in **u** and **v**.

Algorithm 1. TG-SCCA algorithm

Input: Genotype data: $X \in \mathbb{R}^{n \times p}$, imaging phenotype data $Y \in \mathbb{R}^{n \times q}$, and gene expression data $E \in \mathbb{R}^{G \times q}$;

1: Normalize the columns of X and Y to have zero mean and unit Euclidian norm;
2: Choose the tuning parameters c_1, c_2 and λ;
3: Initialize $u \in \mathbb{R}^{p \times 1}$ and $v \in \mathbb{R}^{q \times 1}$;
4: **repeat**
5:    Update u according to Eqs. (9) and (11);
6:    Update v according to Eqs. (13) and (15);
7: **until** convergence.

---

4   Experimental Results and Discussions

We compare the TG-SCCA algorithm with the conventional SCCA algorithm [7] on a real imaging genetics data set to demonstrate its performance. The genotyping and baseline AV-45 PET data of 774 non-Hispanic Caucasian subjects, including 187 healthy control (HC), 76 significant memory concern (SMC), 227 early mild cognitive impairment (MCI), 186 late MCI, and 98 AD participants, were downloaded from the Alzheimer's Disease Neuroimaging Initiative (ADNI) database. One aim of ADNI has been to test whether serial magnetic resonance imaging (MRI), positron emission tomography, other biological markers, and clinical and neuropsychological assessment can be combined to measure the progression of MCI and early AD. For up-to-date information, see www.adni-info.org.

The AV-45 images were aligned to each participant's same visit MRI scan and normalized to the Montreal Neurological Institute (MNI) space. Region-of-interest (ROI) level AV-45 measurements were further extracted based on the MarsBaR AAL atlas. In this study, we focused on the analysis of 1,221 SNPs from 56 AD risk genes and 78 AD related ROIs. Using the regression weights derived from the HC participants, the genotype and imaging measures were preadjusted for removing the effects of the baseline age, gender, education, and handedness. The gene expression data were obtained from the Allen Human Brain Atlas (human.brain-map.org). The data were already normalized via a series of processes to remove non-biological biases and to make those comparable across samples. See Fig. 1 for the expression levels of the studied genes in the studied ROIs.

4.1   Selection of Tuning Parameters λ, c_1 and c_2

Based on our observation that the ℓ_1-sparsity constraints in the SCCA model (1) are not active when $c_1 \geq \|u_1\|_1$ and $c_2 \geq \|v_1\|_1$, where u_1 and v_1 are the left and right singular vectors of $X^T Y$ corresponding to its largest singular value, we propose to set the parameters c_1 and c_2 in the following way: $c_1 = s_1 \|u_1\|_1$ and $c_2 = s_2 \|v_1\|_1$, where $0 < s_1, s_2 < 1$. For the TG-SCCA, we set $c_1 = s_1 [(1 - \lambda) \|u_1\|_1 + \lambda \|u_2\|_1]$ and $c_2 = s_2 [(1 - \lambda) \|v_1\|_1 + \lambda \|v_2\|_1]$, where u_2 and v_2 are the left and right singular vectors of E corresponding to its largest singular

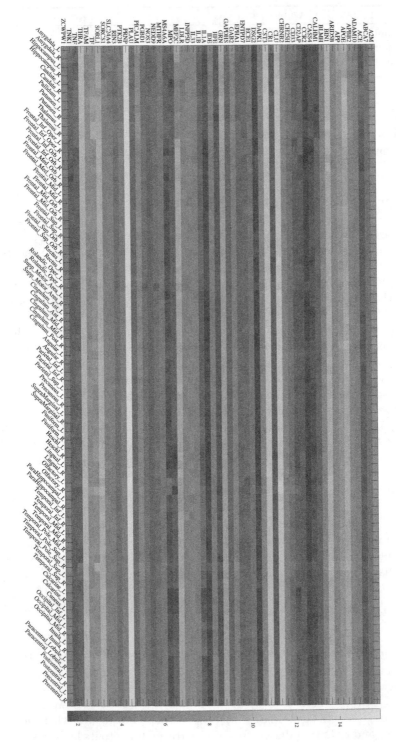

Fig. 1. Brain transcriptome: Map of expression level of the studied genes in the brain regions of interest.

value and E has been scaled to have the same spectral norm as that of $X^{\mathrm{T}}Y$. We set $s_1 = s_2 = 0.5$, and $\lambda = 0.5$. Note that the sparsity level should not affect the relative performance of the SCCA and TG-SCCA algorithms as long as the same sparsity is used for them.

To improve the robustness to the particular choice of the tuning parameters and variable selection accuracy, we employ stability selection [5], which fits the SCCA model to a large number of (100) random subsamples, each of size $n/2$. Variable selection results across all subsamples are integrated to compute the empirical selection probability for each genetic and imaging variable.

4.2   Results

Figure 2 shows the empirical selection probability of the top 25 SNPs and top 10 QTs of the SCCA and TG-SCCA algorithms applied to the AV45 data, and the map of expression profile of the identified genes in the identified brain regions. Six genes (*CLU, CST3, MEF2C, PRNP, SORL1* and *THRA*) are detected by TG-SCCA but not by SCCA. For most of these genes, evidence has been reported

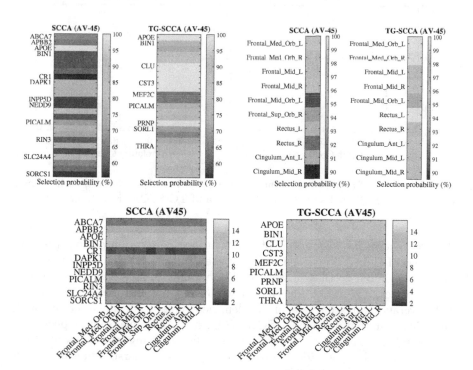

Fig. 2. Comparison of feature selection results between SCCA and TG-SCCA: (a) Selection probability map of top 25 identified SNPs, labelled with their corresponding genes. Each SNP belongs to the nearest gene above it on the heatmap. (b) Selection probability map of top 10 identified imaging biomarkers. (c) Expression level of the identified genes in the identified ROIs.

in the literature on their association with AV-45 measures. For example, *CST3* risk haplotype may account for greater amyloid load or neuronal death and affect resting cortical rhythmicity [1], and the association of *SORL1* gene with hippocampal and cerebral atrophy was reported in [4].

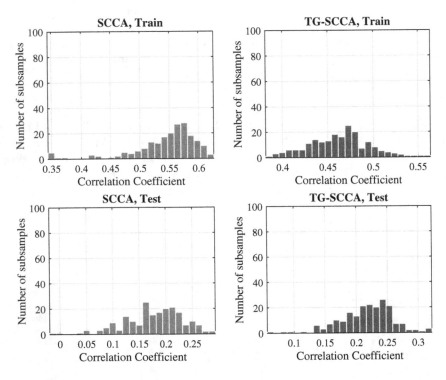

Fig. 3. Histograms of correlation coefficients from analysis of AV45 data, with training (left) and test (right) results of the SCCA (left) and TG-SCCA (right) being shown.

Figure 3 shows the histograms of bootstrapped correlation coefficients from the analysis of the AV45 data, indicating the correlation strength detected by TG-SCCA is similar to that by SCCA. While maintaining a similar correlation discovery power, TG-SCCA identifies a set of imaging and genetic markers so that the average expression level of the identified genes in the identified regions is much higher than that obtained in SCCA (Fig. 2(c)). This meets our expectation. Given these high expression profiles, the identified imaging genetic associations have the potential to provide improved mechanistic understanding of genetic basis of AD-related brain imaging phenotypes.

5 Conclusions

Many existing studies first identify the imaging genetic associations and then go to Allen Human Brain Atlas (AHBA) to look for additional evidence (i.e., the identified gene is expressed in the relevant region). In this work, we have coupled these two steps together and propose a transcriptome-guided sparse canonical correlation analysis (TG-SCCA) framework that directly identifies strong imaging genetic associations with transcriptomic support evidenced in AHBA. To solve the formulated problem, we have developed an efficient algorithm which finds a closed-form global solution for each of the two subproblems. Our study on real imaging genetics data in an AD study has demonstrated that TG-SCCA yields promising and biologically meaningful findings.

References

1. Braskie, M.N., Ringman, J.M., Thompson, P.M.: Neuroimaging measures as endophenotypes in Alzheimer's disease. Int. J. Alzheimer's Dis. **2011**, 1–15 (2011). 490140
2. Chen, J., Bushman, F.D., Lewis, J.D., Wu, G.D., Li, H.: Structure-constrained sparse canonical correlation analysis with an application to microbiome data analysis. Biostatistics **14**(2), 244–258 (2013)
3. Chen, X., Liu, H., Carbonell, J.G.: Structured sparse canonical correlation analysis. In: International Conference on Artificial Intelligence and Statistics, La Palma, Canary Islands, vol. 12, pp. 199–207 (2012)
4. Louwersheimer, E., Ramirez, A., Cruchaga, C., Becker, T., Kornhuber, J., Peters, O., Heilmann, S., Wiltfang, J., Jessen, F., Visser, P.J., Scheltens, P., Pijnenburg, Y.A.L., Teunissen, C.E., Barkhof, F., van Swieten, J.C., Holstege, H., Van der Flier, W.M., Alzheimer's Disease Neuroimaging Initiative and Dementia Competence Network: Influence of genetic variants in SORL1 gene on the manifestation of Alzheimer's disease. Neurobiol. Aging, **36**, 1605.e3–1605.e20 (2015)
5. Meinshausen, N., Bühlmann, P.: Stability selection. J. R. Stat. Soc. Ser. B (Stat. Methodol.) **72**(4), 417–473 (2010)
6. Parkhomenko, E., Tritchler, D., Beyene, J.: Sparse canonical correlation analysis with application to genomic data integration. Stat. Appl. Genet. Mol. Biol. **8**, 1–34 (2009)
7. Witten, D.M., Tibshirani, R., Hastie, T.: A penalized matrix decomposition, with applications to sparse principal components and canonical correlation analysis. Biostatistics **10**(3), 515–34 (2009)
8. Witten, D.M., Tibshirani, R.J.: Extensions of sparse canonical correlation analysis with applications to genomic data. Stat. Appl. Genet. Mol. Biol. **8**(1), 1–27 (2009)
9. Yan, J., Du, L., Kim, S., Risacher, S.L., Huang, H., Moore, J.H., Saykin, A.J., Shen, L.: Transcriptome-guided amyloid imaging genetic analysis via a novel structured sparse learning algorithm. Bioinformatics **30**(17), i564–i571 (2014)

Multilevel Modeling with Structured Penalties for Classification from Imaging Genetics Data

Pascal Lu[1,2](✉), Olivier Colliot[1,2], and
the Alzheimer's Disease Neuroimaging Initiative

[1] Sorbonne Universités, UPMC Université Paris 06, Inserm,
CNRS, Institut du Cerveau et la Moelle (ICM), AP-HP - Hôpital Pitié-Salpêtrière,
Boulevard de l'hôpital, 75013 Paris, France
pascal.lu@inria.fr
[2] INRIA Paris, ARAMIS Project-Team, 75013 Paris, France
olivier.colliot@upmc.fr

Abstract. In this paper, we propose a framework for automatic classification of patients from multimodal genetic and brain imaging data by optimally combining them. Additive models with unadapted penalties (such as the classical group lasso penalty or ℓ_1-multiple kernel learning) treat all modalities in the same manner and can result in undesirable elimination of specific modalities when their contributions are unbalanced. To overcome this limitation, we introduce a multilevel model that combines imaging and genetics and that considers joint effects between these two modalities for diagnosis prediction. Furthermore, we propose a framework allowing to combine several penalties taking into account the structure of the different types of data, such as a group lasso penalty over the genetic modality and a ℓ_2-penalty on imaging modalities. Finally, we propose a fast optimization algorithm, based on a proximal gradient method. The model has been evaluated on genetic (single nucleotide polymorphisms - SNP) and imaging (anatomical MRI measures) data from the ADNI database, and compared to additive models [13,15]. It exhibits good performances in AD diagnosis; and at the same time, reveals relationships between genes, brain regions and the disease status.

1 Introduction

The research area of imaging genetics studies the association between genetic and brain imaging data [8]. A large number of papers studied the relationship between genetic and neuroimaging data by considering that a phenotype can be explained by a sum of effects from genetic variants. These multivariate approaches use partial least squares [16], sparse canonical correlation analysis [17], sparse regularized linear regression with a ℓ_1-penalty [10], group lasso penalty [11,12], or Bayesian model that links genetic variants to imaging regions and imaging regions to the disease status [9].

But another interesting problem is about combining genetic and neuroimaging data for automatic classification of patients. In particular, machine learning

M.J. Cardoso et al. (Eds.): GRAIL/MFCA/MICGen 2017, LNCS 10551, pp. 230–240, 2017.
DOI: 10.1007/978-3-319-67675-3_21

methods have been used to build predictors for heterogeneous data, coming from different modalities for brain disease diagnosis, such as Alzheimer's disease (AD) diagnosis. However, challenging issues are high-dimensional data, small number of observations, the heterogeneous nature of data, and the weight for each modality.

A framework that is commonly used to combine heterogeneous data is multiple kernel learning (MKL) [6]. In MKL, each modality is represented by a kernel (usually a linear kernel). The decision function and weights for the kernel are simultaneously learnt. Moreover, the group lasso [2,3] is a way to integrate structure inside data. However, the standard ℓ_1-MKL and group lasso may eliminate modalities that have a weak contribution. In particular, for AD, imaging data already provides good results for its diagnosis. To overcome this problem, different papers have proposed to use a $\ell_{1,p}$-penalty [7] to combine optimally different modalities [13,14].

These approaches do not consider potential effects between genetic and imaging data for diagnosis prediction, as they only capture brain regions and SNPs separately taken. Moreover, they put on the same level genetic and imaging data, although these data do not provide the same type of information: given only APOE genotyping, subjects can be classified according to their risk to develop AD in the future; on the contrary, imaging data provides a photography of the subject's state at the present time.

Thereby, we propose a new framework that makes hierarchical the parameters and considers interactions between genetic and imaging data for AD diagnosis. We started with the idea that learning AD diagnosis from imaging data already provides good results. Then, we considered that the decision function parameters learnt from imaging data could be modulated, depending on each subject's genetic data. In other words, genes would express themselves through these parameters. Considering a linear regression that links these parameters and the genetic data, it leads to a multilevel model between imaging and genetics. Our method also proposes potential relations between genetic and imaging variables, if both of them are simultaneously related to AD. This approach is different from the modeling proposed by [9], where imaging variables are predicted from genetic variables, and diagnosis is predicted from imaging variables.

Furthermore, current approaches [13–15] do not exploit data structure inside each modality, as it is logical to group SNPs by genes, to expect sparsity between genes (all genes are not linked to AD) and to enforce a smooth regularization over brain regions for imaging modality. Thus, we have imposed specific penalties for each modality by using a ℓ_2-penalty on the imaging modality, and a group lasso penalty over the genetic modality. It models the mapping of variants into genes, providing a better understanding of the role of genes in AD.

To learn all the decision function parameters, a fast optimization algorithm, based on a proximal gradient method, has been developed. Finally, we have evaluated our model on 1,107 genetic (SNP) and 114 imaging (anatomical MRI measures) variables from the ADNI database[1] and compared it to additive models [13,15].

---

[1] http://adni.loni.usc.edu.

2 Model Set-up

2.1 Multilevel Logistic Regression with Structured Penalties

Let $\{(\mathbf{x}_\mathcal{G}^k, \mathbf{x}_\mathcal{I}^k, y^k), k = 1, \ldots, N\}$ be a set of labeled data, with $\mathbf{x}_\mathcal{G}^k \in \mathbb{R}^{|\mathcal{G}|}$ (genetic data), and $\mathbf{x}_\mathcal{I}^k \in \mathbb{R}^{|\mathcal{I}|}$ (imaging data) and $y^k \in \{0, 1\}$ (diagnosis). Genetic, imaging and genetic-imaging cross products training data are assumed centered and normalized.

We propose the following Multilevel Logistic Regression model:

$$p(y = 1 | \mathbf{x}_\mathcal{G}, \mathbf{x}_\mathcal{I}) = \sigma\left(\boldsymbol{\alpha}(\mathbf{x}_\mathcal{G})^\top \mathbf{x}_\mathcal{I} + \alpha_0(\mathbf{x}_\mathcal{G})\right) \quad \text{with } \sigma : x \mapsto \frac{1}{1 + e^{-x}}$$

where $\alpha_0(\mathbf{x}_\mathcal{G})$ is the intercept and $\boldsymbol{\alpha}(\mathbf{x}_\mathcal{G}) \in \mathbb{R}^{|\mathcal{I}|}$ is the parameter vector. On the contrary of the classical logistic regression model, we propose a multilevel model, for which the parameter vector $\boldsymbol{\alpha}(\mathbf{x}_\mathcal{G})$ and the intercept $\alpha_0(\mathbf{x}_\mathcal{G})$ depend on genetic data $\mathbf{x}_\mathcal{G}$.

This is to be compared to an additive model, where the diagnosis is directly deduced from genetic and imaging data put at the same level. We assume that $\boldsymbol{\alpha}$ and α_0 are affine functions of genetic data $\mathbf{x}_\mathcal{G}$:

$$\boldsymbol{\alpha}(\mathbf{x}_\mathcal{G}) = \mathbf{W}\mathbf{x}_\mathcal{G} + \boldsymbol{\beta}_\mathcal{I} \quad \text{and} \quad \alpha_0(\mathbf{x}_\mathcal{G}) = \boldsymbol{\beta}_\mathcal{G}^\top \mathbf{x}_\mathcal{G} + \beta_0$$

where $\mathbf{W} \in \mathcal{M}_{|\mathcal{I}|, |\mathcal{G}|}(\mathbb{R})$, $\boldsymbol{\beta}_\mathcal{I} \in \mathbb{R}^{|\mathcal{I}|}$, $\boldsymbol{\beta}_\mathcal{G} \in \mathbb{R}^{|\mathcal{G}|}$ and $\beta_0 \in \mathbb{R}$. Therefore, the probability becomes $p(y = 1 | \mathbf{x}_\mathcal{G}, \mathbf{x}_\mathcal{I}) = \sigma\left(\mathbf{x}_\mathcal{G}^\top \mathbf{W}^\top \mathbf{x}_\mathcal{I} + \boldsymbol{\beta}_\mathcal{I}^\top \mathbf{x}_\mathcal{I} + \boldsymbol{\beta}_\mathcal{G}^\top \mathbf{x}_\mathcal{G} + \beta_0\right)$. Figure 1 summarizes the relations between parameters.

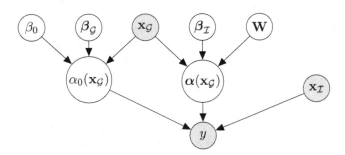

Fig. 1. The disease status y is predicted from imaging data $\mathbf{x}_\mathcal{I}$ and the parameters $\beta_0(\mathbf{x}_\mathcal{G}), \boldsymbol{\beta}(\mathbf{x}_\mathcal{G})$ (which are computed from genetic data $\mathbf{x}_\mathcal{G}$)

The parameters $\mathbf{W}, \boldsymbol{\beta}_\mathcal{I}, \boldsymbol{\beta}_\mathcal{G}, \beta_0$ are obtained by minimizing the objective:

$$S(\mathbf{W}, \boldsymbol{\beta}_\mathcal{I}, \boldsymbol{\beta}_\mathcal{G}, \beta_0) = R_N(\mathbf{W}, \boldsymbol{\beta}_\mathcal{I}, \boldsymbol{\beta}_\mathcal{G}, \beta_0) + \Omega(\mathbf{W}, \boldsymbol{\beta}_\mathcal{I}, \boldsymbol{\beta}_\mathcal{G})$$

with $R_N(\mathbf{W}, \boldsymbol{\beta}_\mathcal{I}, \boldsymbol{\beta}_\mathcal{G}, \beta_0) = \dfrac{1}{N} \sum_{k=1}^{N} \Big\{ -y^k \left((\mathbf{x}_\mathcal{G}^k)^\top \mathbf{W}^\top \mathbf{x}_\mathcal{I}^k + \boldsymbol{\beta}_\mathcal{I}^\top \mathbf{x}_\mathcal{I}^k + \boldsymbol{\beta}_\mathcal{G}^\top \mathbf{x}_\mathcal{G}^k + \beta_0\right)$

$$+ \log\left(1 + e^{(\mathbf{x}_\mathcal{G}^k)^\top \mathbf{W}^\top \mathbf{x}_\mathcal{I}^k + \boldsymbol{\beta}_\mathcal{I}^\top \mathbf{x}_\mathcal{I}^k + \boldsymbol{\beta}_\mathcal{G}^\top \mathbf{x}_\mathcal{G}^k + \beta_0}\right)\Big\}$$

and $\quad \Omega(\mathbf{W}, \boldsymbol{\beta}_\mathcal{I}, \boldsymbol{\beta}_\mathcal{G}) = \lambda_W \Omega_W(\mathbf{W}) + \lambda_\mathcal{I} \Omega_\mathcal{I}(\boldsymbol{\beta}_\mathcal{I}) + \lambda_\mathcal{G} \Omega_\mathcal{G}(\boldsymbol{\beta}_\mathcal{G})$

Ω_W, $\Omega_\mathcal{I}$, $\Omega_\mathcal{G}$ are respectively the penalties for $\mathbf{W}$, $\boldsymbol{\beta}_\mathcal{I}$, $\boldsymbol{\beta}_\mathcal{G}$, whereas $\lambda_W > 0$, $\lambda_\mathcal{I} > 0$, $\lambda_\mathcal{G} > 0$ are respectively the regularization parameters for Ω_W, $\Omega_\mathcal{I}$, $\Omega_\mathcal{G}$.

Genetic data are a sequence of single-polymorphism nucleotides (SNP) counted by minor allele. A SNP can belong (or not) to one gene ℓ (or more) and therefore participate in the production of proteins that interact inside pathways. We decided to group SNPs by genes, and designed a penalty to enforce sparsity between genes and regularity inside genes. Given that some SNPs may belong to multiple genes, the group lasso with overlap penalty [4] is more suitable, with genes as groups. To deal with this penalty, an overlap expansion is performed. Given $\mathbf{x} \in \mathbb{R}^{|\mathcal{G}|}$ a subject's feature vector, a new feature vector is created $\widetilde{\mathbf{x}} = \left(\mathbf{x}_{\mathcal{G}_1}^\top, \ldots, \mathbf{x}_{\mathcal{G}_L}^\top\right)^\top \in \mathbb{R}^{\sum_{\ell=1}^L |\mathcal{G}_\ell|}$, defined by the concatenation of copies of the genetic data restricted by group $\mathcal{G}_\ell$. Similarly, the same expansion is performed on $\boldsymbol{\beta}_\mathcal{G}, \mathbf{W}$ to obtain $\widetilde{\boldsymbol{\beta}}_\mathcal{G} \in \mathbb{R}^{\sum_{\ell=1}^L |\mathcal{G}_\ell|}$ and $\widetilde{\mathbf{W}} \in \mathbb{R}^{|\mathcal{I}| \times (\sum_{\ell=1}^L |\mathcal{G}_\ell|)}$. This group lasso with overlap penalty is used for the matrix $\mathbf{W}$ and for $\boldsymbol{\beta}_\mathcal{G}$.

For imaging variables, the ridge penalty is considered: $\Omega_\mathcal{I}(\boldsymbol{\beta}_\mathcal{I}) = \|\boldsymbol{\beta}_\mathcal{I}\|_2^2$. In particular, brain diseases usually have a diffuse anatomical pattern of alteration throughout the brain and therefore, regularity is usually required for the imaging parameter. Finally, Ω is defined by:

$$\Omega\left(\widetilde{\mathbf{W}}, \widetilde{\boldsymbol{\beta}}_\mathcal{G}, \boldsymbol{\beta}_\mathcal{I}\right) = \lambda_W \sum_{i=1}^{|\mathcal{I}|} \sum_{\ell=1}^{L} \theta_{\mathcal{G}_\ell} \left\|\widetilde{\mathbf{W}}_{i,\mathcal{G}_\ell}\right\|_2 + \lambda_\mathcal{I} \left\|\widetilde{\boldsymbol{\beta}}_\mathcal{I}\right\|_2 + \lambda_\mathcal{G} \sum_{\ell=1}^{L} \theta_{\mathcal{G}_\ell} \left\|\widetilde{\boldsymbol{\beta}}_{\mathcal{G}_\ell}\right\|_2$$

2.2 Minimization of $S(\mathbf{W}\boldsymbol{\beta}_\mathcal{I}, \boldsymbol{\beta}_\mathcal{I}, \beta_0)$

From now on, and for simplicity reasons, $\widetilde{\mathbf{W}}$, $\widetilde{\boldsymbol{\beta}}$ and $\widetilde{\mathbf{x}}$ are respectively denoted as $\mathbf{W}$, $\boldsymbol{\beta}$ and $\mathbf{x}$. Let Φ be the function that reshapes a matrix of $\mathcal{M}_{|\mathcal{I}|,|\mathcal{G}|}(\mathbb{R})$ to a vector of $\mathbb{R}^{|\mathcal{I}| \times |\mathcal{G}|}$ (i.e. $\mathbf{W}_{i,g} = \Phi(\mathbf{W})_{i|\mathcal{G}|+g}$):

$$\Phi : \mathbf{W} \mapsto \left((\mathbf{W}_{1,1}, \ldots, \mathbf{W}_{1,|\mathcal{G}|}), \ldots, (\mathbf{W}_{|\mathcal{I}|,1}, \ldots, \mathbf{W}_{|\mathcal{I}|,|\mathcal{G}|})\right)$$

We will estimate $\Phi(\mathbf{W})$ and then reshape it to obtain $\mathbf{W}$. The algorithm developed is based on a proximal gradient method [1,5].

The parameters $\mathbf{w}^{(t+1)} = \left(\Phi\left(\mathbf{W}^{(t+1)}\right), \beta_\mathcal{I}^{(t+1)}, \beta_\mathcal{G}^{(t+1)}, \beta_0^{(t+1)}\right)$ are updated with:

$$\mathbf{w}^{(t+1)} = \underset{\mathbf{w}}{\arg\min}\, R_N(\mathbf{w}) + \left[\mathbf{w} - \mathbf{w}^{(t)}\right]^\top \nabla R_N\left(\mathbf{w}^{(t)}\right) + \frac{1}{2\varepsilon}\left\|\mathbf{w} - \mathbf{w}^{(t)}\right\|_2^2 + \Omega(\mathbf{w})$$

$$= \underset{\mathbf{w}}{\arg\min}\left\{\frac{1}{2}\left\|\boldsymbol{\omega}^{(t)} - \mathbf{w}^{(t)}\right\|_2^2 + \varepsilon\Omega(\mathbf{w})\right\} \text{ with } \boldsymbol{\omega}^{(t)} = \mathbf{w}^{(t)} - \varepsilon\nabla R_N\left(\mathbf{w}^{(t)}\right)$$

The idea is to update $\mathbf{w}^{(t+1)}$ from $\mathbf{w}^{(t)}$ with a Newton-type algorithm without the constraint Ω given a stepsize ε, and then to project the result onto the compact set defined by Ω. Regarding the stepsize ε, a backtracking line search [5] is performed. Let $\widehat{G}\left(\mathbf{w}^{(t)}, \varepsilon\right) = \frac{1}{\varepsilon}\left[\mathbf{w}^{(t)} - \mathbf{w}^{(t+1)}\right]$ be the step in the proximal gradient update. A line search is performed over ε until the inequality is reached:

$$R_N\left(\mathbf{w}^{(t+1)}\right) \leq R_N\left(\mathbf{w}^{(t)}\right) - \varepsilon\nabla R_N\left(\mathbf{w}^{(t)}\right)^\top \widehat{G}\left(\mathbf{w}^{(t)}, \varepsilon\right) + \frac{\varepsilon}{2}\left\|\widehat{G}\left(\mathbf{w}^{(t)}, \varepsilon\right)\right\|_2^2$$

The minimization algorithm stops when $\left| S\left(\mathbf{w}^{(t+1)}\right) - S\left(\mathbf{w}^{(t)}\right)\right| \leq \eta \left| S\left(\mathbf{w}^{(t)}\right)\right|$, where $\eta = 10^{-5}$. The whole algorithm is summarized below:

Algorithm 1. Training the multilevel logistic regression

---

1 **Input:** $\{(\mathbf{x}_{\mathcal{I}}^k, \mathbf{x}_{\mathcal{G}}^k, y^k), k = 1, \ldots, N\}$, $\delta = 0.8$, $\varepsilon_0 = 1$, $\eta = 10^{-5}$;
2 **Initialization:** $\mathbf{W} = \mathbf{0}$, $\boldsymbol{\beta}_{\mathcal{I}} = \mathbf{0}$, $\boldsymbol{\beta}_{\mathcal{G}} = \mathbf{0}$, $\beta_0 = 0$ and continue = True ;
3 **while** continue **do**
4     $\varepsilon = \varepsilon_0$;
5     $R_N = R_N\left(\mathbf{W}, \boldsymbol{\beta}_{\mathcal{I}}, \boldsymbol{\beta}_{\mathcal{G}}, \beta_0\right)$;
6     $\nabla R_N = \dfrac{1}{N} \displaystyle\sum_{k=1}^{N} \begin{pmatrix} \Phi\left((\mathbf{x}_{\mathcal{I}}^k)^\top \mathbf{x}_{\mathcal{G}}^k\right) \\ \mathbf{x}_{\mathcal{I}}^k \\ \mathbf{x}_{\mathcal{G}}^k \\ 1 \end{pmatrix} \left[\sigma\left((\mathbf{x}_{\mathcal{G}}^k)^\top \mathbf{W}^\top \mathbf{x}_{\mathcal{I}}^k + \boldsymbol{\beta}_{\mathcal{I}}^\top \mathbf{x}_{\mathcal{I}}^k + \boldsymbol{\beta}_{\mathcal{G}}^\top \mathbf{x}_{\mathcal{G}}^k + \beta_0\right) - y^k \right]$
7     $\left(\widehat{\mathbf{W}}, \widehat{\boldsymbol{\beta}}_{\mathcal{I}}, \widehat{\boldsymbol{\beta}}_{\mathcal{G}}, \widehat{\beta}_0, \widehat{G}\right) = \mathbf{Algo\_2}(\mathbf{W}, \boldsymbol{\beta}_{\mathcal{I}}, \boldsymbol{\beta}_{\mathcal{G}}, \beta_0, \nabla R_N, \varepsilon)$;
8   **while** $R_N\left(\widehat{\mathbf{W}}, \widehat{\boldsymbol{\beta}}_{\mathcal{I}}, \widehat{\boldsymbol{\beta}}_{\mathcal{G}}, \widehat{\beta}_0\right) > R_N - \varepsilon \nabla R_N^\top \widehat{G} + \frac{\varepsilon}{2}\|\widehat{G}\|_2^2$ **do**
9       $\varepsilon = \delta\varepsilon$ and $\left(\widehat{\mathbf{W}}, \widehat{\boldsymbol{\beta}}_{\mathcal{I}}, \widehat{\boldsymbol{\beta}}_{\mathcal{G}}, \widehat{\beta}_0, \widehat{G}\right) = \mathbf{Algo\_2}(\mathbf{W}, \boldsymbol{\beta}_{\mathcal{I}}, \boldsymbol{\beta}_{\mathcal{G}}, \beta_0, \nabla R_N, \varepsilon)$;
10   **end**
11   continue $= \left| S\left(\widehat{\mathbf{W}}, \widehat{\boldsymbol{\beta}}_{\mathcal{I}}, \widehat{\boldsymbol{\beta}}_{\mathcal{G}}, \widehat{\beta}_0\right) - S\left(\mathbf{W}, \boldsymbol{\beta}_{\mathcal{I}}, \boldsymbol{\beta}_{\mathcal{G}}, \beta_0\right)\right| >^? \eta \left| S\left(\mathbf{W}, \boldsymbol{\beta}_{\mathcal{I}}, \boldsymbol{\beta}_{\mathcal{G}}, \beta_0\right)\right|$
12     $\mathbf{W} = \widehat{\mathbf{W}}$, $\boldsymbol{\beta}_{\mathcal{I}} = \widehat{\boldsymbol{\beta}}_{\mathcal{I}}$, $\boldsymbol{\beta}_{\mathcal{G}} = \widehat{\boldsymbol{\beta}}_{\mathcal{G}}$, $\beta_0 = \widehat{\beta}_0$;
13 **end**
14 **return** $(\mathbf{W}, \boldsymbol{\beta}_{\mathcal{I}}, \boldsymbol{\beta}_{\mathcal{G}}, \beta_0)$

Algorithm 2. Parameter update

---

1 **Input:** $(\mathbf{W}, \boldsymbol{\beta}_{\mathcal{I}}, \boldsymbol{\beta}_{\mathcal{G}}, \beta_0)$ (parameters), ∇R_N (gradient), ε (stepsize) ;
2 Compute $\boldsymbol{\omega} = \boldsymbol{\beta} - \varepsilon \nabla_{(\mathbf{w}, \boldsymbol{\beta}_{\mathcal{I}}, \boldsymbol{\beta}_{\mathcal{G}})} R_N$;

3 Update $\widehat{\mathbf{W}}_{\mathcal{G}_\ell, i} = \max\left(0, 1 - \dfrac{\varepsilon \lambda_{\mathcal{G}} \theta_{\mathcal{G}_\ell}}{\left\|\boldsymbol{\omega}_{\mathcal{G}_\ell + i|\mathcal{G}|}^{(t)}\right\|_2}\right) \boldsymbol{\omega}_{\mathcal{G}_\ell + i|\mathcal{G}|}$ for $(i, \ell) \in [\![1, |\mathcal{I}|]\!] \times [\![1, L]\!]$;

4 Update $\widehat{\boldsymbol{\beta}}_{\mathcal{I}} = \dfrac{\boldsymbol{\omega}_{\mathcal{I} + |\mathcal{G}||\mathcal{I}|}}{1 + 2\varepsilon\lambda_{\mathcal{I}}}$ (imaging modality) ;

5 Update $\widehat{\boldsymbol{\beta}}_{\mathcal{G}_\ell} = \max\left(0, 1 - \dfrac{\varepsilon \lambda_{\mathcal{G}} \theta_{\mathcal{G}_\ell}}{\left\|\boldsymbol{\omega}_{\mathcal{G}_\ell + (|\mathcal{G}|+1)|\mathcal{I}|}^{(t)}\right\|_2}\right) \boldsymbol{\omega}_{\mathcal{G}_\ell + (|\mathcal{G}|+1)|\mathcal{I}|}$ for $\ell \in [\![1, L]\!]$;

6 Update $\widehat{\beta}_0 = \beta_0 - \varepsilon \dfrac{\partial R_N}{\partial \beta_0}$ and $\widehat{G} = \dfrac{1}{\varepsilon}\left[\begin{pmatrix} \Phi(\mathbf{W}) \\ \boldsymbol{\beta}_{\mathcal{I}} \\ \boldsymbol{\beta}_{\mathcal{G}} \\ \beta_0 \end{pmatrix} - \begin{pmatrix} \Phi(\widehat{\mathbf{W}}) \\ \widehat{\boldsymbol{\beta}}_{\mathcal{I}} \\ \widehat{\boldsymbol{\beta}}_{\mathcal{G}} \\ \widehat{\beta}_0 \end{pmatrix} \right]$;

7 **return** $\left(\widehat{\mathbf{W}}, \widehat{\boldsymbol{\beta}}_{\mathcal{I}}, \widehat{\boldsymbol{\beta}}_{\mathcal{G}}, \widehat{\beta}_0, \widehat{G}\right)$

---

3   Experimental Results

3.1   Dataset

The ADNI1 GWAS dataset from ADNI studied 707 subjects, with 156 Alzheimer's Disease patients (denoted AD), 196 MCI patients at baseline who progressed to AD (denoted pMCI, as progressive MCI), 150 MCI patients who remain stable (denoted sMCI, as stable MCI) and 201 healthy control subjects (denoted CN).

In ADNI1 GWAS dataset, 620,901 SNPs have been genotyped, but we selected 1,107 SNPs based on the 44 first top genes related to AD (from Alz-Gene[2]) and on the Illumina annotation using the Genome build 36.2. Group weighting for genes is based on gene size: for group $\mathcal{G}_\ell$, the weight $\theta_{\mathcal{G}_\ell} = \sqrt{|\mathcal{G}_\ell|}$ ensures that the penalty term is of the order of the number of parameters of the group.

The parameter $\lambda_\mathcal{G}$ influences the number of groups that are selected by the model. In particular, the group $\mathcal{G}_\ell$ enters in the model during the first iteration if $\left\|\nabla_{\boldsymbol{\beta}_{\mathcal{G}_\ell}} R_N(\mathbf{0})\right\|_2 > \lambda_\mathcal{G}\theta_{\mathcal{G}_\ell}$. This inequality gives an upper bound for $\lambda_\mathcal{G}$. The same remark can be done for λ_W. Regarding MRI modality, we used the segmentation of FreeSurfer which gives the volume of subcortical regions (44 features) and the average cortical region thickness (70 features). Therefore, there are $1,107 \times 114 = 126,198$ parameters to infer for $\mathbf{W}$, 114 parameters for $\boldsymbol{\beta}_\mathcal{I}$ and 1,107 parameters for $\boldsymbol{\beta}_\mathcal{G}$.

3.2   Results

We ran our multilevel model and compared it to the logistic regression applied to one single modality with simple penalties (lasso, group lasso, ridge), to additive models ([13,15] EasyMKL with a linear kernel for each modality, and the model $p(y = 1|\mathbf{x}_\mathcal{G}, \mathbf{x}_\mathcal{I}) = \sigma\left(\boldsymbol{\beta}_\mathcal{I}^\top \mathbf{x}_\mathcal{I} + \boldsymbol{\beta}_\mathcal{G}^\top \mathbf{x}_\mathcal{G} + \beta_0\right)$ with our algorithm under the constraint $\boldsymbol{\beta}_\mathcal{G} \neq \mathbf{0}$), and to the multiplicative model with $\mathbf{W}$ only, where $p(y = 1|\mathbf{x}_\mathcal{G}, \mathbf{x}_\mathcal{I}) = \sigma\left(\mathbf{x}_\mathcal{G}^\top \mathbf{W}^\top \mathbf{x}_\mathcal{I} + \beta_0\right)$. We considered two classification tasks: "AD versus CN" and "pMCI versus CN". Four measures are used: the sensitivity (SEN), the specificity (SPE), the precision (PRE) and the balanced accuracy between the sensitivity and the specificity (BACC). A 10-fold cross validation is performed. The parameters $\lambda_W, \lambda_\mathcal{I}, \lambda_\mathcal{G}$ are optimised between $[10^{-3}, 1]$. Classification results for these tasks are shown on Table 1. It typically takes between 5 and 8 min to learn the parameters.

Regarding MRI features, the most important features (in weight) are the left/right hippocampus, the left/right Amygdala, the left/right entorhinal and the left middle temporal cortices. Regarding genetic features, the most important features in weight are SNPs that belong to gene APOE (rs429358) for both tasks "AD versus CN" and "pMCI versus CN".

Regarding the matrix $\mathbf{W}$, the couples (brain region, gene) learnt through the task "pMCI versus CN" are shown on Fig. 2. It can be seen that $\mathbf{W}$ has

---

[2] http://www.alzgene.org.

Table 1. Classification results for different modalities and methods

Modality	Method & Penalty	AD VERSUS CN (%)			
		SEN	SPE	PRE	BACC
SNPs only	logistic regression (lasso ℓ_1)	69.4	77.5	71.1	73.4
SNPs grouped by genes	logistic regression (group lasso)	69.4	77.5	71.1	73.4
MRI (cortical)	logistic regression (ridge ℓ_2)	84.4	89.5	87.1	86.9
MRI (subcortical)	logistic regression (ridge ℓ_2)	80.0	86.0	83.2	83.0
SNP + MRI (all)	[15] EasyMKL, *Aiolli et al.*	89.4	85.0	83.0	87.2
SNP + MRI (all)	[13] *Wang et al.*	89.4	88.0	85.7	88.7
SNP + MRI (all)	additive model ($\boldsymbol{\beta}_{\mathcal{I}}, \boldsymbol{\beta}_{\mathcal{G}}$ only)	88.8	89.5	87.6	89.1
SNP + MRI (all)	multiplicative model ($\mathbf{W}$ only)	89.4	87.0	85.0	88.2
SNP + MRI (all)	multilevel model (all)	90.6	87.0	85.5	88.8

Modality	Method & Penalty	pMCI VERSUS CN (%)			
		SEN	SPE	PRE	BACC
SNPs only	logistic regression (lasso ℓ_1)	72.0	77.0	75.9	74.5
SNPs grouped by genes	logistic regression (group lasso)	72.0	77.0	75.9	74.5
MRI (cortical)	logistic regression (ridge ℓ_2)	74.0	76.0	76.4	75.0
MRI (subcortical)	logistic regression (ridge ℓ_2)	73.0	76.5	76.6	74.7
SNP + MRI (all)	[15] EasyMKL, *Aiolli et al.*	77.0	73.5	75.1	75.3
SNP + MRI (all)	[13] *Wang et al.*	79.5	81.5	82.4	80.5
SNP + MRI (all)	additive model ($\boldsymbol{\beta}_{\mathcal{I}}, \boldsymbol{\beta}_{\mathcal{G}}$ only)	80.5	81.0	82.0	80.8
SNP + MRI (all)	multiplicative model ($\mathbf{W}$ only)	81.0	81.5	82.9	81.3
SNP + MRI (all)	multilevel model (all)	82.5	83.0	84.1	82.8

a sparse structure. Among the couples (brain region, gene) that have non null coefficients for the both tasks "AD versus CN" and "pMCI versus CN", there are (Left Hippocampus, MGMT), (Right Entorhinal, APOE) or (Left Middle Temporal, APOE). Only couples related to AD are selected by the model.

We noticed that genes and brain regions strongly related to AD are captured by the vectors $\boldsymbol{\beta}_{\mathcal{G}}$ and $\boldsymbol{\beta}_{\mathcal{I}}$, whereas genes less strongly related to AD are captured by the matrix $\mathbf{W}$. Coming back to original formulation described in Sect. 2.1, the contribution of the function $\alpha_0 : \mathbf{x}_{\mathcal{G}} \mapsto \boldsymbol{\beta}_{\mathcal{G}}^{\top} \mathbf{x}_{\mathcal{G}} + \beta_0$ is much smaller (in terms of weights) than the function $\boldsymbol{\alpha} : \mathbf{x}_{\mathcal{G}} \mapsto \mathbf{W} \mathbf{x}_{\mathcal{G}} + \boldsymbol{\beta}_{\mathcal{I}}$. Furthermore, Fig. 2 shows that genetic data $\mathbf{x}_{\mathcal{G}}$ tend to express through $\mathbf{W}$, and thereby participate in the modulation of the vector $\boldsymbol{\alpha}(\mathbf{x}_{\mathcal{G}})$.

We compared our approach to [13,15], for which the codes are available. The features that are selected by [13,15] are similar to ours for each modality taken separately. For instance, for [13] and the task "AD versus CN", SNPs that have the most important weights are in genes APOE (rs429358), BZW1 (rs3815501) and MGMT (rs7071424). However, the genetic parameter vector learnt from [13] or [15] is not sparse, in contrary of ours. Furthermore, for [15], the weight for the imaging kernel is nine times much larger than the weight for the genetic kernel. These experiments show that the additive model with adapted penalties for each modality provides better performances than [15], but our additive, multiplicative and multilevel models provide similar performances.

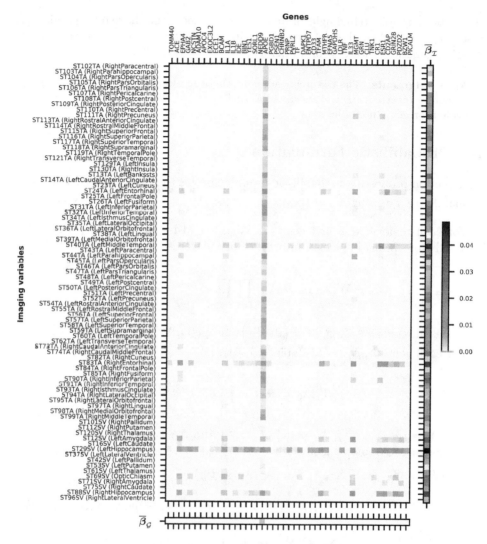

Fig. 2. Overview of the reduced parameters $\overline{\mathbf{W}} \in \mathbb{R}^{|\mathcal{I}| \times L}$, $\overline{\boldsymbol{\beta}}_{\mathcal{I}} \in \mathbb{R}^{|\mathcal{I}|}$ and $\overline{\boldsymbol{\beta}}_{\mathcal{G}} \in \mathbb{R}^L$ (learnt through the task "pMCI vs CN" for the whole model). For brain region i and gene ℓ, $\overline{\mathbf{W}}[i, \ell] = \max_{g \in \mathcal{G}_\ell} |\mathbf{W}[i, g]|$, $\overline{\boldsymbol{\beta}}_{\mathcal{I}}[i] = |\boldsymbol{\beta}_{\mathcal{I}}[i]|$ and $\overline{\boldsymbol{\beta}}_{\mathcal{G}}[\ell] = \max_{g \in \mathcal{G}_\ell} |\boldsymbol{\beta}_{\mathcal{G}}[g]|$. Only some brain regions are shown in this figure.

4   Conclusion

In this paper, we developed a novel approach to integrate genetic and brain imaging data for prediction of disease status. Our multilevel model takes into account potential interactions between genes and brain regions, but also the structure of the different types of data though the use of specific penalties within each modality. When applied to genetic and MRI data from the ADNI database, the model was able to highlight brain regions and genes that have been previously associated with AD, thereby demonstrating the potential of our approach for imaging genetics studies in brain diseases.

Acknowledgments. The research leading to these results has received funding from the program *Investissements d'avenir ANR-10-IAIHU-06*. We wish to thank Theodoros Evgeniou for many useful insights.

A   Probabilistic Formulation

This section proposes a probabilistic formulation for the model. The conditional probability is given by $p(y = 1|\mathbf{x}_\mathcal{G}, \mathbf{x}_\mathcal{I}) = \sigma\left(\mathbf{x}_\mathcal{G}^\top \mathbf{W}^\top \mathbf{x}_\mathcal{I} + \boldsymbol{\beta}_\mathcal{I}^\top \mathbf{x}_\mathcal{I} + \boldsymbol{\beta}_\mathcal{G}^\top \mathbf{x}_\mathcal{G} + \beta_0\right)$.

- For each region $i \in \mathcal{I}$ and gene $\mathcal{G}_\ell$, $\mathbf{W}_{i,\mathcal{G}_\ell} \sim$ M-Laplace$(0, \lambda_W)$ (M-Laplace stands for "Multi-Laplacian prior"). In other words:

$$p(\mathbf{W}; \lambda_W, \mathcal{G}, \boldsymbol{\theta}_\mathcal{G}) \propto \prod_{i=1}^{|\mathcal{I}|} \prod_{\ell=1}^{L} e^{-\lambda_W \theta_{\mathcal{G}_\ell} \|\mathbf{W}_{i,\mathcal{G}_\ell}\|_2}$$

- For each region $i \in \mathcal{I}$, $\boldsymbol{\beta}_i \sim \mathcal{N}\left(0, \frac{1}{2\lambda_\mathcal{I}}\right)$, i.e. $p(\boldsymbol{\beta}_\mathcal{I}; \lambda_\mathcal{I}) \propto e^{-\lambda_\mathcal{I} \|\boldsymbol{\beta}_\mathcal{I}\|_2^2}$
- For each gene $\mathcal{G}_\ell$, $\boldsymbol{\beta}_{\mathcal{G}_\ell} \sim$ M-Laplace$(0, \lambda_\mathcal{G})$, i.e.

$$p(\boldsymbol{\beta}_\mathcal{G}; \lambda_\mathcal{G}, \mathcal{G}, \boldsymbol{\theta}_\mathcal{G}) \propto \prod_{\ell=1}^{L} e^{-\lambda_\mathcal{G} \theta_{\mathcal{G}_\ell} \|\boldsymbol{\beta}_{\mathcal{G}_\ell}\|_2}$$

Let $Y = (y^1, \ldots, y^N)$, $X_\mathcal{I} = (\mathbf{x}_\mathcal{I}^1, \ldots, \mathbf{x}_\mathcal{I}^N)$ and $X_\mathcal{G} = (\mathbf{x}_\mathcal{G}^1, \ldots, \mathbf{x}_\mathcal{G}^N)$.
The generative model is given by:

$$p(\mathbf{W}, \boldsymbol{\beta}_\mathcal{I}, \boldsymbol{\beta}_\mathcal{G}, \beta_0, Y, X_\mathcal{I}, X_\mathcal{G}; \lambda_W, \lambda_\mathcal{I}, \lambda_\mathcal{G}, \mathcal{G}, \boldsymbol{\theta}_\mathcal{G})$$

$$\overset{\text{Bayes}}{=} p(Y, X_\mathcal{I}, X_\mathcal{G}|\mathbf{W}, \boldsymbol{\beta}_\mathcal{I}, \boldsymbol{\beta}_\mathcal{G}) p(\mathbf{W}; \lambda_W, \mathcal{G}, \boldsymbol{\theta}_\mathcal{G}) p(\boldsymbol{\beta}_\mathcal{I}; \lambda_\mathcal{I}) p(\boldsymbol{\beta}_\mathcal{G}; \lambda_\mathcal{G}, \mathcal{G}, \boldsymbol{\theta}_\mathcal{G}) p(\beta_0)$$

$$\overset{\text{obs iid}}{=} \left(\prod_{k=1}^{N} p(y = y^k, \mathbf{x}_\mathcal{I}^k, \mathbf{x}_\mathcal{G}^k | \mathbf{W}, \boldsymbol{\beta}_\mathcal{I}, \boldsymbol{\beta}_\mathcal{G}) \right)$$

$$p(\mathbf{W}; \lambda_W, \mathcal{G}, \boldsymbol{\theta}_\mathcal{G}) p(\boldsymbol{\beta}_\mathcal{I}; \lambda_\mathcal{I}) p(\boldsymbol{\beta}_\mathcal{G}; \lambda_\mathcal{G}, \mathcal{G}, \boldsymbol{\theta}_\mathcal{G}) p(\beta_0)$$

$$\propto \prod_{k=1}^{N} \sigma\left((\mathbf{x}_\mathcal{G}^k)^\top \mathbf{W}^\top \mathbf{x}_\mathcal{I}^k + \boldsymbol{\beta}_\mathcal{I}^\top \mathbf{x}_\mathcal{I}^k + \boldsymbol{\beta}_\mathcal{G}^\top \mathbf{x}_\mathcal{G}^k + \beta_0 \right)^{y^k}$$

$$\prod_{k=1}^{N} \left[1 - \sigma\left((\mathbf{x}_\mathcal{G}^k)^\top \mathbf{W}^\top \mathbf{x}_\mathcal{I}^k + \boldsymbol{\beta}_\mathcal{I}^\top \mathbf{x}_\mathcal{I}^k + \boldsymbol{\beta}_\mathcal{G}^\top \mathbf{x}_\mathcal{G}^k + \beta_0 \right) \right]^{1-y^k}$$

$$\left(\prod_{i=1}^{|\mathcal{I}|} \prod_{\ell=1}^{L} e^{-\lambda_W \theta_{\mathcal{G}_\ell} \|\mathbf{W}_{i,\mathcal{G}_\ell}\|_2} \right) \times e^{-\lambda_\mathcal{I} \|\boldsymbol{\beta}_\mathcal{I}\|_2^2} \times \left(\prod_{\ell=1}^{L} e^{-\lambda_\mathcal{G} \theta_{\mathcal{G}_\ell} \|\boldsymbol{\beta}_{\mathcal{G}_\ell}\|_2} \right)$$

The *maximum a posteriori* estimation is given by:

$$(\widehat{\mathbf{W}}, \hat{\boldsymbol{\beta}}_{\mathcal{I}}, \hat{\boldsymbol{\beta}}_{\mathcal{G}}, \hat{\beta}_0) \in \underset{\mathbf{W}, \boldsymbol{\beta}_{\mathcal{I}}, \boldsymbol{\beta}_{\mathcal{G}}, \beta_0}{\mathrm{argmax}} \ p(\mathbf{W}, \boldsymbol{\beta}_{\mathcal{I}}, \boldsymbol{\beta}_{\mathcal{G}}, \beta_0 | Y, X_{\mathcal{I}}, X_{\mathcal{G}}; \lambda_W, \lambda_{\mathcal{I}}, \lambda_{\mathcal{G}}, \mathcal{G}, \boldsymbol{\theta}_{\mathcal{G}})$$

$$\in \underset{\mathbf{W}, \boldsymbol{\beta}_{\mathcal{I}}, \boldsymbol{\beta}_{\mathcal{G}}, \beta_0}{\mathrm{argmax}} \ p(\mathbf{W}, \boldsymbol{\beta}_{\mathcal{I}}, \boldsymbol{\beta}_{\mathcal{G}}, \beta_0, Y, X_{\mathcal{I}}, X_{\mathcal{G}}; \lambda_W, \lambda_{\mathcal{I}}, \lambda_{\mathcal{G}}, \mathcal{G}, \boldsymbol{\theta}_{\mathcal{G}})$$

It is equivalent to minimize the function S defined by:

$$S(\mathbf{W}, \boldsymbol{\beta}_{\mathcal{I}}, \boldsymbol{\beta}_{\mathcal{G}}, \beta_0) = -\log p(Y, \mathbf{W}, \boldsymbol{\beta}_{\mathcal{I}}, \boldsymbol{\beta}_{\mathcal{G}}, \beta_0, X_{\mathcal{I}}, X_{\mathcal{G}}; \lambda_W, \lambda_{\mathcal{I}}, \lambda_{\mathcal{G}}, \mathcal{G}, \boldsymbol{\theta}_{\mathcal{G}})$$
$$= R_N(\mathbf{W}, \boldsymbol{\beta}_{\mathcal{I}}, \boldsymbol{\beta}_{\mathcal{G}}, \beta_0) + \Omega(\mathbf{W}, \boldsymbol{\beta}_{\mathcal{I}}, \boldsymbol{\beta}_{\mathcal{G}})$$

References

1. Hastie, T., Tibshirani, R., Wainwright, M.: Statistical Learning with Sparsity - The Lasso and Generalizations, vol. 143. CRC Press, Boca Rato (2015)
2. Ming, Y., Yi, L.: Model selection and estimation in regression with grouped variables. J. R. Statist. Soc. B, part 1 **68**, 49–67 (2006)
3. Meier, L., van de Geer, S., Bühlmann, P.: The group lasso for logistic regression. J. R. Statist. Soc. B **70**, 53–71 (2008)
4. Jacob, L., Obozinski, G., Vert. J.-P.: Group lasso with overlap and graph lasso. In: Proceedings of the 26th International Conference on Machine Learning (2009)
5. Beck, A., Teboulle, M.: Gradient-based algorithms with applications to signal recovery problems. In: Palomar, D.P., Eldar, Y.C. (eds.) Convex Optimization in Signal Processing and Communications, pp. 42–88. Cambribge University Press, Cambridge (2010)
6. Gönen, M., Alpaydin, E.: Multiple kernel learning algorithms. J. Mach. Learn. Res. **12**, 2211–2268 (2011)
7. Kloft, M., Brefeld, U., Sonnenburg, S., Zien, A.: ℓ_p-norm multiple kernel learning. J. Mach. Learn. Res. **12**, 953–997 (2011)
8. Liu, J., Calhoun, V.D.: A review of multivariate analyses in imaging genetics. Front. Neuroinform. **8**(29), 1–11 (2014)
9. Batmanghelich, N.K., Dalca, A., Quon, G., Sabuncu, M., Golland, P.: Probabilistic modeling of imaging, genetics and diagnosis. IEEE TMI **35**, 1765–1779 (2016)
10. Kohannim, O., et al.: Discovery and replication of gene influences on brain structure using LASSO regression. Front. Neurosci. **6**(115) (2012)
11. Silver, M., et al.: Fast identification of biological pathways associated with a quantitative trait using group lasso with overlaps. Stat. Appl. Genet. Mol. Biol. **11**(1), 1–40 (2012)
12. Silver, M., Janousova, E., Hua, X., Thompson, P.M., Montana, G., and ADNI: Identification of gene pathways implicated in alzheimer's disease using longitudinal imaging phenotypes with sparse regression. NeuroImage **63**(3), 1681–1694 (2012)
13. Wang, H., Nie, F., Huang, H., Risacher, S.L., Saykin, A.J., Shen, L.: Identifying disease sensitive and quantitative trait-relevant biomarkers from multidimensional heterogeneous imaging genetics data via sparse multimodal multitask learning. Bioinformatics **28**(12), 127–136 (2012)
14. Peng, J., An, L., Zhu, X., Jin, Y., Shen, D.: Structured sparse kernel learning for imaging genetics based Alzheimer's Disease Diagnosis. In: Ourselin, S., Joskowicz, L., Sabuncu, M.R., Unal, G., Wells, W. (eds.) MICCAI 2016. LNCS, vol. 9901, pp. 70–78. Springer, Cham (2016). doi:10.1007/978-3-319-46723-8_9

15. Aiolli, F., Donini, M.: EasyMKL: a scalable multiple kernel learning algorithm. Neurocomputing **169**, 215–224 (2015)
16. Lorenzi, M., Gutman, B., Hibar, D., Altmann, A., Jahanshad, N., Thompson, P.M., Ourselin, S.: Partial least squares modelling for imaging-genetics in Alzheimer's Disease: plausibility and generalization In: IEEE ISBI (2016)
17. Du, L., et al.: A novel structure-aware sparse learning algorithm for brain imaging genetics. In: Golland, P., Hata, N., Barillot, C., Hornegger, J., Howe, R. (eds.) MICCAI 2014. LNCS, vol. 8675, pp. 329–336. Springer, Cham (2014). doi:10.1007/978-3-319-10443-0_42

Coupled Dimensionality-Reduction Model for Imaging Genomics

Pascal Zille$^{(\boxtimes)}$ and Yu-Ping Wang

Tulane University, New Orleans, LA, USA
pzille@tulane.edu

Abstract. Imaging genomics is essentially a multimodal research area whose focus is to analyze the influence of genetic variation on brain function and structure. Due to the high dimensionality of such data, a critical step consists of applying a feature extraction/dimensionality reduction method. Often, unimodal methods are used for each dataset separately, thus failing to properly extract subtle interactions between various modalities. In this paper, we propose a multimodal sparse representation model to jointly extract features of interest by effectively coupling genomic and neuroimaging data. More precisely, we reconstruct neuroimaging data using a sparse linear combination of dictionary atoms, while taking into account contributions from genomic data during such decomposition process. This is achieved by introducing an explicit constraint through the use of a mapping function linking genomic data with the set of subject-wise coefficients associated with the imaging dictionary atoms. The motivation of this work is to extract generative features as well as the intrinsic relationships between the two modalities. This model can be expressed as a constrained optimization problem, for which a complete algorithmic procedure is provided. The proposed method is applied to analyze the differences between two young adult populations whose verbal ability shows significant differences (low/high achievers) by relying on both imaging and genomic data.

1 Introduction

Recent technological progresses in neuroimaging techniques, such as functional magnetic resonance imaging (fMRI), now provide fine scale measures of the brain activity. On the other hand, genome-wide scans obtained with high-throughput genotyping devices allow to analyze the genome more comprehensively. These advances have motivated researchers to investigate the influence of genetic variations over brain development. Since the seminal works of Hariri [1] and Bookheimer [2], imaging genomics has become an emerging research area with an increasing number of publications. One of the main motivations behind imaging genomics is that brain imaging measures could provide reproducible features that can be studied using genetic analysis [3]. As a consequence, the concept of genome-wide association studies (GWAS), which was initially used to study phenotypic values associated with various diseases, has been extended to analyze

© Springer International Publishing AG 2017
M.J. Cardoso et al. (Eds.): GRAIL/MFCA/MICGen 2017, LNCS 10551, pp. 241–248, 2017.
DOI: 10.1007/978-3-319-67675-3_22

neuroimaging data. Stein et al. [4] introduced the concept of voxel-wise genome-wide association study (vGWAS): standard GWAS analysis steps are carried out at multiple brain locations, or even down to single voxel values. Jahanshad et al. [5] proposed to extend such type of analysis to diffusion-base MRI to study the link between genetic variants and aberrant brain connectivity. Besides vGWAS, many other multimodal methods have been designed to extract latent variables from both genetic and imaging data. Liu et al. [6] proposed Parallel Independent Component Analysis (p-ICA) to extract hidden factors/independent components from fMRI and SNP data for the study of schizophrenia. Vounou et al. [7] introduced a sparse regression technique to study genetic associations with brain regions for Alzheimer's disease. Le Floch et al. [8] combined uni-variate filtering and Partial Least Squares (PLS) to identify SNPs co-varying with various neuroimaging phenotypes. More recently, Lin [9] and Jian et al. [10] proposed extesions of canonical correlation analysis (CCA) method based on SNP and fMRI data to extract correlations between genes and brain regions, as well as the resulting differences between schizophrenic and healthy controls. From a modeling perspective within the context of imaging genomics, to our opinion, there are two important factors to take into account:

- Due to the huge amount of data at hand, as well as the number of statistical tests necessary to assess significance, most imaging genomics studies require the use of dimensionality reduction for at least one of the modalities;
- The intrinsically multimodal nature of imaging genomics makes multimodal feature extraction procedures appear more suitable than standard unimodal ones.

In this work, we propose to address these two issues and introduce a model to learn a joint basis for sparse representation of both fMRI and SNP data. Its novelty lies in the fact that an explicit mapping is introduced between the fMRI features and the SNP data, thus enforcing an explicit link between modalities. This model can be re-cast within a general version of dictionary learning [11] which explicitly enforces connection between modalities [12], called Semi-Coupled Dictionary Learning (SCDL). Although increasingly used in computer vision, to our knowledge, such approach hasn't yet been used for genomic or neuroimaging data. In the next section, we briefly review the dictionary learning problem and its extensions, and then propose our **S**emi-**C**oupled Di**c**ionar**y** **L**earning model for **I**maging **G**enomics (SCyLIG).

2   SCyLIG Model for Imaging Genomics

2.1   Dictionary Learning Methods

Let $X \in \mathbb{R}^{p \times n}$ be a data matrix made of $n \in \mathbb{N}$ samples of dimension $p \in \mathbb{N}$. The main motivation behind dictionary learning [11] is to represent X using a linear combination of a few elements called dictionary atoms. Let $D \in \mathbb{R}^{p \times k}$ denote the dictionary, where k is the dimension of the feature space: each column of

D can be seen as a feature. Let $\alpha \in \mathbb{R}^{k \times n}$ denote the associated reconstruction coefficients: the i-th data sample (i.e. i-th column of X) can be represented using coefficients from the i-th row of α and the associated dictionary atoms from D. The dictionary learning problem can be expressed as

$$\underset{D,\alpha}{\arg\min} \quad \|X - D\alpha\|_F^2 + \lambda R(\alpha)$$
$$\text{subject to} \quad \|d_i\|_2^2 \leq 1 \quad \forall i = 1,..,k \tag{1}$$

where d_i denotes the i-th column of D. A usual choice for the penalty term R is such that $R(\alpha) = \sum_{i=1}^{n} \|\alpha_i\|_1$ where $\|\cdot\|_1$ denotes the ℓ_1-norm. Interesting multimodal extensions of Eq. 1 have been proposed to learn coupled dictionaries across modalities. For the sake of simplicity, we will restrict ourself to the case of $M = 2$ modalities here. Suppose we have two data matrices $X \in \mathbb{R}^{p_x \times n}, Y \in \mathbb{R}^{p_y \times n}$. Joint dictionary learning can be expressed in the following way:

$$\underset{D_x,D_y,\alpha_x,\alpha_y}{\arg\min} \quad \sum_{m=1}^{M} \| \begin{pmatrix} X \\ Y \end{pmatrix} - \begin{pmatrix} D_x \\ D_y \end{pmatrix} \alpha \|_F^2 + \lambda R(\alpha) \tag{2}$$

which amounts to a classical dictionary learning problem in the concatenated feature space. Unfortunately, using a single coefficient matrix α is a fairly strong assumption, as it forces the coefficients for both modalities to be equal. An interesting relaxation of this assumption [12], called Semi Coupled Dictionary Learning (SCDL), has recently been proposed. The main idea is to introduce a mapping function between sparse coefficient across modalities in order to learn the dictionaries in a coupled way. The formulation of SCDL is the following:

$$\underset{D_x,D_y,\alpha_x,\alpha_y,W_y}{\arg\min} \quad \|X - D_x\alpha_x\|_F^2 + \|Y - D_y\alpha_y\|_F^2 + \gamma\|\alpha_x - W_y\alpha_y\|_F^2 + \lambda R(\alpha_x,\alpha_y) \tag{3}$$

where W_y defines a linear mapping between the coefficients in both spaces, and $\gamma \in \mathbb{R}$ is a regularization parameter controlling the weight of the coupling assumption. In this work, we propose a model from the family described by Eq. 2 and apply it to imaging genomics.

2.2 SCyLIG Formulation

Given $n \in \mathbb{N}$ subjects for which we have both fMRI and SNP data. Let $X \in \mathbb{R}^{p_x \times n}$ denote the fMRI data matrix made of p_x voxels, and $Y \in \mathbb{R}^{p_y \times n}$ denote the SNP data matrix made of p_y loci. Extracting features for the fMRI modality can be achieved by solving a standard dictionary learning problem minimizing $\|X - D_x\alpha_x\|_F^2$. The columns of D_x can be seen as 'geometrical' fMRI features, while coefficients $\alpha_x \in \mathbb{R}^{k \times n}$ express how much each dictionary atom is expressed in each subject. Variability among subjects can then be looked for within α_x. Additionally, similar to vGWAS studies, one can measure how much of this variability among α_x can be explained using genomic data. This could be achieved through a standard regression framework, i.e., minimizing an error term such as $\|\alpha_x^T - Y^T \alpha_y\|_F^2$, where $\alpha_y \in \mathbb{R}^{p_y \times d}$. Both problems can be combined using the following formulation:

$$\underset{D_x,\alpha_x,\alpha_y}{\arg\min} \quad \frac{1}{2}\|X - D_x\alpha_x\|_F^2 + \gamma\|\alpha_x^T - Y^T\alpha_y\|_F^2 + \sum_{i=1}^{n}(\lambda_x\|\alpha_{x,i}\|_1 + \lambda_y\|\alpha_{y,i}\|_1)$$

$$\text{subject to} \quad \|d_i\|_2^2 \le 1 \quad \forall i = 1,..,k$$

$$(4)$$

where $\gamma \in \mathbb{R}$ is a weight controlling the fit constraint between the fMRI coefficients α_x and the SNP coefficients α_y. Interestingly, Eq. 4 is a special case of the SCDL model from Eq. 3, where $W_y = Y$ and no dictionary is estimated for SNP data. As mentioned earlier, the 'standard' imaging genomics analysis pipeline is made of two steps: (i) feature extraction, usually using imaging data (ii) analysis between subject-wise features and genomic data. In the SCyLIG model, we assume the genomic data influence the imaging feature extraction from the very beginning. The strength of this influence is controlled by the weight parameter γ.

2.3   SCyLIG Optimization

SCyLIG model from Eq. 4 is not convex with respect to $(D_x, \alpha_x, \alpha_y)$. However, it is convex with respect to each variable when others are considered fixed. As a consequence, we can separate Eq. 4 into 3 distinct sub-problems, and solve each of them iteratively until convergence.

- D_x given α_x, α_x: is a quadratically constrained quadratic programming (QCQP) problem with respect to D_x. The solution can be solved using Lagrange dual techniques [13] or projected gradient descent [14].
- α_x given D_x, α_y: This problem can be recast into a set of parallel LASSO estimations of the form $\arg\min_{\alpha_x} \|\tilde{X} - \tilde{D}_x\alpha_x\|_F^2$, using the following notation:

$$\tilde{X} = \begin{pmatrix} X \\ \sqrt{\gamma}\alpha_y^T Y \end{pmatrix}, \quad \tilde{D}_x = \begin{pmatrix} D_x \\ I_{k\times k} \end{pmatrix} \tag{5}$$

  where $I_{k\times k}$ denotes the identity matrix of size k.
- α_y given D_x, α_x: simply amounts to solving k LASSO problems in parallel.

In the next section, we evaluate the proposed model SCyLIG on real imaging genomics data.

3   Experiments

In this work, we are interested in exploring the influence of both brain functionality measures (more precisely, related to working memory) and genomic markers on verbal reasoning ability. More specifically, we will use the proposed SCyLIG model to perform joint feature extraction among a population of young adults (15+ years). This population can be further subdivided into two classes (low/high achievers) based on their verbal reasoning performances, which will allow us to look at group differences.

Data Acquisition and Preprocessing. The Philadelphia Neurodevelopmental Cohort [15] (PNC) is a large-scale collaborative study between the Brain Behaviour Laboratory at the University of Pennsylvania and the Children's Hospital of Philadelphia. It contains, among other modalities, fractal n-back task fMRI, SNP arrays and Computerized Neurocognitive Battery (CNB) performances data for nearly 900 adolescents with age from 8 to 21 years. In order to limit the influence of age over the results, we selected a subset of the full dataset such that the remaining subject's age is above 180 months.

Standard brain imaging preprocessing steps were applied to the fMRI data using SPM12[1], including motion correction, spatial normalization to standard MNI space (adult template) and spatial/temporal smoothing. Stimulus-on versus stimulus-off contrast images were extracted. After removing voxels with too many missing values, $p_x = 85796$ voxels were left for analysis. The n-back task fMRI is one of the most popular experimental paradigm for the study of working memory. As mentioned in previous work [16,17], it is hypothesized that working memory abilities strongly affect verbal reasoning performances.

SNP arrays were acquired using 6 different platforms. We kept subjects genotyped by the 4 most commonly used platforms, all manufactured by Illumina. After standard data cleaning and preprocessing step using PLINK software package[2], $p_y = 98804$ SNP were left for analysis.

Finally, we also relied on performance measures (e.g., ratio of total correct responses) for the Penn Verbal Reasoning Test (PVRT), which measures verbal intellectual ability. In order to divide our population into two distinct groups, we only kept subjects whose absolute z-score value for PVRT test was above $z^* = 1$. Our motivation was to analyze whether the reconstruction coefficients α_x, α_y will show a discriminative behavior between the two groups. After all these steps, we were left with $n = 134$ subjects separated in two groups: low achievers at PVRT (age 16.7 ± 1.91 years 39 females out of 74 subjects) and high achievers (age 17.1 ± 1.92 years, 32 females out of 60 subjects).

Parameters Tuning. There are 4 main parameters that need to be estimated in SCyLIG (see Eq. 4), namely $k, \gamma, \lambda_x, \lambda_y$. To fix the number of dictionary atoms k to be estimated, we simply used SCyLIG within a 10-fold cross validation setup with $\lambda_x = \lambda_y = 0$. For each fold, we can calculate a classification score by feeding the estimated fMRI coefficients α_x into a standard support vector machine (SVM, see [18]) classifier. We display in Fig. 1(left) the evolution of the classification error according to the value of k. We can observe that a minimum is reached for $d \approx 70$, which is the retained value for the rest of our tests. In a similar way, the estimation of $\gamma, \lambda_x, \lambda_y$ is performed using a nested-grid search together with a 10-fold cross validation procedure using an SVM classifier. We display in Fig. 1(right) the evolution of the classification error for different γ values for three different setups: using only the fMRI coefficients α_x as features, using only the SNP coefficients α_y, and using both modalities together $\alpha = [\alpha_x; \alpha_y]$. First of all,

---

[1] http://www.fil.ion.ucl.ac.uk/spm/.

[2] http://pngu.mgh.harvard.edu/~purcell/plink.

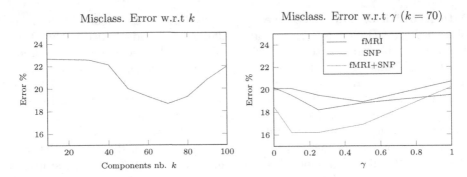

Fig. 1. **(Left)** Classification error according to the number of dictionary atoms k ($\lambda_x = \lambda_y = 0$ here). **(Right)** Classification error associated to the coefficients α_x, α_y according to γ for 3 set ups: (i) fMRI coefficients only (ii) SNP coefficients only (iii) fMRI and SNP coefficients concatenated.

we can observe that combining both modalities lead to the lowest classification error. Also, we can see that the classification error is the lowest for $\gamma \in [0.1, 0.25]$. This is really interesting, as $\gamma = 0$ essentially amounts to using unimodal feature estimation separately on each modality (as the cross modality constraint is not enforced in that case). This illustrates that even though our method is essentially unsupervised, extracting features jointly from both modalities can improve the discriminative ability of these features in some cases.

Analysis on UPenn Data. Besides classification error, we can also analyze the reconstruction errors associated with both fitting terms from Eq. 4. Once again, this is carried out using a 10-fold cross validation procedure, in which the reconstruction error is evaluated on the test set only. Average results for different γ values are displayed in Fig. 2(left). Once again, compared to the standard unimodal approach (i.e. $\gamma = 0$), we can observe that while choosing $\gamma \in [0.1, 0.25]$ slightly increase the fMRI fit error (blue curve), it produces a drastic decrease of the SNP to fMRI fit (red curve). Therefore, this justifies once again in this case the use of a coupled selection scheme compared to the standard unimodal one.

In order to provide some qualitative results, we also display in Fig. 2(right) the imaging coefficients α_x associated with the first atom in D_x (here $\gamma = 0.2$), for each class (i.e., low/high achievers, concatenated results over 50 runs with subsampling). Interestingly, we can observe that the two distributions significantly differ. The first atom is overall less expressed within low achievers (more weights near 0). This atom can be seen in Fig. 3, where the main clusters can be seen in the occipital, frontal and parietal lobes.

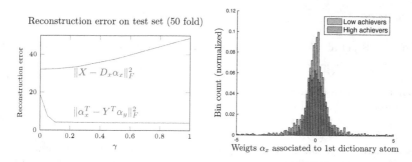

Fig. 2. (Left) Average error for both fit terms from Eq. 4. **(Right)** Ditributions of the fMRI reconstruction coefficents α_x associated to the first atom in D_x for both classes (low/high achievers).

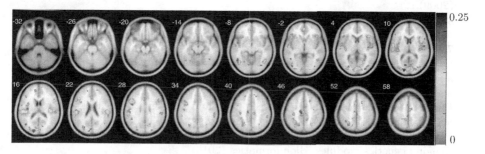

Fig. 3. Slice view of first atom in D_x (i.e. first column of D_x). The main clusters can be seen in the occipital, frontal and parietal lobes

4   Conclusion

The SCyLIG model is proposed in this work for multi-modal feature selection in the context of imaging genomics. We demonstrated that both fMRI and SNP data achieve good prediction performance in analyzing verbal intellectual ability in young adults. Using quantitative measures, we illustrated the benefits of using the proposed multi-modal data based model compared to the standard unimodal approach. Future work includes more experimental results and analysis, especially regarding the sets of SNPs corresponding to each imaging atom. In a multiclass situation such as the one studied in this work, a proper supervised extension of SCyLIG will also be of interest.

Acknowledgment. The work was partially supported by NIH (R01 GM109068, R01 MH104680, R01 MH107354, P20 GM103472, R01 REB020407, 1R01 EB006841) and NSF (#1539067).

References

1. Hariri, A.R., et al.: Serotonin transporter genetic variation and the response of the human amygdala. Science **297**(5580), 400–403 (2002)
2. Bookheimer, S.Y., et al.: Patterns of brain activation in people at risk for alzheimer's disease. N. Engl. J. Med. **343**(7), 450–456 (2000)
3. Thompson, P.M., et al.: Imaging genomics. Curr. Opin. Neurol. **23**(4), 368 (2010)
4. Stein, J.L., et al.: Voxelwise genome-wide association study (vGWAS). Neuroimage **53**(3), 1160–1174 (2010)
5. Jahanshad, N., et al.: Genome-wide scan of healthy human connectome discovers spon1 gene variant influencing dementia severity. Proc. Natl. Acad. Sci. **110**(12), 4768–4773 (2013)
6. Liu, J., et al.: Combining fmri and snp data to investigate connections between brain function and genetics using parallel ICA. Hum. Brain Mapp. **30**(1), 241–255 (2009)
7. Vounou, M., et al.: Sparse reduced-rank regression detects genetic associations with voxel-wise longitudinal phenotypes in alzheimer's disease. Neuroimage **60**(1), 700–716 (2012)
8. Le Floch, É., et al.: Significant correlation between a set of genetic polymorphisms and a functional brain network revealed by feature selection and sparse partial least squares. Neuroimage **63**(1), 11–24 (2012)
9. Lin, D., et al.: Correspondence between fmRI and SNP data by group sparse canonical correlation analysis. Med. Image Anal. **18**(6), 891–902 (2014)
10. Fang, J., et al.: Joint sparse canonical correlation analysis for detecting differential imaging genetics modules. Bioinformatics (2016)
11. Mairal, J., Bach, F., Ponce, J., Sapiro, G.: Online learning for matrix factorization and sparse coding. J. Mach. Learn. Res. **11**, 19–60 (2010)
12. Wang, S., et al.: Semi-coupled dictionary learning with applications to image super-resolution and photo-sketch synthesis. In: 2012 IEEE Conference on Computer Vision and Pattern Recognition (CVPR), pp. 2216–2223. IEEE (2012)
13. Lee, H., et al.: Efficient sparse coding algorithms. Adv. Neural Inf. Process. Syst. **19**, 801 (2007)
14. Yang, M., Zhang, L., Yang, J., Zhang, D.: Metaface learning for sparse representation based face recognition. In: 2010 17th IEEE International Conference on Image Processing (ICIP), 1601–1604. IEEE (2010)
15. Satterthwaite, T.D., et al.: The philadelphia neurodevelopmental cohort: a publicly available resource for the study of normal and abnormal brain development in youth. Neuroimage **124**, 1115–1119 (2016)
16. Hitch, G., Baddeley, A.: Verbal reasoning and working memory. Q. J. Exp. Psychol. **28**(4), 603–621 (1976)
17. Fry, A.F., Hale, S.: Relationships among processing speed, working memory, and fluid intelligence in children. Biol. Psychol. **54**(1), 1–34 (2000)
18. Cortes, C., et al.: Support-vector networks. Mach. Learn. **20**(3), 273–297 (1995)

Author Index

Printed in the United States
By Bookmasters